Injury & Trauma Sour...

Learning Disabilities...

Leukemia Sourcebook

Liver Disorders Sourcebook

Medical Tests Sourcebook, 4th Edition

Men's Health Concerns Sourcebook, 4th Edition

Mental Health Disorders Sourcebook, 5th Edition

Mental Retardation Sourcebook

Movement Disorders Sourcebook, 2nd Edition

Multiple Sclerosis Sourcebook

Muscular Dystrophy Sourcebook

Obesity Sourcebook

Osteoporosis Sourcebook

Pain Sourcebook, 3rd Edition

Pediatric Cancer Sourcebook

Physical & Mental Issues in Aging Sourcebook

Podiatry Sourcebook, 2nd Edition

Pregnancy & Birth Sourcebook, 3rd Edition

Prostate & Urological Disorders Sourcebook

Prostate Cancer Sourcebook

Rehabilitation Sourcebook

Respiratory Disorders Sourcebook, 2nd Edition

Sexually Transmitted Diseases Sourcebook, 5th Edition

Sleep Disorders Sourcebook, 3rd Edition

Smoking Concerns Sourcebook

Sports Injuries Sourcebook, 4th Edition

Stress-Related Disorders Sourcebook, 3rd Edition

Stroke Sourcebook, 2nd Edition

Surgery Sourcebook, 2nd Edition

Thyroid Disorders Sourcebook

Transplantation Sourcebook

Traveler's Health Sourcebook

Urinary Tract & Kidney Diseases & Disorders Sourcebook, 2nd Edition

Vegetarian Sourcebook

Women's Health Concerns Sourcebook, 3rd Edition

Workplace Health & Safety Sourcebook

Worldwide Health Sourcebook

Teen Health Series

Abuse & Violence Information for Teens

Accident & Safety Information for Teens

Alcohol Information for Teens, 2nd Edition

Allergy Information for Teens

Asthma Information for Teens, 2nd Edition

Body Information for Teens

Cancer Information for Teens, 2nd Edition

Complementary & Alternative Medicine Information for Teens

Diabetes Information for Teens, 2nd Edition

Diet Information for Teens, 3rd Edition

Drug Information for Teens, 3rd Edition

Eating Disorders Information for Teens, 2nd Edition

Fitness Information for Teens, 3rd Edition

Learning Disabilities Information for Teens

Mental Health Information for Teens, 3rd Edition

Pregnancy Information for Teens, 2nd Edition

Sexual Health Information for Teens, 3rd Edition

Skin Health Information for Teens, 2nd Edition

Sleep Information for Teens

Sports Injuries Information for Teens, 3rd Edition

Stress Information for Teens

Suicide Information for Teens, 2nd Edition

Tobacco Information for Teens, 2nd Edition

Learning Disabilities

SOURCEBOOK

Fourth Edition

Health Reference Series

Fourth Edition

Learning Disabilities
SOURCEBOOK

Basic Consumer Health Information about Dyslexia, Dyscalculia, Dysgraphia, Speech and Communication Disorders, Auditory and Visual Processing Disorders, and Other Conditions That Make Learning Difficult, Including Attention Deficit Hyperactivity Disorder, Down Syndrome and Other Chromosomal Disorders, Fetal Alcohol Spectrum Disorders, Hearing and Visual Impairment, Autism and Other Pervasive Developmental Disorders, and Traumatic Brain Injury

Along with Facts about Diagnosing Learning Disabilities, Early Intervention, the Special Education Process, Legal Protections, Assistive Technology, and Accommodations, and Guidelines for Life-Stage Transitions, Suggestions for Coping with Daily Challenges, a Glossary of Related Terms, and a Directory of Additional Resources

Edited by
Sandra J. Judd

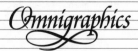

Omnigraphics

155 W. Congress, Suite 200, Detroit, MI 48226

Bibliographic Note
Because this page cannot legibly accommodate all the copyright notices, the Bibliographic Note portion of the Preface constitutes an extension of the copyright notice.

Edited by Sandra J. Judd

Health Reference Series

Karen Bellenir, *Managing Editor*
David A. Cooke, MD, FACP, *Medical Consultant*
Elizabeth Collins, *Research and Permissions Coordinator*
Cherry Edwards, *Permissions Assistant*
EdIndex, Services for Publishers, *Indexers*

* * *

Omnigraphics, Inc.
Matthew P. Barbour, *Senior Vice President*
Kevin M. Hayes, *Operations Manager*

* * *

Peter E. Ruffner, *Publisher*
Copyright © 2012 Omnigraphics, Inc.
ISBN 978-0-7808-1259-8
E-ISBN 978-0-7808-1260-4

Library of Congress Cataloging-in-Publication Data

Learning disabilities sourcebook : basic consumer health information about dyslexia, dyscalculia, dysgraphia, speech and communication disorders, auditory and visual processing disorders, and other conditions that make learning difficult, including attention deficit hyperactivity disorder, down syndrome and other chromosomal disorders, fetal alcohol spectrum disorders, hearing and visual impairment, autism and other pervasive developmental disorders, and traumatic brain Injury; along with facts about diagnosing learning disabilities, early intervention, the special education process, legal protections, assistive technology, and accommodations, and guidelines for life-stage transitions, suggestions for coping with daily challenges, a glossary of related terms, and a directory of additional resources / edited by Sandra J. Judd. -- 4th ed.
     p. cm.
   Includes bibliographical references and index.
   Summary: "Provides basic consumer health information about the signs, symptoms, and diagnosis of various learning disabilities and other conditions that impact learning, along with facts about early intervention and the special education process, advice for coping at home and school, and handling the transition to adulthood. Includes index, glossary of related terms, and other resources"--Provided by publisher.
   ISBN 978-0-7808-1259-8 (hardcover : alk. paper) 1. Learning disabilities--United States--Handbooks, manuals, etc. 2. Learning disabled children--Education--United States--Handbooks, manuals, etc. 3. Learning disabled--Education--United States--Handbooks, manuals, etc. 4. Learning disabilities--United States--Diagnosis--Handbooks, manuals, etc. I. Judd, Sandra J.
   LC4705.L434 2012
   371.9--dc23

                                                                    2012009283

Table of Contents

Visit www.healthreferenceseries.com to view *A Contents Guide to the Health Reference Series*, a listing of more than 16,000 topics and the volumes in which they are covered.

Part II: Types of Learning Disabilities

Part IV: Learning Disabilities and the Educational Process

Part V: Living with Learning Disabilities

Part VI: Additional Help and Information

Preface

About This Book

Learning disabilities are neurological disorders that affect the brain's ability to process, store, and communicate information. They are widespread, affecting as many as one out of every five people in the United States, according to the U.S. Department of Education. More than 2.5 million American children (five percent of all children in public schools) receive some kind of special education support. Learning disabilities directly impact many areas in the lives of those affected, making school difficult, making it hard to obtain and sustain employment, making daily tasks challenging, and even affecting relationships. Yet learning disabilities are invisible obstacles. For this reason they are often misunderstood, and their impact is often underestimated.

Learning Disabilities Sourcebook, Fourth Edition provides information about dyslexia, dyscalculia, dysgraphia, speech and communication disorders, and auditory and visual processing disorders. It also provides details about other conditions that impact learning, including attention deficit hyperactivity disorder, autism and other pervasive developmental disorders, hearing and visual impairment, and Down syndrome and other chromosomal disorders. The book offers facts about diagnosing learning disabilities, the special education process, and legal protections. Guidelines for life-stage transitions and coping with daily challenges, a glossary of related terms, and a directory of resources for additional help and information are also included.

How to Use This Book

This book is divided into parts and chapters. Parts focus on broad areas of interest. Chapters are devoted to single topics within a part.

Part I: Understanding and Identifying Learning Disabilities explains how the brain works, defines what learning disabilities are, and describes theories regarding their potential causes. It explains how learning disabilities are evaluated and provides tips on how to choose an evaluation professional.

Part II: Types of Learning Disabilities describes the most common forms of learning disabilities, including problems with reading, writing, mathematics, speech, language, and communication. It explains what these disorders are, how they are diagnosed, and how they are treated. It also discusses learning disabilities among gifted students, a fairly common—but often unrecognized—phenomenon.

Part III: Other Disorders That Make Learning Difficult discusses common disorders that have a component that affects a child's ability to learn, including attention deficit hyperactivity disorder, epilepsy, fetal alcohol spectrum disorders, pervasive developmental disorders, visual and hearing disabilities, and chromosomal disorders such as Down syndrome.

Part IV: Learning Disabilities and the Educational Process provides information about how learning disabilities are accommodated within the schools. It describes early intervention strategies, explains how the special education process works, and details the legal supports for students with learning disabilities. Specialized teaching techniques and alternative educational options, such as tutoring and home schooling, that are used to help learning-disabled students succeed are described, and it also offers guidelines for successfully negotiating the transitions to high school and to college.

Part V: Living with Learning Disabilities discusses how learning disabilities impact daily life. It includes tips for coping with a learning disability and for parenting a child with a learning disability. The impact of learning disabilities on self-esteem and social skills are discussed, and it offers suggestions to help those with learning disabilities deal with daily tasks, including meal preparation, money management, travel and transportation, and learning to drive. It also provides detailed guidelines for handling the employment issues faced by those with learning disabilities.

Part VI: Additional Help and Information includes a glossary of terms related to learning disabilities, a list of sources of college funding for students with disabilities, and a directory of resources for further help and support.

Bibliographic Note

This volume contains documents and excerpts from publications issued by the following U.S. and other government agencies: Centers for Disease Control and Prevention; Genetics Home Reference; Job Accommodation Network; National Dissemination Center for Children with Disabilities; National Human Genome Research Institute; National Institute of Environmental Health Sciences; National Institute of Mental Health; National Institute of Neurological Disorders and Stroke; National Institute on Alcohol Abuse and Alcoholism; National Institute on Deafness and Other Communication Disorders; Office of Disability Employment Policy, U.S. Department of Labor; and the Wisconsin Department of Public Instruction.

In addition, this volume contains copyrighted documents from the following organizations and individuals: Micaela Bracamonte; Dale S. Brown; Child Welfare League of America; Children's Hearing Institute; Children's Vision Information Network; Collaborative on Health and the Environment; GreatSchools, Inc.; Institutes on Academic Diversity at the University of Virginia Curry School of Education; HelpGuide; International Dyslexia Association; International Reading Association; Learning Disabilities Association of America; Learning Disabilities Worldwide; Aoife Lyons; Massachusetts Institute of Technology News Office; National Center for Learning Disabilities; National Literacy Trust; Nemours Foundation; NYU Child Study Center; Orange County Learning Disabilities Association; PACER Center; Performance Learning Systems; PsychCentral; Smart Kids with Learning Disabilities; Louise Spear-Swerling; St. Louis Learning Disabilities Association; University of Bristol; University of Michigan Health System—Your Child Development and Behavior Resources; University of North Carolina Chapel Hill FPG Child Development Institute; University of Oxford; and the University of Washington DO-IT (Disabilities, Opportunities, Internetworking, and Technology).

Full citation information is provided on the first page of each chapter or section. Every effort has been made to secure all necessary rights to reprint the copyrighted material. If any omissions have been made, please contact Omnigraphics to make corrections for future editions.

Acknowledgements

Thanks go to the many organizations, agencies, and individuals who have contributed materials for this *Sourcebook* and to medical consultant Dr. David Cooke and prepress services provider WhimsyInk. Special thanks go to managing editor Karen Bellenir and permissions coordinator Liz Collins for their help and support.

About the Health Reference Series

The *Health Reference Series* is designed to provide basic medical information for patients, families, caregivers, and the general public. Each volume takes a particular topic and provides comprehensive coverage. This is especially important for people who may be dealing with a newly diagnosed disease or a chronic disorder in themselves or in a family member. People looking for preventive guidance, information about disease warning signs, medical statistics, and risk factors for health problems will also find answers to their questions in the *Health Reference Series*. The *Series*, however, is not intended to serve as a tool for diagnosing illness, in prescribing treatments, or as a substitute for the physician/patient relationship. All people concerned about medical symptoms or the possibility of disease are encouraged to seek professional care from an appropriate healthcare provider.

A Note about Spelling and Style

Health Reference Series editors use *Stedman's Medical Dictionary* as an authority for questions related to the spelling of medical terms and the *Chicago Manual of Style* for questions related to grammatical structures, punctuation, and other editorial concerns. Consistent adherence is not always possible, however, because the individual volumes within the *Series* include many documents from a wide variety of different producers and copyright holders, and the editor's primary goal is to present material from each source as accurately as is possible following the terms specified by each document's producer. This sometimes means that information in different chapters or sections may follow other guidelines and alternate spelling authorities. For example, occasionally a copyright holder may require that eponymous terms be shown in possessive forms (Crohn's disease *vs.* Crohn disease) or that British spelling norms be retained (leukaemia *vs.* leukemia).

Locating Information within the Health Reference Series

The *Health Reference Series* contains a wealth of information about a wide variety of medical topics. Ensuring easy access to all the fact sheets, research reports, in-depth discussions, and other material contained within the individual books of the series remains one of our highest priorities. As the *Series* continues to grow in size and scope, however, locating the precise information needed by a reader may become more challenging.

A Contents Guide to the Health Reference Series was developed to direct readers to the specific volumes that address their concerns. It presents an extensive list of diseases, treatments, and other topics of general interest compiled from the Tables of Contents and major index headings. To access *A Contents Guide to the Health Reference Series*, visit www.healthreferenceseries.com.

Medical Consultant

Medical consultation services are provided to the *Health Reference Series* editors by David A. Cooke, MD, FACP. Dr. Cooke is a graduate of Brandeis University, and he received his M.D. degree from the University of Michigan. He completed residency training at the University of Wisconsin Hospital and Clinics. He is board-certified in Internal Medicine. Dr. Cooke currently works as part of the University of Michigan Health System and practices in Ann Arbor, MI. In his free time, he enjoys writing, science fiction, and spending time with his family.

Our Advisory Board

We would like to thank the following board members for providing guidance to the development of this series:

Dr. Lynda Baker, Associate Professor of Library and Information Science, Wayne State University, Detroit, MI

Nancy Bulgarelli, William Beaumont Hospital Library, Royal Oak, MI

Karen Imarisio, Bloomfield Township Public Library, Bloomfield Township, MI

Karen Morgan, Mardigian Library, University of Michigan-Dearborn, Dearborn, MI

Rosemary Orlando, St. Clair Shores Public Library, St. Clair Shores, MI

Health Reference Series Update Policy

The inaugural book in the *Health Reference Series* was the first edition of *Cancer Sourcebook* published in 1989. Since then, the *Series* has been enthusiastically received by librarians and in the medical community. In order to maintain the standard of providing high-quality health information for the layperson the editorial staff at Omnigraphics felt it was necessary to implement a policy of updating volumes when warranted.

Medical researchers have been making tremendous strides, and it is the purpose of the *Health Reference Series* to stay current with the most recent advances. Each decision to update a volume is made on an individual basis. Some of the considerations include how much new information is available and the feedback we receive from people who use the books. If there is a topic you would like to see added to the update list, or an area of medical concern you feel has not been adequately addressed, please write to:

Editor
Health Reference Series
Omnigraphics, Inc.
155 W. Congress, Suite 200
Detroit, MI 48226
E-mail: editorial@omnigraphics.com

Part One

Understanding and Identifying Learning Disabilities

Chapter 1

The Brain and Learning Disabilities

Chapter Contents

Section 1.1

Brain Basics: How the Brain Works

"Brain Basics: Know Your Brain," National Institute of
Neurological Disorders and Stroke, National Institutes of Health,
NIH Publication No. 01-3440a, August 18, 2010.

Introduction

The brain is the most complex part of the human body. This three-pound organ is the seat of intelligence, interpreter of the senses, initiator of body movement, and controller of behavior. Lying in its bony shell and washed by protective fluid, the brain is the source of all the qualities that define our humanity. The brain is the crown jewel of the human body.

For centuries, scientists and philosophers have been fascinated by the brain, but until recently they viewed the brain as nearly incomprehensible. Now, however, the brain is beginning to relinquish its secrets. Scientists have learned more about the brain in the last ten years than in all previous centuries because of the accelerating pace of research in neurological and behavioral science and the development of new research techniques. As a result, Congress named the 1990s the Decade of the Brain. At the forefront of research on the brain and other elements of the nervous system is the National Institute of Neurological Disorders and Stroke (NINDS), which conducts and supports scientific studies in the United States and around the world.

This section is a basic introduction to the human brain. It may help you understand how the healthy brain works, how to keep it healthy, and what happens when the brain is diseased or dysfunctional.

The Architecture of the Brain

The brain is like a committee of experts. All the parts of the brain work together, but each part has its own special properties. The brain can be divided into three basic units: the forebrain, the midbrain, and the hindbrain.

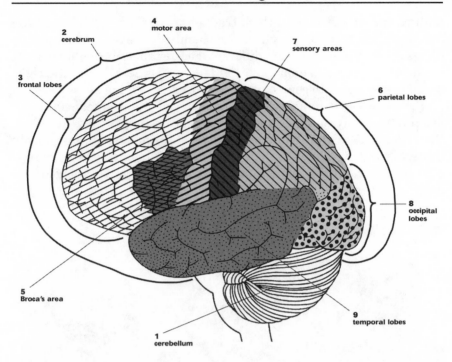

Figure 1.1. *Parts of the brain*

The hindbrain includes the upper part of the spinal cord, the brain stem, and a wrinkled ball of tissue called the cerebellum (1). The hindbrain controls the body's vital functions, such as respiration and heart rate. The cerebellum coordinates movement and is involved in learned rote movements. When you play the piano or hit a tennis ball you are activating the cerebellum. The uppermost part of the brainstem is the midbrain, which controls some reflex actions and is part of the circuit involved in the control of eye movements and other voluntary movements. The forebrain is the largest and most highly developed part of the human brain: it consists primarily of the cerebrum (2) and the structures hidden beneath it.

When people see pictures of the brain it is usually the cerebrum that they notice. The cerebrum sits at the topmost part of the brain and is the source of intellectual activities. It holds your memories, allows you to plan, and enables you to imagine and think. It allows you to recognize friends, read books, and play games.

The cerebrum is split into two halves (hemispheres) by a deep fissure. Despite the split, the two cerebral hemispheres communicate with each other through a thick tract of nerve fibers that lies at the base of this fissure. Although the two hemispheres seem to be mirror images of each other, they are different. For instance, the ability to form words seems to lie primarily in the left hemisphere, while the right hemisphere seems to control many abstract reasoning skills.

For some as-yet-unknown reason, nearly all of the signals from the brain to the body and vice versa cross over on their way to and from the brain. This means that the right cerebral hemisphere primarily controls the left side of the body and the left hemisphere primarily controls the right side. When one side of the brain is damaged, the opposite side of the body is affected. For example, a stroke in the right hemisphere of the brain can leave the left arm and leg paralyzed.

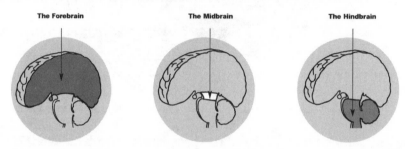

*Figure 1.2.*The forebrain, the midbrain, and the hindbrain, from left to right.

The Geography of Thought

Each cerebral hemisphere can be divided into sections, or lobes, each of which specializes in different functions. To understand each lobe and its specialty we will take a tour of the cerebral hemispheres, starting with the two frontal lobes (3), which lie directly behind the forehead. When you plan a schedule, imagine the future, or use reasoned arguments, these two lobes do much of the work. One of the ways the frontal lobes seem to do these things is by acting as short-term storage sites, allowing one idea to be kept in mind while other ideas are considered. In the rearmost portion of each frontal lobe is a motor area (4), which helps control voluntary movement. A nearby place on the left frontal lobe called Broca area (5) allows thoughts to be transformed into words.

When you enjoy a good meal—the taste, aroma, and texture of the food—two sections behind the frontal lobes called the parietal lobes (6) are at work. The forward parts of these lobes, just behind the motor areas, are the primary sensory areas (7). These areas receive information about temperature, taste, touch, and movement from the rest of the body. Reading and arithmetic are also functions in the repertoire of each parietal lobe.

As you look at the words and pictures on this page, two areas at the back of the brain are at work. These lobes, called the occipital lobes (8), process images from the eyes and link that information with images stored in memory. Damage to the occipital lobes can cause blindness.

The last lobes on our tour of the cerebral hemispheres are the temporal lobes (9), which lie in front of the visual areas and nest under the parietal and frontal lobes. Whether you appreciate symphonies or rock music, your brain responds through the activity of these lobes. At the top of each temporal lobe is an area responsible for receiving information from the ears. The underside of each temporal lobe plays a crucial role in forming and retrieving memories, including those associated with music. Other parts of this lobe seem to integrate memories and sensations of taste, sound, sight, and touch.

The Cerebral Cortex

Coating the surface of the cerebrum and the cerebellum is a vital layer of tissue the thickness of a stack of two or three dimes. It is called the cortex, from the Latin word for bark. Most of the actual information processing in the brain takes place in the cerebral cortex. When people talk about "gray matter" in the brain they are talking about this thin rind. The cortex is gray because nerves in this area lack the insulation that makes most other parts of the brain appear to be white. The folds in the brain add to its surface area and therefore increase the amount of gray matter and the quantity of information that can be processed.

The Inner Brain

Deep within the brain, hidden from view, lie structures that are the gatekeepers between the spinal cord and the cerebral hemispheres. These structures not only determine our emotional state, they also modify our perceptions and responses depending on that state, and allow us to initiate movements that you make without thinking about them. Like the lobes in the cerebral hemispheres, the structures described below come in pairs: each is duplicated in the opposite half of the brain.

The hypothalamus (10), about the size of a pearl, directs a multitude of important functions. It wakes you up in the morning, and gets the adrenaline flowing during a test or job interview. The hypothalamus is also an important emotional center, controlling the molecules that make you feel exhilarated, angry, or unhappy. Near the hypothalamus lies the thalamus (11), a major clearinghouse for information going to and from the spinal cord and the cerebrum.

An arching tract of nerve cells leads from the hypothalamus and the thalamus to the hippocampus (12). This tiny nub acts as a memory indexer—sending memories out to the appropriate part of the cerebral hemisphere for long-term storage and retrieving them when necessary. The basal ganglia (not shown) are clusters of nerve cells surrounding the thalamus. They are responsible for initiating and integrating movements. Parkinson disease, which results in tremors, rigidity, and a stiff, shuffling walk, is a disease of nerve cells that lead into the basal ganglia.

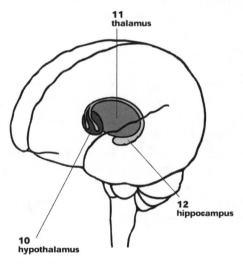

Figure 1.3. The inner brain

Making Connections

The brain and the rest of the nervous system are composed of many different types of cells, but the primary functional unit is a cell called the neuron. All sensations, movements, thoughts, memories, and feelings are the result of signals that pass through neurons. Neurons consist of three parts. The cell body contains the nucleus, where most of the molecules that the neuron needs to survive and function are manufactured. Dendrites extend out from the cell body like the branches of a tree and receive messages from other nerve cells. Signals then pass from the dendrites through the cell body and may travel away from the cell body down an axon to another neuron, a muscle cell, or cells in some other organ. The neuron is usually surrounded by many support cells. Some types of cells wrap around the axon to form an insulating sheath. This sheath can include a fatty molecule called myelin, which provides insulation for the axon and helps nerve signals travel faster and farther. Axons may be very short, such as those that carry signals from one cell in the cortex to another cell less than a hair's width away, or axons may be very long, such as those that carry messages from the brain all the way down the spinal cord.

Scientists have learned a great deal about neurons by studying the synapse—the place where a signal passes from the neuron to another cell. When the signal reaches the end of the axon it stimulates tiny sacs. These sacs release chemicals known as neurotransmitters into the synapse. The neurotransmitters cross the synapse and attach to receptors on the neighboring cell. These receptors can change the properties of the receiving cell. If the receiving cell is also a neuron, the signal can continue the transmission to the next cell.

Some Key Neurotransmitters at Work

Acetylcholine is called an excitatory neurotransmitter because it generally makes cells more excitable. It governs muscle contractions and causes glands to secrete hormones. Alzheimer disease, which initially affects memory formation, is associated with a shortage of acetylcholine.

Gamma-aminobutyric acid (GABA) is called an inhibitory neurotransmitter because it tends to make cells less excitable. It helps control muscle activity and is an important part of the visual system. Drugs that increase GABA levels in the brain are used to treat epileptic seizures and tremors in patients with Huntington disease.

Serotonin is an inhibitory neurotransmitter that constricts blood vessels and brings on sleep. It is also involved in temperature regulation. Dopamine is an inhibitory neurotransmitter involved in mood and the control of complex movements. The loss of dopamine activity in some portions of the brain leads to the muscular rigidity of Parkinson disease. Many medications used to treat behavioral disorders work by modifying the action of dopamine in the brain.

Section 1.2

Executive Function

Executive function is a set of mental processes that helps connect past experience with present action. People use it to perform activities such as planning, organizing, strategizing, paying attention to and remembering details, and managing time and space.

If you have trouble with executive function, these things are more difficult to do. You may also show a weakness with working memory, which is like "seeing in your mind's eye." This is an important tool in guiding your actions.

As with other learning disabilities, problems with executive function can run in families. It can be seen at any age, but it tends to become more apparent as children move through the early elementary grades. This is when the demands of completing schoolwork independently can trigger signs of a problem with executive function.

The brain continues to mature and develop connections well into adulthood. A person's executive function abilities are shaped by both physical changes in the brain and by life experiences, in the classroom and in the world at large. Early attention to developing efficient skills in this area can be very helpful. As a rule, it helps to give direct instruction, frequent reassurance, and explicit feedback.

How does executive function affect learning?

In school, at home, or in the workplace, we're called on all day, every day, to self-regulate behavior. Executive function allows us to:

- make plans;
- keep track of time and finish work on time;
- keep track of more than one thing at once;
- meaningfully include past knowledge in discussions;

- evaluate ideas and reflect on our work;
- change our minds and make mid-course corrections while thinking, reading, and writing;
- ask for help or seek more information when we need it;
- engage in group dynamics;
- wait to speak until we're called on.

What are the warning signs of executive function problems?

A student may have problems with executive function when he or she has trouble:

- planning projects;
- comprehending how much time a project will take to complete;
- telling stories (verbally or in writing), struggling to communicate details in an organized, sequential manner;
- memorizing and retrieving information from memory;
- initiating activities or tasks, or generating ideas independently;
- retaining information while doing something with it, for example, remembering a phone number while dialing.

How are problems with executive function identified?

There is no single test or even battery of tests that identifies all of the different features of executive function. Educators, psychologists, speech-language pathologists, and others use a variety of tests to identify problems. Careful observation and trial teaching are invaluable in identifying and better understanding weaknesses in this area.

What are some strategies to help?

There are many effective strategies to help with the problem of executive function challenges. Here are some methods to try.
General strategies:

- Take step-by-step approaches to work; rely on visual organizational aids.
- Use tools like time organizers, computers, or watches with alarms.

- Prepare visual schedules and review them several times a day.

- Ask for written directions with oral instructions whenever possible.

- Plan and structure transition times and shifts in activities.

Managing time:

- Create checklists and "to do" lists, estimating how long tasks will take.

- Break long assignments into chunks and assign time frames for completing each chunk.

- Use visual calendars at to keep track of long-term assignments, due dates, chores, and activities.

- Use management software such as the Franklin Day Planner, Palm Pilot, or Lotus Organizer.

- Be sure to write the due date on top of each assignment.

Managing space and materials:

- Organize workspace.

- Minimize clutter.

- Consider having separate work areas with complete sets of supplies for different activities.

- Schedule a weekly time to clean and organize the workspace.

Managing work:

- Make a checklist for getting through assignments. For example, a student's checklist could include such items as: get out pencil and paper; put name on paper; put due date on paper; read directions; etc.

- Meet with a teacher or supervisor on a regular basis to review work; troubleshoot problems.

Section 1.3

Sensory and Perceptual Components of Learning

"Sensory and Perceptual Systems" by Joyce Powell Riley, M.A., President, Orange County Learning Disabilities Association. © 2001 Orange County Learning Disabilities Association (www.oclda.org). All rights reserved. Reprinted with permission. Reviewed by David A. Cooke, M.D., FACP, February 2012.

When the neurobiology dysfunctions, it causes distortions in the sensory system of the body. Without proper neurobiological support, the ability to touch, see, and hear can be distorted. When vestibular and proprioceptive systems are inadequate, such perceptions as the ability to know where one is in space, to have a sense of time, and even to have a sense of humor can be distorted in such a way that the individual has difficulty perceiving the world correctly. Visual, auditory, and tactile responses must be able to perceive, interpret, and process information so that a child can learn about the world around him or her. Without good sensory integration, learning and behavior is more difficult and the individual often feels uncomfortable about himself, and cannot easily cope with ordinary demands and stress.[1]

The tactile system is responsible for some of the earliest sensations for an infant. Different kinds of receptors in the skin receive sensations of touch, pressure, texture, heat or cold, and pain. The tactile system is the largest sensory system in the body and plays a vital role in human behavior, both physical and mental. Touch sensations flow throughout the entire nervous system and influence every neural process to some extent. Without a great deal of tactile stimulation of the body, the nervous system tends to become "unbalanced."[2] This helps to explain why the tactile system is involved in most disorders of the human brain.[3]

The proprioceptive system consists of sensory information caused by contraction and stretching of muscles and by bending, straightening, pulling, and compression of the joints between the bones. Because there are so many muscles and joints in the body, the proprioceptive system is almost as large as the tactile system. Most proprioceptive input is processed in areas of the brain that do not produce conscious

13

awareness. Without good automatic responses, such things as eye-hand coordination are very difficult.

The vestibular system is the sensory system that responds to the position of the head in relation to gravity and accelerated or decelerated movement. There are two types of vestibular receptors in the inner ear in a structure called the labyrinth. One type of receptor responds to the force of gravity. The other type of receptor is in the semicircular canals in the ear. These canals are responsible for our sense of movement. The vestibular system is a unifying system. All other types of sensation are processed in reference to this basic vestibular information. The activity in the vestibular system provides a "framework" for the other aspects of our experience. Vestibular input seems to "prime" the entire nervous system to function effectively. When the vestibular does not function in a consistent and accurate way, the interpretation of other sensations will be inconsistent and inaccurate, and the nervous system will have trouble "getting started."

The visual system has become our major means of relating to space, but the vestibular, proprioceptive, and tactile systems must contribute to visual development and function. Together these systems allow us to move about in space, catch a ball, and process the visual body language of others. In order to process more abstract information such as reading, writing, spelling, or calculation, such visual abilities as visual-motor, visual perceptual, visual spatial, visual memory, visual figure-ground and visual closure capacities must be in place. These capacities work well only when the tactile, vestibular, and proprioceptive systems are intact.

The auditory system has lower and higher levels of function. First, the auditory system is closely associated with the vestibular system. These systems deal with gravity and vibration. The higher functions deal with the ability to process information that is heard. This includes auditory memory, auditory sequencing, auditory discrimination, auditory figure-ground and auditory perception. Central auditory processing is a physical response that includes the ability to perceive degraded auditory signals, competing auditory signals, figure-ground and discrimination in noise.

Notes

1. Ayers, A. Jean. Sensory Integration and the Child, Western Psychological Services, 1979, 191pp., p.51.

2. Ibid. pp. 34, 35.

3. Ibid. p. 39.

Section 1.4

Acquisition of Language and Communication Skills

"The Acquisition and Use of Language and Communication Skills" by Joyce Powell Riley, M.A., President, Orange County Learning Disabilities Association. © 2001 Orange County Learning Disabilities Association (www.oclda.org). All rights reserved. Reprinted with permission. Reviewed by David A. Cooke, M.D., FACP, January 2012.

Communication begins at birth with touch, then with vision, and finally with speech and hearing or audition. Each child needs to learn the "codes of his or her culture" because the language of each culture is different. Yet, if a child is to learn about his or her world, the ability to communicate must exist. Even after a baby learns the rudiments of communication through touch, vision, and hearing, those skills need to continue to be refined until, at about age seven, the brain is ready to deal with the abstract concepts involved in reading, writing, comprehension, math "language" or concepts, and body language.

The acquisition and use of language and communication skills is at the heart of learning disabilities. These skills include speech, reading, writing and spelling, comprehension, reasoning, math language, and body language. All of these skills need an intact sensory system to function appropriately.

Language acquisition is divided into several parts:

- **Receptive language:** language that is spoken or written by others and received by an individual, i.e. listening or reading (decoding or getting meaning from spoken words or written symbols). In order to receive language, the individual must be able to attend to, process, comprehend, retain, and/or integrate spoken or written language. In order to do proper auditory processing, the individual needs to have phonemic awareness, the ability to notice, think about, and manipulate the individual sound in words and phonemes (sound-symbol correspondence); and phonological awareness, sound-symbol recognition or the ability to recognize specific sounds, which is necessary for good reading and spelling. Good visual processing demands the ability to interpret visual symbols, to differential visual figures from ground, and to have a functional visual memory and, for writing, good visual-motor activity.

- **Cognitive language:** language that is received, processed into memory, integrated with knowledge already integrated, and made a part of the knowledge of the individual from which new ideas and concepts can be generated. It is a part of the creative process that shapes the thought of each person.

- **Expressive language:** language and communication through speaking, writing, and/or gestures, i.e. selecting words, formulating them into ideas, and producing them through speaking, writing, or gesture (encoding or the process of expressive language). Expressive language involves word retrieval, rules of grammar (syntax), word and sentence structure (morphology), and word meaning (semantics).[1]

By the time a child is five years old, speech skills should be such that the child can be understood 100 percent of the time. The ability to read easy words and comprehend them should be in place for most children by the time a child is seven or eight years old. If children are not ready to read by fourth grade, they will not be able to keep up with the curriculum designated by the state.

Note

1. Moore, Barbara, M.A, CCC. Assessment: What is the Role of the Speech Pathologist in the Assessment of Language/Learning Disordered Students? *OCLDA Newsletter*, Vol. 38, No.6, Nov/Dec, 2000.

Section 1.5

Brain Imaging Reveals How We Learn from Our Competitors

Learning from competitors is a critically important form of learning for animals and humans. A new study has used brain imaging to reveal how people and animals learn from failure and success.

The team from Bristol University led by Dr. Paul Howard-Jones, senior lecturer in education in the Graduate School of Education and Dr. Rafal Bogacz, senior lecturer in the Department of Computer Science, scanned the brains of players as they battled against an artificial opponent in a computer game.

In the game, each player took turns with the computer to select one of four boxes whose payouts were simulating the ebb and flow of natural food sources.

Players were able to learn from their own successful selections but those of their competitor failed completely to increase their neural activity. Instead, it was their competitor's unexpected failures that generated this additional brain activity. Such failures generated both reward signals in the brains of the players and learning signals in regions involved with inhibiting response. This suggests that we benefit from our competitors' failures by learning to inhibit the actions that lead to them.

What's on Your Computer's Mind?

Surprisingly, when players were observing their competitor make selections, the players' brains were activated as if they were performing these actions themselves. Such "mirror neuron" activities occur when we observe the actions of other humans but here the players knew their opponent was just a computer and no animated graphics were used. Previously, it has been suggested that the mirror neuron system supports a type of unconscious mind reading that helps us, for example, judge others' intentions.

Dr. Howard-Jones added: "We were surprised to see the mirror neuron system activating in response to a computer. If the human brain can respond as though a computer has a mind, that's probably good news for those wishing to use the computer as a teacher."

The findings of the study are revealed in a paper published online by the journal *NeuroImage*.

Section 1.6

Recent Research Shows Why We Learn More from Our Successes Than Our Failures

"Why We Learn More from Our Successes Than Our Failures," by Deborah Halber, Picower Institute for Learning and Memory, July 29, 2009. Reprinted with permission from the Massachusetts Institute of Technology News Office. Copyright 2009.

If you've ever felt doomed to repeat your mistakes, researchers at the Massachusetts Institute of Technology's (MIT's) Picower Institute for Learning and Memory may have explained why: Brain cells may only learn from experience when we do something right and not when we fail.

In the July 30, 2009, issue of the journal *Neuron*, Earl K. Miller, the Picower Professor of Neuroscience, and MIT colleagues Mark Histed and Anitha Pasupathy have created for the first time a unique snapshot of the learning process that shows how single cells change their responses in real time as a result of information about what is the right action and what is the wrong one.

"We have shown that brain cells keep track of whether recent behaviors were successful or not," Miller said. Furthermore, when a behavior was successful, cells became more finely tuned to what the animal was learning. After a failure, there was little or no change in the brain—nor was there any improvement in behavior.

The study sheds light on the neural mechanisms linking environmental feedback to neural plasticity—the brain's ability to change in response to experience. It has implications for understanding how we learn, and understanding and treating learning disorders.

Rewarding Success

Monkeys were given the task of looking at two alternating images on a computer screen. For one picture, the animal was rewarded when it shifted its gaze to the right; for another picture it was supposed to look left. The monkeys used trial and error to figure out which images cued which movements.

The researchers found that whether the animals' answers were right or wrong, signals within certain parts of their brains "resonated" with the repercussions of their answers for several seconds. The neural activity following a correct answer and a reward helped the monkeys do better on the trial that popped up a few seconds later.

"If the monkey just got a correct answer, a signal lingered in its brain that said, 'You did the right thing.' Right after a correct answer, neurons processed information more sharply and effectively, and the monkey was more likely to get the next answer correct as well," Miller said, "But after an error there was no improvement. In other words, only after successes, not failures, did brain processing and the monkeys' behavior improve."

Split-Second Influence

The prefrontal cortex orchestrates thoughts and actions in accordance with internal goals while the basal ganglia are associated with motor control, cognition, and emotions. This work shows that these two brain areas, long suspected to play key roles in learning and memory, have full information available to them to do all the neural computations necessary for learning.

The prefrontal cortex and basal ganglia, extensively connected with each other and with the rest of the brain, are thought to help us learn abstract associations by generating brief neural signals when a response is correct or incorrect. But researchers never understood how this transient activity, which fades in less than a second, influenced actions that occurred later.

In this study, the researchers found activity in many neurons within both brain regions that reflected the delivery or withholding of a reward lasted for several seconds, until the next trial. Single neurons in both areas conveyed strong, sustained outcome information for four to six seconds, spanning the entire time frame between trials.

Response selectivity was stronger on a given trial if the previous trial had been rewarded and weaker if the previous trial was an error. This occurred whether the animal was just learning the association or was already good at it.

After a correct response, the electrical impulses coming from neurons in each of the brain areas was more robust and conveyed more information. "The signal-to-noise ratio improved in both brain regions," Miller said. "The heightened response led to them being more likely to get the next trial correct, too. This explains on a neural level why we seem to learn more from our successes than our failures."

Chapter 2

Learning Disabilities Defined

Chapter Contents

Section 2.1

Learning Styles Versus Learning Disabilities

"Learning Styles vs. Learning Disabilities" by Sheldon H. Horowitz, Ed.D. Copyright 2012 by National Center for Learning Disabilities, Inc. All rights reserved. Reprinted with permission. For more information, visit LD.org.

Truth be told, learning disabilities (LD) are not easily explained. While they are "specific" to any number of areas of learning (such as reading, math, and writing) they are also often overlapping or co-occurring, meaning that individuals with LD can have significant challenges in more than one area of skill development and performance. Because learning doesn't take place in a vacuum, social-emotional and behavioral issues often mask or exacerbate the effects of LD. And as individuals are exposed to new information, gain new insights and experience, and build their own menus of strategies to overcome or work around their areas of struggle, the impact of their learning disabilities can change, for better or for worse. Add a person's overall personality and motivation and other factors like opportunities to expand one's repertoire of effective accommodations (trying things out and seeing if they work) to the mix, and it's clear that LD is not just one thing, is not easily captured in a simple explanation, and does not affect all individuals in the same way. Hence the appeal of talking about "learning styles" in the same breath.

Not Everyone with a Preferred Style of Learning Has LD

Look around at the people with whom you have regular contact, think about how they appear to organize themselves for learning, and how they seem to be able to accomplish different tasks with ease or with difficulty:

- "L" is a "phone person," terrific at remembering names of people, and has a knack for keeping calendar dates, appointments, and call-back numbers "in her head."

- "S" dislikes talking on the phone, struggles to retrieve peoples' names but never forgets a face, and writes everything down, most often remembering details without having to refer to his notes.

- "E" is annoyed by long explanations, has little interest in reading, and is a "hands on" person, preferring to ask for information as needed and "getting the job done" without sharing thoughts, pausing for reflection, or asking for feedback.

Question: Do any of these individuals have learning disabilities?

Answer: Maybe.

Determining whether a person has learning disabilities involves formal assessment and very careful documentation, including investigations of prior school experience, response to instruction, skill mastery, information processing strengths and weaknesses, motivation, and more. Information about learning styles can, however, be very helpful in orchestrating opportunities for success in school, at work, and in the community.

Learning Styles Explained

There are too many theories about learning styles, each with unique features, to summarize in this brief section. The core principle they share, however, is almost always the same: individuals respond to and use different types of information and approaches when engaged in learning. The most common terms that are used to describe these language styles are shown in Table 2.1.

Table 2.1. Types of Learning Styles

Key "Style" Terms	Some Underlying Assumptions and Characteristics
Auditory (linguistic)	Spoken language is a preferred way of taking in and responding to information.
Visual (spatial)	Visual information (e.g., printed words, maps, charts, environmental cues) are needed for ease of learning.
Kinesthetic	Engaging in hands-on activity and getting feedback from physical sensations are important and helpful in facilitating learning and in demonstrating mastery of skills.

As mentioned earlier, no one uses only one approach to learning all the time, and having strong preferences for how information is presented and how feedback (or performance) is required and evaluated is not, by itself, a sure sign of learning disabilities.

Self-knowledge of Learning Styles Can Lead to Success

Knowing how an individual learns best, in a variety of subject areas and given a variety of different performance tasks, can be very helpful:

- Students can (and should!) speak with teachers about the features of instruction that work best for them and request that classroom practices be adjusted to enable them to achieve success.

- Parents can support school efforts and provide the types of practice, structure, and support at home that reflect learning style preferences and that lead to greater independence and school success. Be sure to engage in discussion about learning style preferences during teacher conferences and at Individualized Education Program (IEP) meetings.

- Educators can tailor and modify instruction to ensure that the needs of students with highly stylized learning preferences are being met (in addition to providing services and supports that address the challenges posed by specific learning disabilities).

Section 2.2

Federal Definitions and Criteria for Specific Learning Disabilities

"Federal Definition/Criteria for Specific Learning Disabilities," Wisconsin Department of Public Instruction, September 5, 2008.

34 CFR 300.7 Children with Disabilities

(c) Definitions of disability terms. The terms used in this definition are defined as follows:

(10) Specific learning disability is defined as follows:

(i) General. The term means a disorder in one or more of the basic psychological processes involved in understanding or in using language, spoken or written, that may manifest itself in an imperfect ability to listen, think, speak, read, write, spell, or to do mathematical calculations, including conditions such as perceptual disabilities, brain injury, minimal brain dysfunction, dyslexia, and developmental aphasia.

(ii) Disorders not included. The term does not include learning problems that are primarily the result of visual, hearing, or motor disabilities, of mental retardation, of emotional disturbance, or of environmental, cultural, or economic disadvantage.

34 CFR 300.540 Additional Team Members

The determination of whether a child suspected of having a specific learning disability is a child with a disability as defined in § 300.7, must be made by the child's parents and a team of qualified professionals which must include:

(a)(1) The child's regular teacher; or

(2) If the child does not have a regular teacher, a regular classroom teacher qualified to teach a child of his or her age; or

(3) For a child of less than school age, an individual qualified by the State Education Agency (SEA) to teach a child of his or her age; and

(b) At least one person qualified to conduct individual diagnostic examinations of children, such as a school psychologist, speech-language pathologist, or remedial reading teacher.

34 CFR 300.541 Criteria for Determining the Existence of a Specific Learning Disability

(a) A team may determine that a child has a specific learning disability if:

(1) The child does not achieve commensurate with his or her age and ability levels in one or more of the areas listed in paragraph (a)(2) of this section, if provided with learning experiences appropriate for the child's age and ability levels; and

(2) The team finds that a child has a severe discrepancy between achievement and intellectual ability in one or more of the following areas:

(i) Oral expression

(ii) Listening comprehension

(iii) Written expression

(iv) Basic reading skill

(v) Reading comprehension

(vi) Mathematics calculation

(vii) Mathematics reasoning

(b) The team may not identify a child as having a specific learning disability if the severe discrepancy between ability and achievement is primarily the result of:

(1) a visual, hearing, or motor impairment;

(2) mental retardation;

(3) emotional disturbance; or

(4) environmental, cultural, or economic disadvantage.

34 CFR 300.542 Observation

(a) At least one team member other than the child's regular teacher shall observe the child's academic performance in the regular classroom setting.

(b) In the case of a child of less than school age or out of school, a team member shall observe the child in an environment appropriate for a child of that age.

34 CFR 300.543 Written Report

(a) For a child suspected of having a specific learning disability, the documentation of the team's determination of eligibility, as required by § 300.543 (a)(2), must include a statement of:

(1) whether the child has a specific learning disability;

(2) the basis for making the determination;

(3) the relevant behavior noted during the observation of the child;

(4) the relationship of that behavior to the child's academic functioning;

(5) the educationally relevant medical findings, if any;

(6) whether there is a severe discrepancy between achievement and ability that is not correctable without special education and related services; and

(7) the determination of the team concerning the effects of environmental, cultural, or economic disadvantage.

(b) Each team member shall certify in writing whether the report reflects his or her conclusion. If it does not reflect his or her conclusion, the team member must submit a separate statement presenting his or her conclusions.

Section 2.3

What Learning Disabilities Are and What They Are Not

"Exceptional Children: Navigating Learning Disabilities and Special Education" by Sheldon H. Horowitz, *Children's Voice*, December 2005. © 2005 Child Welfare League of America (www.cwla.org). Reprinted with permission. Reviewed by David A. Cooke, M.D., FACP, January 2012.

Even though some three million school-age children are classified as having specific learning disabilities (LD), this category of special need is often widely misunderstood. Surveys of both parents and educators confirm that many people mistakenly link LD with mental retardation and disorders of mental health and believe that, left alone, children are likely to outgrow LD over time.

Let's set the record straight:

- The term specific learning disability refers to one or more of the basic psychological processes involved in understanding or using language, spoken or written, and affects a person's ability to listen, think, speak, read, write, spell, or do mathematical calculations.

- LD does not include problems primarily due to visual, hearing, or motor disabilities, although students with such diagnoses can also have learning disabilities.

- LD does not include problems that result primarily from mental retardation or emotional disturbance, although, again, children who experience such difficulties can also have learning disabilities.

- LD does not include problems that result primarily from cultural, environmental, or economic disadvantage.

- Learning disabilities are real! Although they often aren't observed until a child is doing school-related tasks, a proven biological basis for LD exists, including emerging data that document genetic links for LD within families.

- LD is common, affecting an estimated 4 to 6 percent of the public school population. And if you include individuals who, for a number of reasons, struggle with reading, the numbers are considerably higher.

- Learning disabilities are lifelong. That said, individuals with LD can learn to compensate for areas of weakness and, with early, effective support, can be highly successful and productive members of society.

Serving Students with LD: It's the law!

The quality of services and supports children receive in school are key to their learning success. Working together, general and special educators are charged with ensuring that all children receive a free and appropriate public education in the least restrictive setting.

Although states and school districts have considerable latitude in how they meet this challenge, a few important federal laws underlie their efforts.

The Individuals with Disabilities Education Act (IDEA) provides for special education services for children and youth, ages three to twenty-one, with disabilities. It ensures each child receives a free, appropriate public education based on his or her individual needs, and it specifies thirteen possible educational disabling conditions, including specific learning disabilities. It also guarantees a number of important rights—timely evaluation, access to all meetings and paperwork, transition planning, and related services—for children with disabilities and their parents or guardians. Most children with LD are served under IDEA.

Section 504 of the Rehabilitation Act of 1973 is a civil rights law prohibiting discrimination on the basis of disability in programs and activities that receive federal funding. It does not provide funding for these programs, but it does permit the government to withdraw funds from programs that do not comply with the law. To qualify for services under Section 504, a person must have a physical or mental impairment that substantially limits one or more major life activities. Some schools use this law to support students with LD who need only simple accommodations or modifications. It is also frequently used for children with attention deficit/hyperactivity disorder who do not need more comprehensive special education support.

The Americans with Disabilities Act (ADA) is also a civil rights law that protects individuals with LD from discrimination in schools, the workplace, and other settings. ADA does not provide funding for services and accommodations, and, as with Section 504, persons must have a physical or mental impairment that substantially limits one or more major life activities. Learning is considered a major life activity under ADA, so if a student qualifies for services under IDEA, he or she is also protected under ADA.

No Child Left Behind (NCLB) is the current version of the Elementary and Secondary Education Act, first passed in 1965, which affects all public education, from kindergarten through grade twelve. The power of NCLB is that it holds schools accountable for student progress by demanding clearly defined content standards (what students should be learning) and achievement standards (how well they should be learning). It also requires schools to measure student progress to see whether all students are making adequate yearly progress. NCLB ensures that schools report overall student progress data as well as progress for various student subgroups, including students with disabilities.

Chapter 3

Causes of Learning Disabilities

Chapter Contents

Section 3.1

Neurobiology of Learning Disabilities

"The Neurobiology" by Joyce Powell Riley, M.A., President, Orange County Learning Disabilities Association. © 2001 Orange County Learning Disabilities Association (www.oclda.org). All rights reserved. Reprinted with permission. Edited by David A. Cooke, MD, FACP, February 2012.

The underlying medical disorder in learning disabilities is a dysfunction of the central nervous system, which includes the brain. When the brain dysfunctions it affects the neurobiology of the body. The neurobiology involves the interaction of the central nervous system with the immune system and the endocrine system. There are many reasons for the dysfunctions:

- Genetics play a part. Many times the disorder comes down the father's line from grandfather, father to son. Fragile X, XYY, or Tourette may be involved. Depression, particularly bipolar, may be involved. There is a need for much more research in this field.

- Pre-natal, peri-natal, and post-natal problems such as maternal measles during gestation, problems of birthing such as brain damage from the use of forceps, or the use of soy-based formula with excessive manganese after birth, can be responsible for the onset of learning disabilities. Certain vaccinations may also cause problems.

- Structural problems of the brain, many times caused by the use of substances by the mother during gestation, can cause dysfunction of the brain after birth. When the fetus gets hit with a load of cocaine, whatever brain function was in development at that moment may be damaged. There are many substances and circumstances that can cause structural defects in a developing fetus's brain.

- Toxic substances can be very dangerous to brain function. Concern about lead depressing children's IQ led to the elimination of lead in gasoline and paint. Mercury and cadmium, pesticides, and petrochemical-based products can have a devastating effect on brain function.

- Infections such as encephalitis, meningitis, pneumonia, severe influenza, measles, and other childhood diseases that overwhelm the individual's immune system make it difficult for the central nervous system to function properly.

- Brain trauma can be the result of many things. Specific head injury can impair thought even when the doctor finds no problem. Abuse and neglect can affect the brain directly or indirectly because of malnutrition. Abandonment and loss situations, such as the death of a parent or a divorce in the family, can cause grief and the grief cycle. Feelings of anger and depression can look like learning disabilities but may clear when the time of grief has passed.

A knowledgeable physician is necessary to diagnose the medical aspects of learning disabilities.

Section 3.2

Genetic Causes of Learning Disabilities

"Genetic Changes Involved in Learning Disability,"
June 26, 2009. Reprinted with permission from the University
of Oxford (www.ox.ac.uk). Copyright 2009.

The first comprehensive effort to pinpoint the genetic causes of learning disability has narrowed down the genes involved from a potential list of thousands to several dozen key genes.

The study by scientists at Oxford University and Radboud University Nijmegen Medical Centre in The Netherlands could lead to diagnostic testing and genetic counseling being offered as an option to people with learning difficulties and their families.

The seventy-eight genes identified by the research are involved in the nervous system. This is the first time that evidence from across the human genome has shown that learning disability is a disorder of the brain and nervous system. The study was funded by the Medical Research Council and the Netherlands Organisation for Health Research and Development, and the findings are published in the journal *PLoS Genetics*.

"We have found a set of key genes in which changes or variations could lead to learning disability," says Professor Chris Ponting of the MRC Functional Genomics Unit at the University of Oxford. "This could be a first step towards offering people the option of having a genetic diagnostic test for learning difficulties, should they want it."

"For example, if I had a child with learning difficulties, I might choose to know whether I had passed on a genetic change or if such a change had arisen spontaneously by chance. Such knowledge might remove worries I might have about wanting further kids. But proper genetic counseling and support would be needed to help in making such choices."

People with learning difficulties can have problems with skills needed for daily life, social interaction, and communication. It can result from different environmental causes (such as injuries in car crashes or childhood illness) and genetic factors.

The genetic causes of learning disability are poorly understood. Because the condition is so generally defined, the symptoms are so broad, and the brain is so complex, it is estimated that thousands of genes could be associated with learning difficulties. However, there is little evidence available to back up this assumption.

The team from Oxford University and Radboud University Nijmegen Medical Centre set out to identify the types of genes that, when changed, can result in learning disability.

First, they looked at large-scale changes in the deoxyribonucleic acid (DNA) of over one thousand people with learning disabilities. These were deletions or duplications of whole chunks of DNA that had arisen spontaneously and were not found in their unaffected parents, with each chunk often containing as many as forty individual genes.

To understand which of the many genes in these long lengths of DNA might be involved in learning disability, the researchers turned to the vast amount of genetic information available from mice. Over five thousand genes have been individually disrupted in mice to see what role they play in the body. This means that data exist on the mouse equivalents of roughly one in four human genes.

Putting all this together, the researchers found that the DNA changes associated with learning disability contained greater than expected numbers of genes whose loss in mice affected the nervous system. This suggests that the loss or disruption of these genes could result in learning difficulties.

"Essentially, we've gone along every missing chunk of DNA, checking to see which type of genes continually comes up," explains Professor Ponting. "Wherever possible, we've then looked to mice to see what happens if each of the genes is disrupted."

The genes that have been identified can now be scrutinized further to aid understanding of what processes in the body break down and result in learning difficulties.

"Now that we have shown how powerful this technique of combining human and mouse genetic data can be, we intend to look at the genetic basis of autism and schizophrenia next," says Dr. Caleb Webber, also of the MRC Functional Genomics Unit at Oxford University.

Section 3.3

Environmental Contaminants and Learning Disabilities

Excerpted from "Scientific Consensus Statement on Environmental Agents Associated with Neurodevelopmental Disorders," developed by the Collaborative on Health and the Environment's Learning and Developmental Disabilities Initiative, 2008. © 2008 Collaborative on Health and the Environment. All rights reserved. Reprinted with permission. For additional information including the complete text of this consensus statement, visit www.healthandenvironment.org.

High-Confidence Conclusions

Many environmental contaminants have been conclusively shown to affect the developing nervous system, causing a range of performance deficits.[1,2]

Alcohol

The effects of ethyl alcohol on brain development and function are well established. Fetal alcohol syndrome (FAS), now considered part of fetal alcohol spectrum disorder (FASD), is the most preventable form of behavioral and learning disabilities. In the United States, FASD is estimated to affect 9.1 per 1,000 infants[3], with even higher rates in other parts of the world.[4] Even low or moderate consumption of alcohol during pregnancy can cause subtle and permanent performance deficits.[5,6] Specific genetic polymorphisms enhance the risk of FASD.[7]

35

Lead

Lead is probably the most studied of environmental contaminants in both humans and animals. Its effects on learning and development are undisputed. Recent research indicates that there is no safe level of lead exposure for children.[8-10] Lead exposure impairs overall intelligence as measured by intelligence quotient (IQ), learning, and memory and is associated with attention deficit hyperactivity disorder (ADHD) even at minute exposures. Efforts to prevent lead exposure provide an outstanding example of the struggle when science meets policy.[11-13] This debate is still unfolding: the U.S. Centers for Disease Control and Prevention (CDC) has not adjusted the blood-lead action level since 1990 despite scientific evidence of behavioral effects well below 10 micrograms per deciliter (µg/dL). Arguments have been made to reduce the CDC blood-lead action level to 2 µg/dL.[11]

Mercury

There is no doubt that mercury exposure causes learning and developmental disorders; the controversy regards the level of exposure. We are all exposed to some form of mercury. Inorganic mercury is the liquid silver form and is used in dental amalgams. Mercury is also present in coal, and coal-burning electric utilities facilities are a significant source of atmospheric environmental mercury. While much of the mercury falls close to the facility, mercury can be carried long distances to pollute water supplies and, ultimately, contaminate the food supply. Inorganic mercury is converted to the organic methylmercury and bioaccumulates in the flesh of fish, being biomagnified up the food chain. Methylmercury contamination often results in fish-consumption advisories, particularly for women and children. The knowledge (and concern) that methylmercury exposures affect the developing nervous system resulted in several very sophisticated studies designed to assess the effects of very low level exposures on a range of learning and memory tests and on other performance-based tests.[14-24] These tests typically included age-related assessment of learning and memory, reading, IQ, and other neurological functions.

Polychlorinated Biphenyls (PCBs)

PCBs are mixtures of chlorinated compounds that were once used as cooling and insulating fluids in electrical transformers and other electronic components. Because they are very persistent, PCBs have become widely distributed in the environment despite being banned in the 1970s.

Because PCBs bioaccumulate in fat, human exposure continues through the food supply, and infant exposure continues through contaminated breast milk. Numerous studies have documented that PCB exposure can adversely affect motor skills, learning, and memory as shown in lower full-scale and verbal IQ scores and reading ability.[19, 25-31]

Polybrominated Diphenyl Ethers (PBDEs)

PBDEs have been used commonly as flame-retardant chemicals for several decades. PBDEs, structurally similar to PCBs, bioaccumulate in animals and humans, and are excreted in human breast milk. Recent studies have left little doubt that PBDEs are developmental neurotoxicants in animals and lead to changes in motor activity and reduced performance on learning and memory tests.[32,33]

Manganese

Manganese is a trace element which is necessary in small amounts for growth and development. Recent studies indicate that high levels of manganese exposure, either from inhalation (welding fumes)[34,35] or through drinking water, can damage the developing nervous system[36,37] as measured in full-scale IQ and verbal tests.[36, 38-43] For example, a case study documented memory effects in a child exposed to manganese in drinking water[39], and a more recent study confirmed similar effects.[37] The U.S. Environmental Protection Agency (EPA) advises that water levels of manganese should not exceed 300 µg Mn/L, but approximately 6 percent of domestic household wells exceed this level.[43]

Arsenic

Arsenic is commonly found in drinking water around the world, sometimes in concentrations high enough to cause cancer.[44] Recent studies have found a dose-response relationship between exposure to arsenic and intellectual impairment.[38, 45-48] While additional studies assessing the impact of low levels of arsenic in drinking water are needed, it is clear that arsenic affects the neurodevelopment of children.

Solvents

Solvents include a broad array of different compounds including toluene, benzene, alcohol, turpentine, acetone, and tetrachloroethylene (TCE) (see Table 3.1), with more than fifty million metric tons used in the United States and more than ten million people exposed in the workplace. Solvent neurotoxicity is well recognized in adult workers.[49] Ethyl alcohol is a widely used and consumed solvent with clear learning and developmental effects (see above). Recent studies indicate that occupational exposure to solvents in salons and laboratories can result in visual deficits in offspring.[50-53] Several reports have documented that the adverse developmental effects of maternal toluene exposure include low birth weight, decreased head circumference, and developmental delays.[54,55] Awareness of developmental effects of solvent exposure has resulted in increasing concern for women working in nail and beauty salons. Some solvents, such as toluene, have also been abused by pregnant women who purposely sniff them.

Table 3.1. Examples of Solvents

Products that are mostly solvent	Partially solvent-based
Gasoline	Glues
Diesel fuel	Adhesives
Charcoal lighter fluid	Oil-based paints
Lantern fuel	Fingernail polish
Grease	Furniture polishes
Lubricating oils	Floor polishes and waxes
Degreasing agents	Spot removers
Paint strippers	Metal and wood cleaners
Paint thinner	Correction fluid
Turpentine	Computer disk cleaners
Nail polish remover	Varnishes and shellacs
Rubbing alcohol	Wood and concrete stains

Polycyclic Aromatic Hydrocarbons (PAHs)

Polycyclic aromatic hydrocarbons (PAHs) are widely distributed air pollutants and well-recognized human mutagens and carcinogens. PAHs are generated during combustion of fuels from motor vehicles, coal-fired power plants, residential heating and cooking, and are also present in tobacco smoke. Recent studies have indicated that elevated exposure to PAHs results in lower birth weight[56] and affects cognitive development.[57]

Pesticides

Major classes of pesticides are specifically designed to kill insects, plants, fungi, or animals. Agricultural and residential application of pesticides in the United States totals more than one billion pounds per year, with thousands of people exposed every year. Data from acute exposure incidents leave no doubt that some pesticides, particularly insecticides, are neurotoxic. There is now evidence that childhood exposure to pesticides, such as organophosphates, enhances the risk for developmental disorders including deficits in memory[58], poorer motor performance[59,60], and an array of other conditions.[61-69] A recent study documented the developmental effects of the pesticide chlorpyrifos on inner-city children.[70] There is also evidence of specific genetic susceptibility to pesticide exposure and related health effects.[71-73, 61]

Nicotine and Environmental Tobacco Smoke

Many studies link maternal smoking during pregnancy to behavioral disorders in children[74-77], and developmental delays caused by environmental tobacco smoke (ETS, also known as secondhand smoke) are costly and preventable.[78] Furthermore, new data indicates that childhood exposure to ETS is associated with neurobehavioral effects.[79] There is growing recognition of subsequent behavioral disorders in young adults following exposures either prenatally or as children.[77,80,81] The CDC reported in 2002 that 11.4 percent of all women giving birth in the United States smoked during pregnancy.[82] Clearly this highly preventable form of developmental disorder requires that parents, both male and female, be educated about the harmful effects of tobacco.

Other Contributors and Emerging Evidence

It is not possible to address all the chemicals that might be associated with causing learning and developmental disorders. A more comprehensive assessment of developmental neurotoxicity of chemicals was undertaken by Grandjean and Landrigan1 in which they pointed out that, for the majority of chemicals, we do not have the data necessary to conclude there are no adverse developmental effects. They estimate that more than two hundred chemicals are known to cause neurotoxic effects in adults and that, for many of these chemicals, developmental effects have not been examined. In addition, very few studies have focused on the potential synergistic impacts of chemicals in mixtures. Highlighted below are just a few agents that are of significant concern.

Endocrine Disruptors

Animal studies have documented that a wide range of chemicals have the ability to disrupt endocrine function in animals and affect cognitive function.[83] Endocrine disruptors include phthalates, PCBs and polychlorinated dibenzodioxins, brominated flame retardants, dioxins, dichlorodiphenyltrichloroethane (DDT), perfluorinated compounds (PFCs), organochlorine pesticides, bisphenol A, and some metals. The controversy around the effects of endocrine disruptors is perhaps best illustrated by research on bisphenol A,[84,85] whose estrogenic activity was first reported in 1936. It was subsequently found to stabilize polycarbonates and resins and is now widely used in many products including food-can liners. There is a growing body of evidence related to the very low dose effects of bisphenol A.[86–88] The very low dose effects of endocrine disruptors cannot be predicted from high-dose studies, which contradicts the standard "dose makes the poison" rule of toxicology. Nontraditional dose-response curves are referred to as nonmonotonic dose-response curves.

Fluoride

Fluoride is commonly added to municipal drinking water across the United States based on strong data that it reduces dental decay. This practice is supported by the U.S. Centers for Disease Control (CDC).[89,90] In addition to drinking water, fluoride is also present in a range of consumer products including toothpaste (1,000–1,500 parts per million or ppm), mouthwashes, and fluoride supplements. The drinking water standards were established prior to the introduction of fluoride into many consumer products and the direct application of fluoride by dentists.

The central question, which is still unresolved, is what level of exposure results in harmful health effects to children. Children's small size means that, pound-for-pound of body weight, they receive a greater dose of fluoride than adults. The CDC estimates that up to 33 percent of children may have dental fluorosis because of the excessive intake of fluoride either through drinking water or through other sources—an estimate which is supported by other studies.[91] This concern has resulted in CDC issuing a recommendation to limit fluoride exposure in children under eight years of age and to use fluoride-free water when preparing infant milk formula.

In addition, some recent studies suggest that excessive ingestion of fluoride lowers thyroid hormone levels, which is particularly critical for women with subclinical hypothyroidism. Decreased maternal thyroid levels are known to adversely affect fetal neurodevelopment.[92] A study in China, for example, reported decreased child IQ levels associated with fluoride in drinking water. (Children in this study were also exposed to arsenic in drinking water, which may have confounded the results).[89,90] The same year, in *Fluoride in Drinking Water: A Scientific Review of EPA's Standards*, a report produced by the National Academy of Sciences (NAS)[89], researchers analyzed the appropriateness of EPA's four ppm maximum contaminant level goal for fluoride in drinking water. The NAS was not directed to conduct a risk assessment of the effects of low-level fluoride exposure nor analyze other sources of exposure to fluoride. Referring to human and animal studies related to neurobehavioral effects, the NAS reports states "the consistency of the results appears significant enough to warrant additional research on the effects of fluoride on intelligence." The primary question remains as to whether exposures to fluoride via multiple routes of exposure, from drinking water, food, and dental-care products, may result in a high enough cumulative exposure to contribute to developmental effects.

While it is clear that fluoride has beneficial effects on dental health, emerging science suggests we need to further study the dose at which fluoridation may increase risks of neurodevelopment disorders, cancer, and skeletal or dental fluorosis, particularly for sensitive individuals.

Food Additives

Artificial or synthetic food colors and additives are ubiquitous in the food supply and have long been suspected of causing conduct disorders. Their use has encouraged treatments such as the Feingold diet,[93,94] in which many food additives are removed from the diet of individuals with ADHD. Previous and recent carefully conducted double-blind human studies have confirmed that artificial food colorings such as sunset yellow, tartrazine, carmoisine, and ponceau, as well as the preservative sodium benzoate, can cause conduct disorders.[93-99] Recent studies using well-designed randomized, double-blind, placebo-controlled, crossover trials show that artificial food colors and additives cause increased hyperactivity in three-year-old children.[97] This has the potential to become a serious issue given the large number of children diagnosed with ADHD.

References

1. Grandjean P, Landrigan PJ. Developmental neurotoxicity of industrial chemicals. *Lancet* 2006; 368(9553): 2167–78.

2. Schettler T. Toxic threats to neurologic development of children. *Environ Health Perspect* 2001; 109 Suppl 6:813–166.

3. Sokol RJ, Delaney-Black V, Nordstrom B. Fetal alcohol spectrum disorder. *JAMA* 2003; 290(22): 2996–99.

4. Warren KR, Calhoun FJ, May PA, Viljoen DL, Li TK, Tanaka H, et al. Fetal alcohol syndrome: an international perspective. *Alcohol Clin Exp Res* 2001; 25(5 Suppl ISBRA): 202S–206S.

5. Streissguth AP, Barr HM, Sampson PD. Moderate prenatal alcohol exposure: effects on child IQ and learning problems at age 7 1/2 years. *Alcohol Clin Exp Res* 1990; 14(5): 662–69.

6. Streissguth AP, Barr HM, Sampson PD, Bookstein FL. Prenatal alcohol and offspring development: the first fourteen years. *Drug Alcohol Depend* 1994; 36(2): 89–99.

7. Warren KR, Li TK. Genetic polymorphisms: impact on the risk of fetal alcohol spectrum disorders. *Birth Defects Res A Clin Mol Teratol* 2005; 73(4): 195–203.

8. Lanphear BP, Hornung R, Khoury J, Yolton K, Baghurst P, Bellinger DC, et al. Low-level environmental lead exposure and children's intellectual function: an international pooled analysis. *Environ Health Perspect* 2005; 113(7): 894–99.

9. Canfield RL, Henderson CR, Jr., Cory-Slechta DA, Cox C, Jusko TA, Lanphear BP. Intellectual impairment in children with blood lead concentrations below 10 microg per deciliter. *N Engl J Med* 2003; 348(16): 1517–26.

10. Miranda ML, Kim D, Galeano MA, Paul CJ, Hull AP, Morgan SP. The Relationship between early childhood blood lead levels and performance on end-of-grade tests. *Environ Health Perspect* 2007; 115(8): 1242–47.

11. Gilbert SG, Weiss B. A rationale for lowering the blood lead action level from 10 to 2 microg/dL. *Neurotoxicology* 2006; 27(5): 693–701.

12. Bellinger DC, Bellinger AM. Childhood lead poisoning: the torturous path from science to policy. *J Clin Invest* 2006; 116(4): 853–57.

13. Gilbert SG. Ethical, legal, and social issues: our children's future. *Neurotoxicology* 2005; 26(4): 521–30.

14. Gilbert SG, Grant-Webster KS. Neurobehavioral effects of developmental methylmercury exposure. *Environ Health Perspect* 1995; 103 Suppl 6: 135–42.

15. Grandjean P, Weihe P, White RF, Debes F, Araki S, Yokoyama K, et al. Cognitive deficit in 7-year-old children with prenatal exposure to methylmercury. *Neurotoxicol Teratol* 1997; 19(6): 417–28.

16. Grandjean P, White RF. Effects of methylmercury exposure on neurodevelopment. *JAMA* 1999; 281(10): 896; author reply 897.

17. Clarkson TW. Mercury: major issues in environmental health. *Environ Health Perspect* 1992; 100: 31–38.

18. Rice DC, Neurotoxicity of lead, methylmercury, and PCBs in relation to the Great Lakes. *Environ Health Perspect* 1995; 103 Suppl 9: 71–87.

19. Grandjean P, Weihe P, Burse VW, Needham LL, Storr-Hansen E, Heinzow B, et al. Neurobehavioral deficits associated with PCB in 7-year-old children prenatally exposed to seafood neurotoxicants. *Neurotoxicol Teratol* 2001; 23(4): 305–17.

20. Davidson PW, Myers GJ, Weiss B, Shamlaye CF, Cox C. Prenatal methylmercury exposure from fish consumption and child development: a review of evidence and perspectives from the Seychelles Child Development Study. *Neurotoxicology* 2006; 27(6): 1106–9.

21. Davidson PW, Myers GJ, Cox C, Wilding GE, Shamlaye CF, Huang LS, et al. Methylmercury and neurodevelopment: longitudinal analysis of the Seychelles child development cohort. *Neurotoxicol Teratol* 2006; 28(5): 529–35.

22. Trasande L, Landrigan PJ, Schechter C. Public health and economic consequences of methylmercury toxicity to the developing brain. *Environ Health Perspect* 2005; 113(5): 590–96.

23. Goldman LR, Farland WH. Methylmercury risks. *Science* 1998; 279(5351): 640–41; author reply 641.

24. Grandjean P, White RF, Nielsen A, Cleary D, de Oliveira Santos EC. Methylmercury neurotoxicity in Amazonian children downstream from gold mining. *Environ Health Perspect* 1999; 107(7): 587–91.

25. ATSDR. Toxicological Profile For Polychlorinated Biphenyls (PCBs): Agency for Toxic Substances and Disease Registry. Available at http://www.atsdr.cdc.gov/toxprofiles/tp17.pdf; 2000.

26. Jacobson JL, Jacobson SW. Intellectual impairment in children exposed to polychlorinated biphenyls in utero. *N Engl J Med* 1996; 335(11): 783–89.

27. Jacobson JL, Jacobson SW. Dose-response in perinatal exposure to polychlorinated biphenyls (PCBs): the Michigan and North Carolina cohort studies. *Toxicol Ind Health* 1996; 12(3–4): 435–45.

28. Nakajima S, Saijo Y, Kato S, Sasaki S, Uno A, Kanagami N, et al. Effects of prenatal exposure to polychlorinated biphenyls and dioxins on mental and motor development in Japanese children at 6 months of age. *Environ Health Perspect* 2006; 114(5): 773–78.

29. Vreugdenhil HJ, Van Zanten GA, Brocaar MP, Mulder PG, Weisglas-Kuperus N. Prenatal exposure to polychlorinated biphenyls and breastfeeding: opposing effects on auditory P300 latencies in 9-year-old Dutch children. *Dev Med Child Neurol* 2004; 46(6): 398–405.

30. Schantz SL, Gasior DM, Polverejan E, McCaffrey RJ, Sweeney AM, Humphrey HE, et al. Impairments of memory and learning in older adults exposed to polychlorinated biphenyls via consumption of Great Lakes fish. *Environ Health Perspect* 2001; 109(6): 605–11.

31. Schantz SL, Widholm JJ, Rice DC. Effects of PCB exposure on neuropsychological function in children. Environ Health Perspect 2003; 111(3): 357–576.

32. Costa LG, Giordano G. Developmental neurotoxicity of poly-brominated diphenyl ether (PBDE) flame retardants. *Neurotoxicology* 2007.

33. Rice DC, Reeve EA, Herlihy A, Zoeller RT, Thompson WD, Markowski VP. Developmental delays and locomotor activity in the C57BL6/J mouse following neonatal exposure to the fully brominated PBDE, decabromodiphenyl ether. *Neurotoxicol Teratol* 2007; 29(4): 511–20.

34. Bowler RM, Nakagawa S, Drezgic M, Roels HA, Park RM, Diamond E, et al. Sequelae of fume exposure in confined space welding: a neurological and neuropsychological case series. *Neurotoxicology* 2007; 28(2): 298–311.

35. Bowler RM, Roels HA, Nakagawa S, Drezgic M, Diamond E, Park R, et al. Dose-effect relationships between manganese exposure and neurological, neuropsychological and pulmonary

function in confined space bridge welders. *Occup Environ Med* 2007; 64(3): 167–77.

36. ATSDR. Toxicological Profile For Manganese: Agency for Toxic Substances and Disease Registry. Available at http://www.atsdr .cdc.gov/toxprofiles/tp17.pdf; 2000.

37. Bouchard M, Laforest F, Vandelac L, Bellinger D, Mergler D. Hair manganese and hyperactive behaviors: pilot study of school-age children exposed through tap water. *Environ Health Perspect* 2007; 115(1): 122–27.

38. Wasserman GA, Liu X, Parvez F, Ahsan H, Factor-Litvak P, Kline J, et al. Water arsenic exposure and intellectual function in 6-year-old children in Araihazar, Bangladesh. *Environ Health Perspect* 2007; 115(2): 285–89.

39. Woolf AD, Wright RO, Amarasiriwardena C, Bellinger DC. A child with chronic manganese exposure from drinking water. *Environ Health Perspect* 2002; 110(6): 613–16.

40. Wright RO, Amarasiriwardena C, Woolf AD, Jim R, Bellinger DC. Neuropsychological correlates of hair arsenic, manganese, and cadmium levels in school-age children residing near a hazardous waste site. *Neurotoxicology* 2006; 27(2): 210–16.

41. Pal PK, Samii A, Calne DB. Manganese neurotoxicity: a review of clinical features, imaging and pathology. *Neurotoxicology* 1999; 20(2–3): 227–38.

42. Mergler D, Baldwin M, Belanger S, Larribe F, Beuter A, Bowler R, et al. Manganese neurotoxicity, a continuum of dysfunction: results from a community based study. *Neurotoxicology* 1999; 20(2–3): 327–42.

43. Wasserman GA, Liu X, Parvez F, Ahsan H, Levy D, Factor-Litvak P, et al. Water manganese exposure and children's intellectual function in Araihazar, Bangladesh. *Environ Health Perspect* 2006; 114(1): 124–29.

44. Ahsan H, Chen Y, Parvez F, Zablotska L, Argos M, Hussain I, et al. Arsenic exposure from drinking water and risk of premalignant skin lesions in Bangladesh: baseline results from the Health Effects of Arsenic Longitudinal Study. *Am J Epidemiol* 2006; 163(12): 1138–48.

45. Wasserman GA, Liu X, Parvez F, Ahsan H, Factor-Litvak P, van Geen A, et al. Water arsenic exposure and children's intellectual

function in Araihazar, Bangladesh. *Environ Health Perspect* 2004; 112(13): 1329–33.

46. Hafeman DM, Ahsan H, Louis ED, Siddique AB, Slavkovich V, Cheng Z, et al. Association between arsenic exposure and a measure of subclinical sensory neuropathy in Bangladesh. *J Occup Environ Med* 2005; 47(8): 778–84.

47. Golub MS, Macintosh MS, Baumrind N. Developmental and reproductive toxicity of inorganic arsenic: animal studies and human concerns. *J Toxicol Environ Health B Crit Rev* 1998; 1(3): 199–241.

48. ATSDR. Toxicological Profile For Arsenic: Agency for Toxic Substances and Disease Registry. Available at http://www.atsdr.cdc.gov/toxprofiles/tp17.pdf; 2005.

49. White RF, Proctor SP. Solvents and neurotoxicity. *Lancet* 1997; 349(9060): 1239–43.

50. Eskenazi B, Gaylord L, Bracken MB, Brown D. In utero exposure to organic solvents and human neurodevelopment. *Dev Med Child Neurol* 1988; 30(4): 492–501.

51. Laslo-Baker D, Barrera M, Knittel-Keren D, Kozer E, Wolpin J, Khattak S, et al. Child neurodevelopmental outcome and maternal occupational exposure to solvents. *Arch Pediatr Adolesc Med* 2004; 158(10): 956–61.

52. Till C, Westall CA, Koren G, Nulman I, Rovet JF. Vision abnormalities in young children exposed prenatally to organic solvents. *Neurotoxicology* 2005; 26(4): 599–613.

53. Till C, Westall CA, Rovet JF, Koren G. Effects of maternal occupational exposure to organic solvents on offspring visual functioning: a prospective controlled study. *Teratology* 2001; 64(3): 134–41.

54. Arnold GL, Kirby RS, Langendoerfer S, Wilkins-Haug L. Toluene embryopathy: clinical delineation and developmental follow-up. *Pediatrics* 1994; 93(2): 216–20.

55. Hersh JH, Podruch PE, Rogers G, Weisskopf B. Toluene embryopathy. *J Pediatr* 1985; 106(6): 922–27.

56. Choi H, Jedrychowski W, Spengler J, Camann DE, Whyatt RM, Rauh V, et al. International studies of prenatal exposure to polycyclic aromatic hydrocarbons and fetal growth. *Environ Health Perspect* 2006; 114(11): 1744–50.

57. Perera FP, Rauh V, Whyatt RM, Tsai WY, Tang D, Diaz D, et al. Effect of prenatal exposure to airborne polycyclic aromatic hydrocarbons on neurodevelopment in the first 3 years of life among inner city children. *Environ Health Perspect* 2006; 114(8): 1287–92.

58. Guillette EA, Meza MM, Aquilar MG, Soto AD, Garcia IE. An anthropological approach to the evaluation of preschool children exposed to pesticides in Mexico. *Environ Health Perspect* 1998; 106(6): 347–53.

59. Rohlman DS, Anger WK, Tamulinas A, Phillips J, Bailey SR, McCauley L. Development of a neurobehavioral battery for children exposed to neurotoxic chemicals. *Neurotoxicology* 2001; 22(5): 657–65.

60. Rohlman DS, Arcury TA, Quandt SA, Lasarev M, Rothlein J, Travers R, et al. Neurobehavioral performance in preschool children from agricultural and non-agricultural communities in Oregon and North Carolina. *Neurotoxicology* 2005; 26(4): 589–98.

61. Berkowitz GS, Wetmur JG, Birman-Deych E, Obel J, Lapinski RH, Godbold JH, et al. In utero pesticide exposure, maternal paraoxonase activity, and head circumference. *Environ Health Perspect* 2004; 112(3): 388–91.

62. Grandjean P, Harari R, Barr DB, Debes F. Pesticide exposure and stunting as independent predictors of neurobehavioral deficits in Ecuadorian school children. *Pediatrics* 2006; 117(3): e546–56.

63. Ruckart PZ, Kakolewski K, Bove FJ, Kaye WE. Long-term neurobehavioral health effects of methyl parathion exposure in children in Mississippi and Ohio. *Environ Health Perspect* 2004; 112(1): 46–51.

64. Whyatt RM, Garfinkel R, Hoepner LA, Holmes D, Borjas M, Williams MK, et al. Within- and between-home variability in indoor-air insecticide levels during pregnancy among an inner-city cohort from New York City. *Environ Health Perspect* 2007; 115(3): 383–89.

65. Whyatt RM, Rauh V, Barr DB, Camann DE, Andrews HF, Garfinkel R, et al. Prenatal insecticide exposures and birth weight and length among an urban minority cohort. *Environ Health Perspect* 2004; 112(10): 1125–32.

66. Young JG, Eskenazi B, Gladstone EA, Bradman A, Pedersen L, Johnson C, et al. Association between in utero organophosphate pesticide exposure and abnormal reflexes in neonates. *Neurotoxicology* 2005; 26(2): 199–209.

67. Handal AJ, Lozoff B, Breilh J, Harlow SD. Effect of community of residence on neurobehavioral development in infants and young children in a flower-growing region of Ecuador. *Environ Health Perspect* 2007; 115(1): 128–33.

68. Handal AJ, Lozoff B, Breilh J, Harlow SD. Neurobehavioral development in children with potential exposure to pesticides. *Epidemiology* 2007; 18(3): 312–20.

69. Handal AJ, Lozoff B, Breilh J, Harlow SD. Sociodemographic and nutritional correlates of neurobehavioral development: a study of young children in a rural region of Ecuador. *Rev Panam Salud Publica* 2007; 21(5): 292–300.

70. Rauh VA, Garfinkel R, Perera FP, Andrews HF, Hoepner L, Barr DB, et al. Impact of prenatal chlorpyrifos exposure on neurodevelopment in the first 3 years of life among inner-city children. *Pediatrics* 2006; 118(6): e1845–59.

71. Furlong CE, Cole TB, Jarvik GP, Pettan-Brewer C, Geiss GK, Richter RJ, et al. Role of paraoxonase (PON1) status in pesticide sensitivity: genetic and temporal determinants. *Neurotoxicology* 2005; 26(4): 651–59.

72. Furlong CE, Holland N, Richter RJ, Bradman A, Ho A, Eskenazi B. PON1 status of farmworker mothers and children as a predictor of organophosphate sensitivity. *Pharmacogenet Genomics* 2006; 16(3): 183–90.

73. Holland N, Furlong C, Bastaki M, Richter R, Bradman A, Huen K, et al. Paraoxonase polymorphisms, haplotypes, and enzyme activity in Latino mothers and newborns. *Environ Health Perspect* 2006; 114(7): 985–91.

74. Linnet KM, Dalsgaard S, Obel C, Wisborg K, Henriksen TB, Rodriguez A, et al. Maternal lifestyle factors in pregnancy risk of attention deficit hyperactivity disorder and associated behaviors: review of the current evidence. *Am J Psychiatry* 2003; 160(6): 1028–40.

75. Orlebeke JF, Knol DL, Verhulst FC. Child behavior problems increased by maternal smoking during pregnancy. *Arch Environ Health* 1999; 54(1): 15–19.

76. Thapar A, Fowler T, Rice F, Scourfield J, van den Bree M, Thomas H, et al. Maternal smoking during pregnancy and attention deficit hyperactivity disorder symptoms in offspring. *Am J Psychiatry* 2003; 160(11): 1985–89.

77. Wakschlag LS, Pickett KE, Cook E, Jr., Benowitz NL, Leventhal BL. Maternal smoking during pregnancy and severe antisocial behavior in offspring: a review. *Am J Public Health* 2002; 92(6): 966–74.

78. Miller T, Rauh VA, Glied SA, Hattis D, Rundle A, Andrews H, et al. The economic impact of early life environmental tobacco smoke exposure: early intervention for developmental delay. *Environ Health Perspec* 2006; 114(10): 1585–88.

79. Gatzke-Kopp LM, Beauchaine TP. Direct and Passive Prenatal Nicotine Exposure and the Development of Externalizing Psychopathology. *Child Psychiatry Hum Dev* 2007.

80. Wakschlag LS, Pickett KE, Leventhal BL. The association between maternal cigarette smoking and psychiatric diseases or criminal outcome in the offspring. *Reprod Toxicol* 2000; 14(6): 579–80.

81. Brennan PA, Grekin ER, Mortensen EL, Mednick SA. Relationship of maternal smoking during pregnancy with criminal arrest and hospitalization for substance abuse in male and female adult offspring. *Am J Psychiatry* 2002; 159(1): 48–54.

82. MMWR. Smoking During Pregnancy—United States, 1990–2002. In: Center for Disease Control and Prevention. Available at http://www.cdc.gov/MMWR/preview/mmwrhtml/mm5339a1.htm; 2004. p. 911–15.

83. Schantz SL, Widholm JJ. Cognitive effects of endocrine-disrupting chemicals in animals. *Environ Health Perspect* 2001; 109(12): 1197–206.

84. Gross L. The toxic origins of disease. *PLoS Biol* 2007; 5(7):e193.

85. Kuehn BM. Expert panels weigh bisphenol-A risks. *JAMA* 2007; 298(13): 1499–503.

86. vom Saal FS, Hughes C. An extensive new literature concerning low-dose effects of bisphenol A shows the need for a new risk assessment. *Environ Health Perspect* 2005; 113(8): 926–33.

87. vom Saal FS, Nagel SC, Timms BG, Welshons WV. Implications for human health of the extensive bisphenol A literature showing adverse effects at low doses: a response to attempts to mislead the public. *Toxicology* 2005; 212(2–3): 244–52, author reply 253–54.

88. vom Saal FS, Cooke PS, Buchanan DL, Palanza P, Thayer KA, Nagel SC, et al. A physiologically based approach to the study of bisphenol A and other estrogenic chemicals on the size of reproductive organs, daily sperm production, and behavior. *Toxicol Ind Health* 1998; 14(1–2): 239–60.

89. NRC. Fluoride in Drinking Water: A Scientific Review of EPA's Standards. In: National Research Council of the National Academies. Available at http://books.nap.edu/openbook .php?record_id=11571&page=R1; 2006.

90. Wang SX, Wang ZH, Cheng XT, Li J, Sang ZP, Zhang XD, et al. Arsenic and fluoride exposure in drinking water: children's IQ and growth in Shanyin county, Shanxi province, China. *Environ Health Perspect* 2007; 115(4): 643–47.

91. Erdal S, Buchanan SN. A quantitative look at fluorosis, fluoride exposure, and intake in children using a health risk assessment approach. *Environ Health Perspect* 2005; 113(1): 111–17

92. LaFranchi SH, Haddow JE, Hollowell JG. Is thyroid inadequacy during gestation a risk factor for adverse pregnancy and developmental outcomes? *Thyroid* 2005; 15 (1): 60–71.

93. Weiss B, Williams JH, Margen S, Abrams B, Caan B, Citron LJ, et al. Behavioral responses to artificial food colors. *Science* 1980; 207(4438): 1487–89.

94. Schab DW, Trinh NH. Do artificial food colors promote hyperactivity in children with hyperactive syndromes? A meta-analysis of double-blind placebo-controlled trials. *J Dev Behav Pediatr* 2004; 25(6): 423–34.

95. Bateman B, Warner JO, Hutchinson E, Dean T, Rowlandson P, Gant C, et al. The effects of a double blind, placebo controlled, artificial food colourings and benzoate preservative challenge on hyperactivity in a general population sample of preschool children. In: *Arch Dis Child*; 2004. pp. 506–11.

96. Boris M, Mandel FS. Foods and additives are common causes of the attention deficit hyperactive disorder in children. *Ann Allergy* 1994; 72(5): 462–68.

97. McCann D, Barrett A, Cooper A, Crumpler D, Dalen L, Grimshaw K, et al. Food additives and hyperactive behaviour in 3-year-old and 8/9-year-old children in the community: a randomised, doubleblinded, placebo-controlled trial. *Lancet* 2007; 370(9598): 1560–67.

98. Rowe KS, Briggs DR. Food additives and behaviour. *Med J Aust* 1994; 161(10): 581–82.

99. Rowe KS, Rowe KJ. Synthetic food coloring and behavior: a dose response effect in a doubleblind, placebo-controlled, repeated-measures study. *J Pediatr* 1994; 125(5 Pt 1): 691–98.

Section 3.4

Infectious Agents and Learning Disabilities

Excerpted from "New Thinking on Neurodevelopment," National Institute of Environmental Health Sciences, National Institutes of Health, February 1, 2006. Updated by David A. Cooke, M.D., FACP, January 2012.

Exposure to a neurotoxicant may not be the only way to disrupt the natural growth of the brain. Scientists are now looking at the subtle physiological effects of immunotoxicants and infectious agents on biological events during development.

It turns out that mothers who experience an infection during pregnancy are at a greater risk of having a child with a neurodevelopmental disorder such as autism or schizophrenia. For example, prenatal exposure to the rubella virus is associated with neuromotor and behavioral abnormalities in childhood and an increased risk of schizophrenia spectrum disorders in adulthood, according to an article in the March 2001 issue of *Biological Psychiatry*. Rubella has also been linked to autism: some 8 to 13 percent of children born during the 1964 rubella pandemic developed the disorder, according to a report in the March 1967 *Journal of Pediatrics*. The same study also noted a connection between the rubella virus and mental retardation.

Some epidemiologic studies have found an increased risk of schizophrenia among the children of women who were exposed to the influenza virus during the second trimester of pregnancy, according to a report in the February 2002 *Current Opinion in Neurobiology*. In the August 2004 *Archives of General Psychiatry*, Ezra Susser, head of epidemiology at Columbia University's Mailman School of Public Health, and his colleagues reported that the risk of the mental disorder was increased sevenfold if the schizophrenic patient's mother had influenza during her first trimester of pregnancy. A prospective birth cohort study in the April 2001 *Schizophrenia Bulletin* found that second-trimester exposure to the diphtheria bacterium also significantly increased the risk of schizophrenia.

How might infectious agents cause these disorders? According to John Gilmore, a professor of psychiatry at the University of North Carolina at Chapel Hill, maternal infections during pregnancy can alter the development of fetal neurons in the cerebral cortex of rats. The mechanism is far from clear, but signaling molecules in the mother's immune system, called cytokines, have been implicated. Speaking at the XXII International Neurotoxicology Conference, Gilmore described in vitro experiments showing that elevated levels of certain cytokines—interleukin-1ß, interleukin-6 and tumor necrosis factor-alpha (TNF-α)—reduce the survival of cortical neurons and decrease the complexity of neuronal dendrites in the cerebral cortex. "I believe that the weight of the data to date indicates [that the maternal immune response] can have harmful effects," says Gilmore.

Inflammatory responses in the mother may not be the only route to modifying the fetal brain. The University of California, Davis, Center for Children's Environmental Health and Disease Prevention is conducting a large study of autistic children in California called CHARGE (Childhood Autism Risks from Genetics and the Environment), which suggests that the child's immune system may also be involved. According to Isaac Pessah, the study principal investigator, children with autism appear to have a unique immune system. "Autistic children have a significant reduction in plasma immunoglobulins and a skewed profile of plasma cytokines compared to other children," he says. "We think that an immune system dysfunction may be one of the etiological cores of autism."

Such problems might extend to the central nervous system. The brains of individuals who have a neurodevelopmental disorder also show evidence of inflammation. In the January 2005 issue of the *Annals of Neurology*, Carlos Pardo, an assistant professor of neurology and pathology at the Johns Hopkins University School of Medicine, and his colleagues report finding high levels of inflammatory cytokines (interleukin-6, interleukin-8, and interferon-gamma) in the cerebrospinal fluid of autistic patients. Glial cells, which serve as the brain's innate immune system, are the primary sources of cytokines in the central nervous system. So it may not be surprising that Pardo's team also discovered that glia are activated—showing both morphological and physiological changes—in postmortem brains of autistic patients.

The recognition that the immune system is involved in neurodevelopmental disorders is changing people's perceptions of these conditions. "Historically, scientists have focused on the role of neurons in all kinds of neurological diseases," Pardo says, "but they have generally been ignoring the [glia]." He adds, "In autism, it could be that the [glia] are responding to some external insult, such as an infection, an intrauterine injury, or a neuro-toxicant."

According to Pardo, it's still not clear whether the neuroimmune responses associated with autism contribute to the dysfunction of the brain or whether they are secondary reactions to some neural abnormality. "John Gilmore's work [showing that cytokines can be harmful to brain cells] is quite interesting and important," he says. "However, in vitro studies may produce results that don't reflect what occurs under in vivo conditions. Cytokines like TNF-α may be beneficial for some neurobiological functions at low concentrations, but may be extremely neurotoxic at high concentrations."

Chapter 4

Signs and Symptoms of Learning Disabilities

Common Characteristics of Dyslexia

Most of us have one or two of these characteristics. That does not mean that everyone has dyslexia. A person with dyslexia usually has several of these characteristics that persist over time and interfere with his or her learning.

Oral Language

- Late learning to talk
- Difficulty pronouncing words
- Difficulty acquiring vocabulary or using age-appropriate grammar
- Difficulty following directions
- Confusion with before/after, right/left, and so on
- Difficulty learning the alphabet, nursery rhymes, or songs
- Difficulty understanding concepts and relationships
- Difficulty with word retrieval or naming problems

Reading

- Difficulty learning to read
- Difficulty identifying or generating rhyming words, or counting syllables in words (phonological awareness)
- Difficulty with hearing and manipulating sounds in words (phonemic awareness)
- Difficulty distinguishing different sounds in words (phonological processing)
- Difficulty in learning the sounds of letters (phonics)
- Difficulty remembering names and shapes of letters, or naming letters rapidly
- Transposing the order of letters when reading or spelling
- Misreading or omitting common short words
- "Stumbles" through longer words
- Poor reading comprehension during oral or silent reading, often because words are not accurately read
- Slow, laborious oral reading

Written Language

- Difficulty putting ideas on paper
- Many spelling mistakes
- May do well on weekly spelling tests, but may have many spelling mistakes in daily work
- Difficulty proofreading

Other Common Symptoms That Occur with Dyslexia

- Difficulty naming colors, objects, and letters rapidly, in a sequence (RAN: rapid automatized naming)
- Weak memory for lists, directions, or facts
- Needs to see or hear concepts many times to learn them
- Distracted by visual or auditory stimuli
- Downward trend in achievement test scores or school performance

- Inconsistent schoolwork
- Teacher says, "If only she would try harder," or "He's lazy."
- Relatives may have similar problems

Common Characteristics of Other Related Learning Disorders

Dysgraphia (Handwriting)

- Unsure of handedness
- Poor or slow handwriting
- Messy and unorganized papers
- Difficulty copying
- Poor fine motor skills
- Difficulty remembering the kinesthetic movements to form letters correctly

Dyscalculia (Math)

- Difficulty counting accurately
- May misread numbers
- Difficulty memorizing and retrieving math facts
- Difficulty copying math problems and organizing written work
- Many calculation errors
- Difficulty retaining math vocabulary and concepts

ADHD—Attention-Deficit/Hyperactivity Disorder (Attention)

- Inattention
- Variable attention
- Distractibility
- Impulsivity
- Hyperactivity

Dyspraxia (Motor skills)

- Difficulty planning and coordinating body movements
- Difficulty coordinating facial muscles to produce sounds

Executive Function/Organization

- Loses papers
- Poor sense of time
- Forgets homework
- Messy desk
- Overwhelmed by too much input
- Works slowly

If your child is having difficulties learning to read and you have noted several of these characteristics in your child, he or she may need to be evaluated for dyslexia or a related disorder.

What Kind of Instruction Does My Child Need?

Dyslexia and other related learning disorders cannot be cured. Proper instruction promotes reading success and alleviates many difficulties associated with dyslexia. Instruction for individuals with reading and related learning disabilities should be:

- **Intensive:** given every day or very frequently for sufficient time.

- **Explicit:** component skills for reading, spelling, and writing are explained, directly taught, and modeled by the teacher. Children are discouraged from guessing at words.

- **Systematic and cumulative:** has a definite, logical sequence of concept introduction; concepts are ordered from simple to more complex; each new concept builds upon previously introduced concepts, with built in review to aid memory and retrieval.

- **Structured:** has step-by-step procedures for introducing, reviewing, and practicing concepts.

- **Multisensory:** links listening, speaking, reading, and writing together; involves movement and "hands on" learning.

Suggested Readings

Moats, L. C., and Dakin, K. E. (2007). Basic facts about dyslexia and other reading problems. Baltimore: The International Dyslexia Association.

Shaywitz, S. (2003). Overcoming dyslexia: A new and complete science-based program for reading problems at any level. New York: Knopf.

Tridas, E. Q. (Ed.). (2007). From ABC to ADHD: What every parent should know about dyslexia. Baltimore: The International Dyslexia Association.

Chapter 5

Diagnosing Learning Disabilities

Chapter Contents

Section 5.1

What to Do If You Suspect Your Child Has a Learning Disability

"What Do I Do If I Suspect a Learning Disability?" by Margy Davidson, M.A. © 2011 Learning Disabilities Worldwide, Inc. All rights reserved. Reprinted with permission from Teresa Allissa Citro, CEO of Learning Disabilities Worldwide, Inc. For additional information and resources, visit www.ldworldwide.org.

If your child is struggling with learning in school and at home, there a number of things you can do:

1. Talk with your child's doctor. You will want to rule out any medical problems that may contribute to your child's difficulty.

2. Talk with your child's teacher. You will want to understand the types of difficulties your child is experiencing in the classroom.

3. Have your child evaluated. An evaluation will help you and your child understand how he or she learns best, what his or her strengths and weaknesses are, and what should be done to help your child. In the United States, you have the right to ask the school district, in writing, to evaluate your child for learning disabilities.

4. Learn everything you can about learning disabilities and any associated disorders that are impacting your child. The more knowledge you have, the more you will be able to help your child.

5. Learn to how to be a good advocate for your child:

   • Understand the laws that determine the rights of an individual with disabilities. In the United States, Parent Training and Information Centers (PTI) provide this type of information.

   • Develop respectful, positive relationships and regular communication with your child's teacher and other staff members at school.

6. Take care of your child's mental health. Having learning disabilities can cause frustration and poor self-concept. Counseling can help with these issues and teach good social skills.

7. Connect with other parents of children with learning disabilities and associated disorders. Such connections provide opportunities to exchange advice and support.

8. Take good care of you! Exercise, eat right, get good sleep, and most of all, set aside "me" time. Taking good care of you helps you take good care of your child.

Section 5.2

How to Choose an Evaluation Professional

An evaluation of your child's learning needs determines eligibility for special education services—and equally important, what those services will be. But not all evaluations are up to the mark. Following are some guidelines to help you find your way to an evaluation that will serve your child well.

How skillful is the evaluator?

A psychoeducational evaluation includes tests for cognitive abilities, usually including an intelligence test; tests to assess your child's level of achievement; and an evaluation of your child's social and emotional functioning, in addition to your child's developmental history. Most important is the evaluator's skill in determining the exact nature of the child's difficulties, often via additional tests, direct observation, and anecdotal input from teachers and parents.

An evaluation must provide a clear understanding of both strengths and weaknesses and offer detailed recommendations on the help your child needs.

Where can you find a good evaluator?

In school, learning disabilities specialists may administer achievement tests. Intelligence tests must be given by a qualified school psychologist. Getting a reliable diagnosis from testing demands substantial skill that may not be readily available within the school setting.

There is also the chance for a conflict of interest in school testing: Recommending intensive services translates into higher costs to the school system.

Finding a qualified outside evaluator requires the same effort as finding a doctor in a medical specialty. Ask other parents, teachers, regional or state learning disabilities associations, doctors, or therapists. Conduct phone interviews with the candidates and ask for a sample report.

What is the bottom line?

An evaluation by an outside educational diagnostician or a clinical or educational psychologist costs between $2,000 and $3,500. The cost can be recovered from your school district if the school agrees in advance or if the school changes your child's Individualized Education Program (IEP) as a result of the new evaluation, indicating their acceptance of the findings.

Regardless of the route you chose, it's critical that interventions are based on an evaluation that provides the correct diagnosis of the problems and reliable recommendations for what needs to be done.

Section 5.3

Questions to Ask When Selecting an Evaluation Professional

What to Ask

1. Which types of tests or measurements do you use?

2. How long will an assessment take?

3. How do you diagnose a learning disability? (The psychologist should utilize more than one method.)

4. What does an assessment include (i.e., feedback session, consultation with professionals who work with my child)?

5. Do you take insurance?

6. If you confirm a diagnosis of a learning disability or another disability, would you be willing to write a letter to the school or speak to a school official?

7. What age range do you assess?

8. Are you familiar with the types of services provided at public schools for children with learning or behavioral difficulties?

9. What other professionals if any will be involved in the assessment?

Section 5.4

Evaluating Children for Learning Disabilities

"Evaluation: What Does It Mean for Your Child?" Used with permission from PACER Center Inc., Minneapolis, MN, 952-838-9000, www.pacer.org. © 2006. All rights reserved. Reviewed by David A. Cooke, M.D., FACP, February 2012.

What is an evaluation?

Evaluation is the process for determining whether a child has a disability and needs special education and related services. It's the first step in developing an educational program that will help the child learn. A full and individual initial evaluation must be done before the initial provision of any special education or related services to a child with a disability, and students must be reevaluated at least once every three years.

Evaluation involves gathering information from a variety of sources about a child's functioning and development in all areas of suspected disability, including information provided by the parent. The evaluation may look at cognitive, behavioral, physical, and developmental factors, as well as other areas. All this information is used to determine the child's educational needs.

Why have an evaluation?

A full and individual educational evaluation serves many important purposes:

1. Identification. It can identify children who have delays or learning problems and may need special education and related services as a result.

2. Eligibility. It can determine whether your child is a child with a disability under the Individuals with Disabilities Education Act (IDEA) and qualifies for special education and related services.

3. Planning an Individualized Education Program (IEP). It provides information that can help you and the school develop an appropriate IEP for your child.

4. Instructional strategies. It can help determine what strategies may be most effective in helping your child learn.

5. Measuring progress. It establishes a baseline for measuring your child's educational progress.

The evaluation process establishes a foundation for developing an appropriate educational program. The school must provide a copy of the evaluation report and the documentation of determination of eligibility to the parent. Even if the evaluation results show that your child does not need special education and related services, the information may still be used to help your child in a regular education program.

What measures are used to evaluate a child?

No single test may be used as the sole measure for determining whether a child has a disability or for determining an appropriate educational program for your child. Both formal and informal tests and other evaluation measures are important in determining the special education and related services your child needs.

Testing measures a child's ability or performance by scoring the child's responses to a set of questions or tasks. It provides a snapshot of a child and the child's performance on a particular day. Formal test data is useful in predicting how well a child might be expected to perform in school. It also provides information about unique learning needs.

Other measures of a child's growth and development, such as observation or interviews with parents and others who know the child, provide vital information on how the child functions in different settings and circumstances.

The school must conduct a full and individual evaluation consistent with the IDEA that uses information from diverse sources, including formal and informal data. Tests are important, but evaluation also includes other types of information, such as:

- medical information;

- comparisons of the child's progress to typical expectations of child development;

- observations of how the child functions in school, at home, or in the community;

- interviews with parents and school staff.

As a parent, you have a wealth of information about the development and needs of your child. When combined with the results of tests and other evaluation materials, this information can be used to make decisions about your child's appropriate educational program.

What types of tests are available?

There are many types of tests that schools use to measure student progress. Here are a few important terms parents may need to know.

Group tests: Group achievement tests may not be used to determine eligibility for special services. They furnish information about how a child performs in relation to others of the same age or grade level, but they do not identify an individual student's pattern of strengths and needs.

Individual tests: Tests administered individually to your child can clarify the special education and related services your child needs to progress in school.

Curriculum-based assessments (CBAs) or curriculum-based measurements (CBMs): These types of tests are developed by school staff to examine the progress a child has made in learning the specific materials the teacher has presented to the class. They can be useful tools for teachers and parents in determining whether learning is taking place, but they must never be used to determine eligibility for services.

Standardized tests: Standardized tests are rigorously developed by experts to be used with large populations of students. The tests are administered according to specific standards. Standardized tests can evaluate what a child has already learned (achievement), or predict what a child may be capable of doing in the future (aptitude).

Norm-referenced tests: Norm-referenced tests are standardized tests that compare a child's performance to that of peers. They can tell you where your child stands in relation to other children of the same age or grade.

Criterion-referenced tests: These tests measure what the child is able to do or the specific skills a child has mastered. Criterion-referenced tests do not assess a child's standing in a group but the child's performance measured against standard criteria. They may compare a child's present performance with past performance as a way of measuring progress.

What criteria are used in selecting tests?

Schools should look at many factors when selecting tests to use in evaluation. Here are a few:

- Tests must be reliable. A test is reliable if it offers consistent results when taken at different times and/or given by different evaluators. You should feel comfortable asking for the reliability of the tests given to your child if this information isn't discussed along with the test results.

- Tests must be valid. A test is valid if it actually measures what it was designed to measure. Tests must accurately reflect the child's aptitude or achievement level. Any standardized tests your child is given must have been validated for the specific testing purpose and administered by trained and knowledgeable personnel.

- Tests and other evaluation materials must not discriminate against a child on a racial or cultural basis. They must be administered in the child's native language or other mode of communication unless it is clearly not feasible to do so.

- Factors such as your child's attentiveness, motivation, anxiety, and understanding of the test directions can affect the score.

What is functional assessment?

While tests are an important part of a full and individual evaluation, sometimes what children can do or need to learn is not reflected in their scores. A functional assessment looks at how a child actually functions at home, at school, and in the neighborhood.

Functional assessment for some students includes looking at reading, writing, and math skills. For others, evaluating whether the student is able to ride the city bus, dress independently, or handle money might be more appropriate.

What is functional behavioral assessment?

When a child has behavior problems that do not respond to standard interventions, a functional behavioral assessment can provide additional information to help the team plan more effective interventions.

A typical functional behavioral assessment includes the following:

- A clear description of the problem behavior.

- Observations of the child at different times and in different settings. These observations should record (1) what was happening in the environment before the behavior occurred, (2) what the actual behavior was, and (3) what the student achieved as a result of the behavior.

- Positive behavioral interventions, strategies, and supports to address that behavior, and to teach behavior skills.

Once the functional behavior assessment has been completed, the results may be used to write a behavior intervention plan or to develop behavior goals for the individualized education program.

How are evaluation results used?

After your child's evaluation is complete, you'll meet with a group of qualified professionals to discuss the results and determine whether your child has a disability under IDEA. The school must provide you with a copy of the evaluation report and a written determination of eligibility.

If the team determines, based on the evaluation results, that your child is eligible for special education and related services, the next step is to develop an IEP to meet your child's needs.

The goals and objectives the IEP team develops relate directly to the strengths and needs that were identified through evaluation.

It's important for you to understand the results of your child's evaluation before beginning to develop an IEP. Parents should ask to have the evaluation results explained to them in plain language by a qualified professional.

You will want to request the evaluation summary report before meeting with other members of the IEP team to develop the IEP. Reviewing the results in a comfortable environment before developing the IEP can reduce stress for parents and provide time to consider whether the results fit their own observations and experiences with their child.

When are students reevaluated?

Students receiving special education services must be evaluated not more often than once a year, unless the parent and the local educational agency agree otherwise; and at least once every three years, unless the parent and the local educational agency agree that a reevaluation is unnecessary to make educational decisions.

The reevaluation will include a review of existing evaluation data and information you provide, classroom assessments, and observations consistent with the IDEA. The IEP team then decides if any additional data is needed to determine if the child continues to have a disability and continues to need special education and related services.

If the IEP team decides no additional data are needed, you will be informed in writing that the team has sufficient information to determine whether your child continues to be eligible for special education and related services. At this point, the team is not required to conduct additional assessments unless parents or the child's teacher request them.

What questions should I consider when evaluation or re-evaluation is proposed?

1. What tests and other evaluation materials are being considered for my child? Why? How will the information be used to plan my child's education?

2. Will the evaluator observe my child in the classroom and talk to my child's teachers?

3. Has the evaluator had experience testing children whose problems may be similar to my child's?

4. Will my child's disability interfere with obtaining valid test scores in any area?

5. Will a translator or an interpreter be available if my child needs one? Testing must be done in a child's native language or sign language if needed.

6. Is my child similar to the group on which the test was normed (the children used when the test was developed)? Is the person responsible for conducting the test familiar with my child's culture?

7. Will test scores be based on my child's grade or age? If my child was retained, how will that be considered in evaluating the test results?

8. What kind of information will I be asked to contribute to the evaluation?

9. What will be done to help my child feel comfortable during the testing session?

What if I disagree with the school's evaluation?

If you disagree with the results of an evaluation, you have the right to obtain an independent educational evaluation (IEE) at public expense. An IEE is conducted by qualified examiners not employed by the school. The school district must provide parents with a list of names of possible examiners and provide the evaluation at no cost to the parents.

If the school district denies a request for an IEE at public expense, the district must initiate a due process hearing to show that its evaluation was appropriate.

When the school arranges for the provision of an IEE, the evaluation must be accomplished under the same criteria that the school district uses for its evaluations. The school may not unreasonably delay an IEE, and it must consider the results of the IEE when determining eligibility or developing your child's IEP.

If the result of the hearing is that the agency's evaluation is appropriate, you still have the right to obtain an IEE at your own expense. If the IEE meets the school's criteria, those results, too, must be considered by the IEP team in determining your child's placement and special education and related services.

When the IEE evaluation is complete, ask for a written report. Be sure that any recommendations for services or specific kinds of programs are in writing. When you receive the report, contact your child's school to arrange an IEP meeting.

Section 5.5

Evaluating Adults for Learning Disabilities

Introduction

When adults suspect they have a learning disability, or that someone they care about does, they need information. They often have questions such as: What can I do? Whom can I call? How can I obtain information? Where are available services?

Assessing the Problem

Those adults who suspect they may have a learning disability can begin to find assistance by having an assessment conducted by qualified professionals. Qualified professionals are individuals trained to conduct assessments. Often the professionals have been certified to select, administer, and interpret a variety of neurological, psychological, educational, and vocational assessment instruments.

Different assessment procedures may be appropriate in various settings such as community colleges, adult basic education programs, and through vocational rehabilitation agencies. It is important for the adult not only to be actively involved in the assessment process, but also to have confidence in the professional with whom he or she is working.

An assessment refers to the gathering of relevant information that can be used to help an adult make decisions, and provides a means for assisting an adult to live more fully. An adult is assessed because of problems in employment, education, and/or life situations. An assessment involves more than just taking tests. An assessment includes an evaluation, a diagnosis, and recommendations.

The first stage of an evaluation is usually a screening. Screening tools use abbreviated, informal methods to determine if an individual is at risk for a learning disability. Examples of informal methods include, but are not limited to: an interview; reviews of medical, school, or employment histories; written answers to a few questions; or a brief test. It is important to understand, however, that being screened for a learning disability is different from undergoing a thorough evaluation. When conducting a thorough evaluation, qualified professionals may first refer to the results of the screening in order to plan which tests to administer. Such tests may include, but are not limited to, those that provide information on intelligence, aptitude, achievement, and vocational interests. During the evaluation stage of the assessment process, all relevant information about an individual should be gathered.

A diagnosis is a statement of the specific type of learning disability that an individual may have, based on an interpretation of the information gathered during the evaluation. A diagnosis serves a useful purpose if it explains an individual's particular strengths and weaknesses, as well as determines eligibility for resources or support services that have not been otherwise available. Through a careful examination and analysis of all the information gathered during the evaluation, qualified professionals use the diagnostic stage of the assessment process to explain the information gathered and to offer recommendations.

Recommendations should provide direction in employment, education, and daily living. Specific recommendations may be made regarding the instructional strategies that an individual will find most successful, as well as other ways to compensate for and/or overcome some of the effects of the disability. Based on specific strengths and areas for development identified during the evaluation and diagnostic stages of the assessment process, recommendations should also suggest possible accommodations that an individual can use to be more successful and feel less frustrated in everyday life.

Adults should be assessed according to their age, experience, and career objectives. This is the only way appropriate, helpful, and conclusive information can be provided to adults. As a result of an assessment, adults will have new information that can help them plan how to obtain the assistance they need. Regardless of their diagnosis, individuals will know more about themselves, have a greater understanding of their strengths and weaknesses, and feel better about themselves.

Locating a Qualified Professional

In addition to the resources listed here, there are agencies in most areas that can refer inquirers to diagnosticians or professionals qualified to conduct assessments appropriate for adults. Check your telephone directory for the following:

- Learning Disabilities Association of America, often listed with the name of the city or county first

- Adult education in the public school system

- Adult literacy programs or literacy councils

- Community mental health agencies

- Counseling or study skills center at a local college or university

- Educational therapists or learning specialists in private practice

- Guidance counselors in high schools

- International Dyslexia Association

- Private schools or institutions specializing in learning disabilities

- Special education departments and/or disability support service offices in colleges or universities

- State Vocational Rehabilitation Agency

- University-affiliated hospitals

Questions to Ask Qualified Professionals

- Have you tested many adults with learning disabilities?

- How long will the assessment take?

- What will the assessment cover?

- Will there be a written and an oral report of the assessment?

- Will our discussion give me more information regarding why I am having trouble with my job or job training, school, or daily life?

- Will you also give me ideas on how to improve my skills and how to compensate for my disability?

- Will the report make recommendations about where to go for immediate help?

- What is the cost? What does the cost cover?

- What are possibilities and costs for additional consultation?

- Can insurance cover the costs? Are there other funding sources? Can a payment plan be worked out?

A Learning Disabilities Checklist

A checklist is a guide. It is a list of characteristics. It is difficult to provide a checklist of typical characteristics of adults with learning disabilities because their most common characteristics are their unique differences. In addition, most adults exhibit or have exhibited some of these characteristics. In other words, saying yes to anyone item on this checklist does not mean you are a person with a learning disability. Even if a number of the following items sound familiar to you, you are not necessarily an individual with a learning disability. However, if you say that's me for most of the items, and if you experience these difficulties to such a degree that they cause problems in employment, education, and/or daily living, it might be useful for you to obtain an assessment by qualified professionals experienced in working with adults with learning disabilities.

There are many worthwhile checklists available from a number of organizations. The following checklist was adapted from lists of learning disabilities' characteristics developed by the following organizations: Learning Disabilities Association of America, *For Employers . . . A Look at Learning Disabilities*; ERIC Clearinghouse on Disabilities and Gifted Education, *Examples of Learning Disability Characteristics*; The International Dyslexia Association's *Annals of Dyslexia*; and the Council for Learning Disabilities, Infosheet.

While individuals with learning disabilities have average or above average intelligence, they do not excel in employment, education, and/ or life situations at the same level as their peers. Identified characteristics are as follows:

• May perform similar tasks differently from day to day

• May read well but not write well, or write well but not read well

• May be able to learn information presented in one way, but not in another

• May have a short attention span, be impulsive, and/or be easily distracted

• May have difficulty telling or understanding jokes

• May misinterpret language, have poor comprehension of what is said

• May have difficulty with social skills, may misinterpret social cues

• May find it difficult to memorize information

- May have difficulty following a schedule, being on time, or meeting deadlines
- May get lost easily, either driving and/or in large buildings
- May have trouble reading maps
- May often misread or miscopy
- May confuse similar letters or numbers, reverse them, or confuse their order
- May have difficulty reading the newspaper, following small print, and/or following columns
- May be able to explain things orally, but not in writing
- May have difficulty writing ideas on paper
- May reverse or omit letters, words, or phrases when writing
- May have difficulty completing job applications correctly
- May have persistent problems with sentence structure, writing mechanics, and organizing written work
- May experience continuous problems with spelling the same word differently in one document
- May have trouble dialing phone numbers and reading addresses
- May have difficulty with math, math language, and math concepts
- May reverse numbers in checkbook and have difficulty balancing a checkbook
- May confuse right and left, up and down
- May have difficulty following directions, especially multiple directions
- May be poorly coordinated
- May be unable to tell you what has just been said
- May hear sounds, words, or sentences imperfectly or incorrectly

As mentioned previously, an adult with learning disabilities may exhibit some of these characteristics, but not necessarily all of them. If an individual exhibits several or many of these characteristics to such a degree that they cause problems in work, school, or everyday life, he or she might benefit from an assessment by a qualified professional.

Section 5.6

Response to Intervention as an Evaluation Tool

Response to intervention (RTI) is an assessment tool aimed at early identification of children with learning issues. Based on the notion that students who receive intensive, effective interventions at the earliest point possible are most likely to succeed, RTI is being heralded as a potential game-changer for special education.

Before RTI, children with learning disabilities qualified for services based upon a discrepancy model: a child with average or above-average intelligence had to perform two years below grade level in order to establish a discrepancy between intelligence and achievement. This wait-to-fail approach discouraged early identification and prevention, which are the most successful interventions for children with reading and other learning disabilities.

Only by employing individual, comprehensive assessments can students with true learning disabilities be distinguished from those students whose learning difficulties stem from other causes.

What Is RTI?

RTI is an individualized, comprehensive assessment and intervention process that utilizes a problem-solving framework to identify and address academic difficulties through effective, research-based instruction.

The goal of RTI is to separate children with true learning disabilities from those who perform poorly as a result of poor instruction.

How Does RTI Work?

In the RTI process, students who show signs of learning difficulties are provided with a series of increasingly intensive and individualized instruction. The research-based intervention process is designed and delivered by general education staff in collaboration with special educators and school psychologists and includes systematic monitoring of the student's progress.

If a child does not respond to instruction that is effective for the majority of children (not responsive to a series of interventions—RTI) that child is considered to have a learning disability and to be in need of special education services.

In order for RTI to be successful, all students must receive high-quality, research-based instruction in the general education environment. The model reorients service delivery to provide early intervention—particularly valuable in the area of early reading acquisition, where there is a wealth of research and interventions based on that research.

Part Two

Types of
Learning Disabilities

Chapter 6

Auditory
Processing Disorder

About Auditory Processing Disorder

Auditory processing disorder (APD), also known as central auditory processing disorder (CAPD), is a complex problem affecting about 5 percent of school-aged children. These kids can't process the information they hear in the same way as others because their ears and brain don't fully coordinate. Something adversely affects the way the brain recognizes and interprets sounds, most notably the sounds composing speech.

Kids with APD often do not recognize subtle differences between sounds in words, even when the sounds are loud and clear enough to be heard. These kinds of problems usually occur in background noise, which is a natural listening environment. So kids with APD have the basic difficulty of understanding any speech signal presented under less than optimal conditions.

Detecting APD

Kids with APD are thought to hear normally because they can usually detect pure tones that are delivered one by one in a very quiet environment (such as a sound-treated room). Those who can normally detect sounds and recognize speech in ideal listening conditions are not considered to have hearing difficulties.

However, the ability to detect the presence of sounds is only one part of the processing that occurs in the auditory system. So, most kids with APD do not have a loss of hearing sensitivity, but have a hearing problem in the sense that they do not process auditory information normally.

If the auditory deficits aren't identified and managed early, many of these kids will have speech and language delays and academic problems.

Symptoms of APD can range from mild to severe and can take many different forms. If you think your child might have a problem processing sounds, consider these questions:

- Is your child easily distracted or unusually bothered by loud or sudden noises?

- Are noisy environments upsetting to your child?

- Does your child's behavior and performance improve in quieter settings?

- Does your child have difficulty following directions, whether simple or complicated?

- Does your child have reading, spelling, writing, or other speech-language difficulties?

- Is abstract information difficult for your child to comprehend?

- Are verbal (word) math problems difficult for your child?

- Is your child disorganized and forgetful?

- Are conversations hard for your child to follow?

APD is an often misunderstood problem because many of the behaviors noted above also can appear in other conditions like learning disabilities, attention deficit hyperactivity disorder (ADHD), and even depression. Although APD is often confused with ADHD, it is possible to have both. It is also possible to have APD and specific language impairment or learning disabilities.

Causes

The causes of APD are unknown. But evidence suggests links to head trauma, lead poisoning, and chronic ear infections. Because there are many different possibilities—even combinations of causes—each child must be assessed individually.

Diagnosis

Audiologists (hearing specialists) can determine if a child has APD. Although speech-language pathologists can get an idea by interacting with the child, only audiologists can perform auditory processing testing and determine if there really is a problem.

Some of the skills a child needs to be evaluated for auditory processing disorder don't develop until age seven or eight. Younger kids' brains just haven't matured enough to accept and process a lot of information. So, many kids diagnosed with APD can develop better skills with time.

Once diagnosed, kids with APD usually work with a speech therapist. The audiologist will also recommend that they return for yearly follow-up evaluations.

Problem Areas for Kids With CAPD

The five main problem areas that can affect both home and school activities in kids with APD are:

1. **Auditory figure-ground problems:** when a child can't pay attention if there's noise in the background. Noisy, low-structured classrooms could be very frustrating.

2. **Auditory memory problems:** when a child has difficulty remembering information such as directions, lists, or study materials. It can be immediate ("I can't remember it now") and/or delayed ("I can't remember it when I need it for later").

3. **Auditory discrimination problems:** when a child has difficulty hearing the difference between words or sounds that are similar (COAT/BOAT or CH/SH). This can affect following directions, and reading, spelling, and writing skills, among others.

4. **Auditory attention problems:** when a child can't stay focused on listening long enough to complete a task or requirement (such as listening to a lecture in school). Kids with CAPD often have trouble maintaining attention, although health, motivation, and attitude also can play a role.

5. **Auditory cohesion problems:** when higher-level listening tasks are difficult. Auditory cohesion skills—drawing inferences from conversations, understanding riddles, or comprehending verbal math problems—require heightened auditory processing and language levels. They develop best when all the other skills (levels 1 through 4 above) are intact.

85

How Can I Help My Child?

Strategies applied at home and school can ease some of the problem behaviors associated with APD. Because it's common for kids with CAPD to have difficulty following directions, for example, these tactics might help:

- Since most kids with APD have difficulty hearing amid noise, it's very important to reduce the background noise at home and at school.

- Have your child look at you when you're speaking.

- Use simple, expressive sentences.

- Speak at a slightly slower rate and at a mildly increased volume.

- Ask your child to repeat the directions back to you and to keep repeating them aloud (to you or to himself or herself) until the directions are completed.

- For directions that are to be completed at a later time, writing notes, wearing a watch, and maintaining a household routine also help. General organization and scheduling also can be beneficial.

It's especially important to teach your child to notice noisy environments, for example, and move to quieter places when listening is necessary.

Other strategies that might help:

- Provide your child with a quiet study place (not the kitchen table).

- Maintain a peaceful, organized lifestyle.

- Encourage good eating and sleeping habits.

- Assign regular and realistic chores, including keeping a neat room and desk.

- Build your child's self-esteem.

Be sure to keep in regular contact with school officials about your child's progress. Kids with APD aren't typically put in special education programs. Instead, teachers can make it easier by:

- altering seating plans so the child can sit in the front of the room or with his or her back to the window;

- providing additional aids for study, like an assignment pad or a tape recorder.

One of the most important things that both parents and teachers can do is to acknowledge that CAPD is real. Symptoms and behaviors are not within the child's control. What is within the child's control is recognizing the problems associated with APD and applying the strategies recommended both at home and school.

A positive, realistic attitude and healthy self-esteem in a child with APD can work wonders. And kids with APD can go on to be just as successful as other classmates. Although some children do grow up to be adults with APD, by using coping strategies as well as techniques learned in speech therapy, they can be very successful adults.

Chapter 7

Dyscalculia

Dyscalculia refers to a wide range of lifelong learning disabilities involving math. There is no single type of math disability. Dyscalculia can vary from person to person. And, it can affect people differently at different stages of life.

Two major areas of weakness can contribute to math learning disabilities:

- Visual-spatial difficulties, which result in a person having trouble processing what the eye sees

- Language processing difficulties, which result in a person having trouble processing and making sense of what the ear hears

Using alternate learning methods, people with dyscalculia can achieve success.

What Are the Effects of Dyscalculia?

Disabilities involving math vary greatly. So, the effects they have on a person's development can vary just as much. For instance, a person who has trouble processing language will face different challenges in math than a person who has trouble with visual-spatial relationships. Another person may have trouble remembering facts and keeping a sequence of steps in order. This person will have yet a different set of math-related challenges to overcome.

For individuals with visual-spatial troubles, it may be hard to visualize patterns or different parts of a math problem. Language processing problems can make it hard for a person to get a grasp of the vocabulary of math. Without the proper vocabulary and a clear understanding of what the words represent, it is difficult to build on math knowledge.

When basic math facts are not mastered earlier, teens and adults with dyscalculia may have trouble moving on to more advanced math applications. These require that a person be able to follow multi-step procedures and be able to identify critical information needed to solve equations and more complex problems.

What Are the Warning Signs of Dyscalculia?

Having trouble learning math skills does not necessarily mean a person has a learning disability. All students learn at different paces. It can take young people time and practice for formal math procedures to make practical sense. So how can you tell if someone has dyscalculia? If a person continues to display trouble with the areas listed below, consider testing for dyscalculia. Extra help may be beneficial.

Dyscalculia: Warning signs by Age

Young children:

- Difficulty learning to count

- Trouble recognizing printed numbers

- Difficulty tying together the idea of a number (4) and how it exists in the world (four horses, four cars, four children)

- Poor memory for numbers

- Trouble organizing things in a logical way—putting round objects in one place and square ones in another

School-age children:

- Trouble learning math facts (addition, subtraction, multiplication, division)

- Difficulty developing math problem-solving skills

- Poor long-term memory for math functions

- Not familiar with math vocabulary
- Difficulty measuring things
- Avoiding games that require strategy

Teenagers and adults:

- Difficulty estimating costs like groceries bills
- Difficulty learning math concepts beyond the basic math facts
- Poor ability to budget or balance a checkbook
- Trouble with concepts of time, such as sticking to a schedule or approximating time
- Trouble with mental math
- Difficulty finding different approaches to one problem

How Is Dyscalculia Identified?

When a teacher or trained professional evaluates a student for learning disabilities in math, the student is interviewed about a full range of math-related skills and behaviors. Pencil-and-paper math tests are often used, but an evaluation needs to accomplish more. It is meant to reveal how a person understands and uses numbers and math concepts to solve advanced-level, as well as everyday, problems. The evaluation compares a person's expected and actual levels of skill and understanding while noting the person's specific strengths and weaknesses. Below are some of the areas that may be addressed:

- Ability with basic math skills like counting, adding, subtracting, multiplying, and dividing
- Ability to predict appropriate procedures based on understanding patterns—knowing when to add, subtract, multiply, divide, or do more advanced computations
- Ability to organize objects in a logical way
- Ability to measure—telling time, using money
- Ability to estimate number quantities
- Ability to self-check work and find alternate ways to solve problems.

How Is Dyscalculia Treated?

Helping a student identify his or her strengths and weaknesses is the first step to getting help. Following identification, parents, teachers, and other educators can work together to establish strategies that will help the student learn math more effectively. Help outside the classroom lets a student and tutor focus specifically on the difficulties that student is having, taking pressure off moving to new topics too quickly. Repeated reinforcement and specific practice of straightforward ideas can make understanding easier. Other strategies for inside and outside the classroom include:

- Use graph paper for students who have difficulty organizing ideas on paper.

- Work on finding different ways to approach math facts; i.e., instead of just memorizing the multiplication tables, explain that 8 x 2 = 16, so if 16 is doubled, 8 x 4 must = 32.

- Practice estimating as a way to begin solving math problems.

- Introduce new skills beginning with concrete examples and later moving to more abstract applications.

- For language difficulties, explain ideas and problems clearly and encourage students to ask questions as they work.

- Provide a place to work with few distractions and have pencils, erasers, and other tools on hand as needed.

Help students become aware of their strengths and weaknesses. Understanding how a person learns best is a big step in achieving academic success and confidence.

Chapter 8

Dysgraphia

What is dysgraphia?

Dysgraphia is a specific learning disability that affects how easily children acquire written language and how well they use written language to express their thoughts.

Dysgraphia is a Greek word. The base word graph refers both to the hand's function in writing and to the letters formed by the hand. The prefix *dys* indicates that there is impairment. *Graph* refers to producing letter forms by hand. The suffix *ia* refers to having a condition. Thus, *dysgraphia* is the condition of impaired letter writing by hand, that is, disabled handwriting and sometimes spelling. Impaired handwriting can interfere with learning to spell words in writing. Occasionally, but not very often, children have just spelling problems and not handwriting or reading problems.

What causes dysgraphia?

Research to date has shown orthographic coding in working memory is related to handwriting. Orthographic coding refers to the ability to store unfamiliar written words in working memory while the letters in the word are analyzed during word learning or the ability to create permanent memory of written words linked to their pronunciation and meaning. Children with dysgraphia do not have primary developmental motor disorder, another cause of poor handwriting, but they may have difficulty planning sequential finger movements such as the touching of the thumb to successive fingers on the same hand.

Does dysgraphia occur alone or with other specific learning disabilities?

Children with impaired handwriting may also have attention deficit hyperactivity disorder (ADHD)—inattentive, hyperactive, or combined inattentive and hyperactive subtypes. Children with this kind of dysgraphia may respond to a combination of explicit handwriting instruction plus stimulant medication, but appropriate diagnosis of ADHD by a qualified professional and monitoring of response to both instruction and medication are needed.

Dysgraphia may occur alone or with dyslexia (impaired reading disability) or with oral and written language learning disability (OWL LD, also referred to as selective language impairment, SLI).

Dyslexia is a disorder that includes poor word reading, word decoding, oral reading fluency, and spelling. Children with dyslexia may have impaired orthographic and phonological coding and rapid automatic naming and switching. Phonological coding refers to coding sounds in spoken words in working memory. Phonological coding is necessary for developing phonological awareness—analyzing the sounds in spoken words that correspond to alphabet letters. If children have both dysgraphia and dyslexia, they may also have difficulty in planning sequential finger movements.

OWL LD (SLI) are disorders of language (morphology—word parts that mark meaning and grammar; syntax—structures for ordering words and understanding word functions; finding words in memory, and/or making inferences that go beyond what is stated in text). These disorders affect spoken as well as written language. Children with these language disorders may also exhibit the same writing and reading and related disorders as children with dysgraphia or dyslexia.

Why is diagnosis of dysgraphia and related learning disabilities important?

Without diagnosis, children may not receive early intervention or specialized instruction in all the relevant skills that are interfering with their learning of written language. Considering that many schools do not have systematic instructional programs in handwriting and spelling, it is important to assess whether children need explicit, systematic instruction in handwriting and spelling in addition to word reading and decoding. Many schools offer accommodations in testing and teaching to students with dysgraphia, but these students also need ongoing, explicit instruction in handwriting, spelling, and composition. It is also important to determine if a child with dysgraphia may also have dyslexia and require special help with reading or OWL LD (SLI) and need special help with oral as well as written language.

What kinds of instructional activities improve the handwriting of children with dysgraphia?

Initially, children with impaired handwriting benefit from activities that support learning to form letters:

- Playing with clay to strengthen hand muscles
- Keeping lines within mazes to develop motor control
- Connecting dots or dashes to create complete letter forms
- Tracing letters with index finger or eraser end of pencil
- Imitating the teacher modeling sequential strokes in letter formation
- Copying letters from models

Subsequently, once children learn to form legible letters, they benefit from instruction that helps them develop automatic letter writing, using the following steps to practice each of the twenty-six letters of the alphabet in a different order daily:

- Studying numbered arrow cues that provide a consistent plan for letter formation.
- Covering the letter with a 3 x 5 card and imaging the letter in the mind's eye.
- Writing the letter from memory after interval that increases in duration over the handwriting lessons.
- Writing letters from dictation (spoken name to letter form).
- Writing letters during composing for five minutes on a teacher-provided topic.

Students benefit from explicit instruction in spelling throughout K–12:

- Initially in high frequency Anglo-Saxon words

- Subsequently in coordinating the phonological, orthographic, and morphological processes relevant for the spelling of longer, more complex, less frequent words

- At all grade levels in the most common and important words used for the different academic domains of the curriculum

Throughout K-12, students benefit from strategies for composing:

- Planning, generating, reviewing/evaluating, and revising compositions of different genre including narrative, informational, compare and contrast, and persuasive.

- Self-regulation strategies for managing the complex executive functions involved in composing.

Do children with dysgraphia make reversals or other letter production errors?

Some children do make reversals (reversing direction letter faces along a vertical axis), inversions (flipping letters along a horizontal axis so that the letter is upside down), or transpositions (sequence of letters in a word is out of order). These errors are symptoms rather than causes of handwriting problems. The automatic letter writing instruction described earlier has been shown to reduce reversals, which are less likely to occur when retrieval of letters from memory and production of letters have become automatic.

What kind of instructional strategies improve spelling of children with dysgraphia?

If children have both handwriting and spelling problems, the kinds of handwriting instruction described earlier should be included along with the spelling instruction.

Are educators in public schools identifying children with dysgraphia and providing appropriate instruction in public schools?

In general, no. Although federal law specifies written expression as one of the areas in which students with learning disabilities may be affected, it does not clearly identify the transcription problems that are the causal factors in dysgraphia—impaired handwriting and/or spelling—for impaired written expression of ideas. Some of the tests used to assess written expression are not scored for handwriting or spelling problems and mask the nature of the disability in dysgraphia. Content or ideas may not be impaired. All too often, the poor writing or failure to complete writing assignments in a timely fashion or at all is misattributed to lack of motivation, laziness, or other issues unrelated to the real culprit—dysgraphia. Children who are twice exceptional—gifted and dysgraphic—are especially underdiagnosed and underserved. Teachers mistakenly assume that if a student is bright and cannot write it is because the student is not trying.

Are there research-supported assessment tools for diagnosing dysgraphia?

Yes. See Berninger (2007a) and Milone (2007) below for assessing handwriting problems associated with dysgraphia. Also, see Berninger (2007b) and Berninger, O'Donnell, and Holdnack (2008) for using these tests and other evidence-based assessment procedures in early identification, prevention, and diagnosis for treatment planning and linking them to evidence-based handwriting and spelling instruction (also see Troia 2008).

In summary, dysgraphia is a specific learning disability that can be diagnosed and treated. Children with dysgraphia usually have other problems such as difficulty with spelling and written expression, as well as dyslexia and, in some cases, oral language problems. It is important that a thorough assessment of handwriting and related skill areas be carried out in order to plan specialized instruction in all deficient skills that may be interfering with a student's learning of written language. For example, a student may need instruction in both handwriting and oral language skills to improve written expression. Although early intervention is, of course, desirable, it is never too late to intervene to improve a student's deficient skills and provide appropriate accommodations.

References

Berninger, V. (2007a). *Process Assessment of the Learner, 2nd Edition. Diagnostic for Reading and Writing (PAL-II RW)*. San Antonio, TX: The Psychological Corporation.

Berninger, V. (2007b). *Process Assessment of the Learner II User's Guide*. San Antonio, TX: Harcourt/PsyCorp. (CD format) ISBN 0158661818. Second Edition issued August, 2008.

Berninger, V. (2007). Evidence-based written language instruction during early and middle childhood. In R. Morris and N. Mather (Eds.),

Evidence-based interventions for students with learning and behavioral challenges. Philadelphia: Lawrence Erlbaum Associates.

Berninger, V., O'Donnell, L., and Holdnack, J. (2008). Research-supported differential diagnosis of specific learning disabilities and implications for instruction and response to instruction (RTI). In A. Prifitera, D. Saklofske, and L. Weiss (Eds.), *WISC-IV Clinical Assessment and Intervention, Second Edition* (pp. 69–108). San Diego, CA: Academic Press (Elsevier).

Berninger, V., and Wolf, B. (in press-a). Teaching students with dyslexia and dysgraphia: Lessons from teaching and science. Baltimore: Paul H. Brookes.

Berninger, V., and Wolf, B. (in press-b). Helping students with dyslexia and dysgraphia make connections: Differentiated instruction lesson plans in reading and writing. Baltimore: Paul H. Brookes. [Spiral-bound book with teaching plans from University of Washington Research Program.]

Graham, S., Harris, K., and Loynachan, C. (1994). The spelling for writing list. *Journal of Learning Disabilities*, 27, 210–14.

Henry, M. (2003). *Unlocking literacy. Effective decoding and spelling instruction.* Baltimore: Paul H. Brookes Publishing.

Milone, M. (2007). *Test of Handwriting Skills-Revised.* Novato, CA: Academic Therapy. Distributed by ProEd, Austin, TX.

Moats, L. C. (Winter, 2005/2006). How spelling supports reading: And why it is more regular and predictable than you think. *American Educator*, 12–22, 42–43.

Troia, G. (Ed.). (2008). *Instruction and assessment for struggling writers: Evidence-based practices.* New York: Guilford.

Yates, C., Berninger, V., and Abbott, R. (1994). Writing problems in intellectually gifted children. *Journal for the Education of the Gifted*, 18, 131–55.

Chapter 9

Dyslexia

Chapter Contents

Section 9.1

Dyslexia Basics

What is dyslexia?

Dyslexia is a language-based learning disability. Dyslexia refers to a cluster of symptoms, which result in people having difficulties with specific language skills, particularly reading. Students with dyslexia usually experience difficulties with other language skills such as spelling, writing, and pronouncing words. Dyslexia affects individuals throughout their lives; however, its impact can change at different stages in a person's life. It is referred to as a learning disability because dyslexia can make it very difficult for a student to succeed academically in the typical instructional environment, and in its more severe forms will qualify a student for special education, special accommodations, or extra support services.

What causes dyslexia?

The exact causes of dyslexia are still not completely clear, but anatomical and brain imagery studies show differences in the way the brain of a dyslexic person develops and functions. Moreover, most people with dyslexia have been found to have problems with identifying the separate speech sounds within a word and/or learning how letters represent those sounds, a key factor in their reading difficulties. Dyslexia is not due to either lack of intelligence or desire to learn; with appropriate teaching methods, dyslexics can learn successfully.

How widespread is dyslexia?

About 13 to 14 percent of the school population nationwide has a handicapping condition that qualifies them for special education. Current studies indicate that one-half of all the students who qualify for special education are classified as having a learning disability (LD) (six to seven percent). About 85 percent of those LD students have a primary learning disability in reading and language processing. Nevertheless, many more people—perhaps as many as 15 to 20 percent of the population as a whole—have some of the symptoms of dyslexia, including slow or inaccurate reading, poor spelling, poor writing, or mixing up similar words. Not all of these will qualify for special education, but they are likely to struggle with many aspects of academic learning and are likely to benefit from systematic, explicit, instruction in reading, writing, and language.

Dyslexia occurs in people of all backgrounds and intellectual levels. People who are very bright can be dyslexic. They are often capable or even gifted in areas that do not require strong language skills, such as art, computer science, design, drama, electronics, math, mechanics, music, physics, sales, and sports.

In addition, dyslexia runs in families; dyslexic parents are very likely to have children who are dyslexic. Some people are identified as dyslexic early in their lives, but for others, their dyslexia goes unidentified until they get older.

What are the effects of dyslexia?

The impact that dyslexia has is different for each person and depends on the severity of the condition and the effectiveness of instruction or remediation. The core difficulty is with word recognition and reading fluency, spelling, and writing. Some dyslexics manage to learn early reading and spelling tasks, especially with excellent instruction, but later experience their most debilitating problems when more complex language skills are required, such as grammar, understanding textbook material, and writing essays.

People with dyslexia can also have problems with spoken language, even after they have been exposed to good language models in their homes and good language instruction in school. They may find it difficult to express themselves clearly, or to fully comprehend what others mean when they speak. Such language problems are often difficult to recognize, but they can lead to major problems in school, in the workplace, and in relating to other people. The effects of dyslexia reach well beyond the classroom.

Dyslexia can also affect a person's self-image. Students with dyslexia often end up feeling "dumb" and less capable than they actually are. After experiencing a great deal of stress due to academic problems, a student may become discouraged about continuing in school.

How is dyslexia diagnosed?

Schools may use a new process called Response to Intervention (RTI) to identify children with learning disabilities. Under an RTI model, schools provide those children not readily progressing with the acquisition of critical early literacy skills with intensive and individualized supplemental reading instruction. If a student's learning does not accelerate enough with supplemental instruction to reach the established grade-level benchmarks, and other kinds of developmental disorders are ruled out, he or she may be identified as learning disabled in reading. The majority of students thus identified are likely dyslexic and they will probably qualify for special education services. Schools are encouraged to begin screening children in kindergarten to identify any child who exhibits the early signs of potential reading difficulties.

For children and adults who do not go through this RTI process, an evaluation to formally diagnose dyslexia is needed. Such an evaluation traditionally has included intellectual and academic achievement testing, as well as an assessment of the critical underlying language skills that are closely linked to dyslexia. These include receptive (listening) and expressive language skills, phonological skills including phonemic awareness, and also a student's ability to rapidly name letters and names. A student's ability to read lists of words in isolation, as well as words in context, should also be assessed. If a profile emerges that is characteristic of dyslexic readers, an individualized intervention plan should be developed, which should include appropriate accommodations, such as extended time. The testing can be conducted by trained school or outside specialists.

What are the signs of dyslexia?

The problems displayed by individuals with dyslexia involve difficulties in acquiring and using written language. It is a myth that dyslexic individuals "read backwards," although spelling can look quite jumbled at times because students have trouble remembering letter symbols for sounds and forming memories for words. Other problems experienced by dyslexics include the following:

- Learning to speak
- Learning letters and their sounds
- Organizing written and spoken language
- Memorizing number facts
- Reading quickly enough to comprehend

- Persisting with and comprehending longer reading assignments
- Spelling
- Learning a foreign language
- Correctly doing math operations

Not all students who have difficulties with these skills are dyslexic. Formal testing of reading, language, and writing skills is the only way to confirm a diagnosis of suspected dyslexia.

How is dyslexia treated?

Dyslexia is a lifelong condition. With proper help, many people with dyslexia can learn to read and write well. Early identification and treatment is the key to helping dyslexics achieve in school and in life. Most people with dyslexia need help from a teacher, tutor, or therapist specially trained in using a multisensory, structured language approach. It is important for these individuals to be taught by a systematic and explicit method that involves several senses (hearing, seeing, touching) at the same time. Many individuals with dyslexia need one-on-one help so that they can move forward at their own pace. In addition, students with dyslexia often need a great deal of structured practice and immediate, corrective feedback to develop automatic word recognition skills. When students with dyslexia receive academic therapy outside of school, the therapist should work closely with classroom teachers, special education providers, and other school personnel.

Schools can implement academic accommodations and modifications to help dyslexic students succeed. For example, a student with dyslexia can be given extra time to complete tasks, help with taking notes, and work assignments that are modified appropriately. Teachers can give taped tests or allow dyslexic students to use alternative means of assessment. Students can benefit from listening to books on tape and using the computer for text reading programs and for writing.

Students may also need help with emotional issues that sometimes arise as a consequence of difficulties in school. Mental health specialists can help students cope with their struggles.

What are the rights of a dyslexic person?

The Individuals with Disabilities Education Act 2004 (IDEA), Section 504 of the Rehabilitation Act of 1973, and the Americans with Disabilities Act (ADA) define the rights of students with dyslexia and other specific learning disabilities. These individuals are legally entitled to special services to help them overcome and accommodate their learning problems. Such services include education programs designed to meet the needs of these students. The Acts also protect people with dyslexia against unfair and illegal discrimination.

Section 9.2

Dyslexia and the Brain: What Current Research Tells Us

Excerpted from "Dyslexia and the Brain: What Does Current Research Tell Us?" by Roxanne F. Hudson, Leslie High, and Stephanie Al Otaiba. *The Reading Teacher*, Volume 60, Issue 6, pages 506–15, March 2007. © 2007 International Reading Association. Reprinted with permission of John Wiley and Sons, via Copyright Clearance Center. Reviewed by David A. Cooke, M.D., FACP, February 2012.

Developmental dyslexia and how it relates to brain function are complicated topics that researchers have been studying since dyslexia was first described over a hundred years ago.

W. Pringle Morgan (cited in Shaywitz, 1996), a doctor in Sussex, England, described the puzzling case of a boy in the *British Medical Journal*: "Percy ... aged 14 ... has always been a bright and intelligent boy, quick at games, and in no way inferior to others of his age. His great difficulty has been—and is now—his inability to read" (p. 98).

Almost every teacher in the United States has at least one student who could fit the same description written so many years ago. This situation leads many school personnel to wonder why their articulate, clearly bright student has so many problems with what appears to be a simple task—reading a text that everyone else seems to easily comprehend.

Having information about the likely explanation for and potential cause of the student's difficulties often relieves teachers' fears and uncertainties about how to teach the student and how to think about providing instruction that is relevant and effective. Current research on dyslexia and the brain provide the most up-to-date information available about the problems faced by over 2.8 million school-aged children.

When talking with teachers about their students who struggle with reading, we have encountered similar types of questions from teachers. They often wonder, what is dyslexia? What does brain research tell us about reading problems, and what does this information mean for classroom instruction?

The purpose of this section is to explain the answers to these questions and provide foundational knowledge that will lead to a firmer understanding of the underlying characteristics of students with dyslexia. A greater understanding of the current brain research and how it relates to students with dyslexia is important in education and will help teachers understand and evaluate possible instructional interventions to help their students succeed in the classroom.

What Is Dyslexia?

Dyslexia is an often-misunderstood, confusing term for reading problems. The word *dyslexia* is made up of two different parts: *dys*, meaning not or difficult, and *lexia*, meaning words, reading, or language. So quite literally, dyslexia means difficulty with words (Catts & Kamhi, 2005).

Despite the many confusions and misunderstandings, the term *dyslexia* is commonly used by medical personnel, researchers, and clinicians. One of the most common misunderstandings about this condition is that dyslexia is a problem of letter or word reversals (b/d, was/saw) or of letters, words, or sentences "dancing around" on the page (Rayner, Foorman, Perfetti, Pesetsky, & Seidenberg, 2001).

In fact, writing and reading letters and words backwards are common in the early stages of learning to read and write among average and dyslexic children alike, and the presence of reversals may or may not indicate an underlying reading problem. See Table 9.1 for explanations of this and other common misunderstandings.

One of the most complete definitions of dyslexia comes from over twenty years of research:

> Dyslexia is a specific learning disability that is neurobiological in origin. It is characterized by difficulties with accurate and/or fluent word recognition and by poor spelling and decoding abilities. These difficulties typically result from a deficit in the phonological component of language that is often unexpected in relation to other cognitive abilities and the provision of effective classroom instruction. (Lyon, Shaywitz, & Shaywitz, 2003, p. 2)

Dyslexia is a specific learning disability in reading that often affects spelling as well. In fact, reading disability is the most widely known

105

and most carefully studied of the learning disabilities, affecting 80 percent of all those designated as learning disabled. Because of this, we will use the terms *dyslexia* and *reading disabilities (RD)* interchangeably in this section to describe the students of interest.

It is neurobiological in origin, meaning that the problem is located physically in the brain. Dyslexia is not caused by poverty, developmental delay, speech or hearing impairments, or learning a second language, although those conditions may put a child more at risk for developing a reading disability (Snow, Burns, & Griffin, 1998).

Children with dyslexia will often show two obvious difficulties when asked to read text at their grade level. First, they will not be able to read as many of the words in a text by sight as average readers. There will be many words on which they stumble, guess at, or attempt to "sound out." This is the problem with "fluent word recognition" identified in the previous definition.

Table 9.1. Common Misunderstandings about Students with Reading Disabilities

Writing letters and words backwards are symptoms of dyslexia.
Writing letters and words backwards are common in the early stages of learning to read and write among average and dyslexic children alike. It is a sign that orthographic representations (i.e., letter forms and spellings of words) have not been firmly established, not that a child necessarily has a reading disability (Adams, 1990).

Reading disabilities are caused by visual perception problems.
The current consensus based on a large body of research (e.g., Lyon et al., 2003; Morris et al., 1998; Rayner et al., 2001; Wagner & Torgesen, 1987) is that dyslexia is best characterized as a problem with language processing at the phoneme level, not a problem with visual processing.

If you just give them enough time, children will outgrow dyslexia.
There is no evidence that dyslexia is a problem that can be outgrown. There is, however, strong evidence that children with reading problems show a continuing persistent deficit in their reading rather than just developing later than average children (Francis, Shaywitz, Stuebing, Shaywitz, & Fletcher, 1996). More strong evidence shows that children with dyslexia continue to experience reading problems into adolescence and adulthood (Shaywitz et al., 1999, 2003).

More boys than girls have dyslexia.
Longitudinal research shows that as many girls as boys are affected by dyslexia (Shaywitz, Shaywitz, Fletcher, & Escobar, 1990). There are many possible

Second, they will often show decoding difficulties, meaning that their attempts to identify words they do not know will produce many errors. They will not be very accurate in using letter-sound relationships in combination with context to identify unknown words.

These problems in word recognition are due to an underlying deficit in the sound component of language that makes it very difficult for readers to connect letters and sounds in order to decode. People with dyslexia often have trouble comprehending what they read because of the great difficulty they experience in accessing the printed words.

What Areas of the Brain Relate to Language and Reading?

The human brain is a complex organ that has many different functions. It controls the body and receives, analyzes, and stores information.

Table 9.1. Common Misunderstandings about Students with Reading Disabilities (*continued*)

reasons for the overidentification of males by schools, including greater behavioral acting out and a smaller ability to compensate among boys. More research is needed to determine why.

Dyslexia only affects people who speak English.
Dyslexia appears in all cultures and languages in the world with written language, including those that do not use an alphabetic script such as Korean and Hebrew. In English, the primary difficulty is accurate decoding of unknown words. In consistent orthographies such as German or Italian, dyslexia appears more often as a problem with fluent reading—readers may be accurate, but very slow (Ziegler & Goswami, 2005).

People with dyslexia will benefit from colored text overlays or lenses.
There is no strong research evidence that intervention using colored overlays or special lenses has any effect on the word reading or comprehension of children with dyslexia (American Optometric Association, 2004; Lovino, Fletcher, Breitmeyer, & Foorman, 1998).

A person with dyslexia can never learn to read.
This is simply not true. The earlier children who struggle are identified and provided systematic, intense instruction, the less severe their problems are likely to be (National Institute of Child Health and Human Development, 2000; Torgesen, 2002). With adequately intensive instruction, however, even older children with dyslexia can become accurate, albeit slow readers (Torgesen et al., 2001).

The brain can be divided down the middle lengthwise into a right and a left hemisphere. Most of the areas responsible for speech, language processing, and reading are in the left hemisphere, and for this reason we will focus all of our descriptions and figures on the left side of the brain. Within each hemisphere, we find the following four brain lobes:

- The frontal lobe is the largest and responsible for controlling speech, reasoning, planning, regulating emotions, and consciousness. In the nineteenth century, Paul Broca was exploring areas of the brain used for language and noticed a particular part of the brain that was impaired in a man whose speech became limited after a stroke. This area received more and more attention, and today we know that the Broca area, located here in the frontal lobe, is important for the organization, production, and manipulation of language and speech (Joseph, Noble, & Eden, 2001). Areas of the frontal lobe are also important for silent reading proficiency (Shaywitz et al., 2002).

- The parietal lobe is located farther back in the brain and controls sensory perceptions as well as linking spoken and written language to memory to give it meaning so we can understand what we hear and read.

- The occipital lobe, found at the back of the head, is where the primary visual cortex is located. Among other types of visual perception, the visual cortex is important in the identification of letters.

- The temporal lobe is located in the lower part of the brain, parallel with the ears, and is involved in verbal memory. The Wernicke area, long known to be important in understanding language (Joseph et al., 2001), is located here. This region, identified by Carl Wernicke at about the same time and using the same methods as Broca, is critical in language processing and reading.

In addition, converging evidence suggests that two other systems, which process language within and between lobes, are important for reading.

The first is the left parietotemporal system that appears to be involved in word analysis—the conscious, effortful decoding of words (Shaywitz et al., 2002). This region is critical in the process of mapping letters and written words onto their sound correspondences—letter sounds and spoken words (Heim & Keil, 2004). This area is also important for comprehending written and spoken language (Joseph et al., 2001).

The second system that is important for reading is the left occipito-temporal area. This system seems to be involved in automatic, rapid access to whole words and is a critical area for skilled, fluent reading (Shaywitz et al., 2002, 2004).

What Does Brain Imaging Research Tell Us about Dyslexia?

Structural Brain Differences

Studies of structural differences in the brains of people of all ages show differences between people with and without reading disabilities.

The brain is chiefly made up of two types of material: gray matter and white matter. Gray matter is what we see when we look at a brain and is mostly composed of nerve cells. Its primary function is processing information.

White matter is found within the deeper parts of the brain, and is composed of connective fibers covered in myelin, the coating designed to facilitate communication between nerves. White matter is primarily responsible for information transfer around the brain.

Booth and Burman (2001) found that people with dyslexia have less gray matter in the left parietotemporal area than nondyslexic individuals. Having less gray matter in this region of the brain could lead to problems processing the sound structure of language (phonological awareness).

Many people with dyslexia also have less white matter in this same area than average readers, which is important because more white matter is correlated with increased reading skill (Deutsch, Dougherty, Bammer, Siok, Gabrieli, & Wandell, 2005). Having less white matter could lessen the ability or efficiency of the regions of the brain to communicate with one another.

Other structural analyses of the brains of people with and without RD have found differences in hemispherical asymmetry. Specifically, most brains of right-handed, nondyslexic people are asymmetrical with the left hemisphere being larger than the same area on the right.

In contrast, Heim and Keil (2004) found that right-handed people with dyslexia show a pattern of symmetry (right equals left) or asymmetry in the other direction (right larger than left). The exact cause of these size differences is the subject of ongoing research, but they seem to be implicated in the reading and spelling problems of people with dyslexia.

Functional Brain Differences

We lack space here for a detailed explanation of imaging techniques. For excellent descriptions of several techniques, readers are directed to Papanicolaou, Pugh, Simos, and Mencl (2004) and Richards (2001).

One commonly used method for imaging brain function is functional magnetic resonance imaging (fMRI), a noninvasive, relatively new method that measures physiological signs of neural activation using a strong magnet to pinpoint blood flow. This technique is called "functional" because participants perform tasks while in (or under) the magnet, allowing measurement of the functioning brain rather than the activity of the brain at rest.

Several studies using functional imaging techniques that compared the brain activation patterns of readers with and without dyslexia show potentially important patterns of differences. We might expect that readers with RD would show underactivation in areas where they are weaker and overactivation in other areas in order to compensate, and that is exactly what many researchers have found (e.g., Shaywitz et al., 1998).

This type of functional imaging research has just begun to be used with children. This is in part because of the challenges involved in imaging children, including the absolute need for the participant's head to remain motionless during the scanning.

We will present the largest, best-specified study as an example of these new findings with children. Shaywitz et al. (2002) studied 144 right-handed children with and without RD on a variety of in- and out-of-magnet tasks. They compared brain activation between the two groups of children on tasks designed to tap several component processes of reading:

- Identifying the names or sounds of letters

- Sounding out nonsense words

- Sounding out and comparing meanings of real words

The nonimpaired readers had more activation in all of the areas known to be important for reading than the children with dyslexia.

Shaywitz et al. (2002) also found that the children who were good decoders had more activation in the areas important for reading in the left hemisphere and less in the right hemisphere than the children with RD.

They suggested that for children with RD, disruption in the rear reading systems in the left hemisphere that are critical for skilled,

110

fluent reading leads the children to try and compensate by using other, less efficient systems.

This finding could explain the common experience in school that even as children with dyslexia develop into accurate readers, their reading in grade-level text is often still slow and labored without any fluency (e.g., Torgesen, Rashotte, & Alexander, 2001).

In summary, the brain of a person with dyslexia has a different distribution of metabolic activation than the brain of a person without reading problems when accomplishing the same language task. There is a failure of the left hemisphere rear brain systems to function properly during reading.

Furthermore, many people with dyslexia often show greater activation in the lower frontal areas of the brain. This leads to the conclusion that neural systems in frontal regions may compensate for the disruption in the posterior area (Shaywitz et al., 2003). This information often leads educators to wonder whether brain imaging can be used as a diagnostic tool to identify children with reading disabilities in school.

Can We Screen Everyone Who Has Reading Difficulties?

Not yet. It is an appealing vision of putting a child we are concerned about in an fMRI machine to quickly and accurately identify his or her problem, but research has not taken us that far.

There are several reasons why a clinical or school-based use of imaging techniques to identify children with dyslexia is not currently feasible. One is the enormous cost of fMRI machines, the computers, and the software needed to run them. Another part of the cost is the staff that is needed to run and interpret the results.

Also, in order for this technology to be used for diagnosis, it needs to be accurate for individuals. Currently, results are reliable and reported for groups of participants, but not necessarily for individuals within each group (Richards, 2001; Shaywitz et al., 2002).

The number of children who would be identified as being average when they really have a problem (false negatives) or as having a problem when they are average (false positives) would need to be significantly lower for imaging techniques to be used for diagnosis of individual children.

Can Dyslexia Be Cured?

In a word, no. Dyslexia is a lifelong condition that affects people into old age. However, that does not mean that instruction cannot remediate some of the difficulties people with dyslexia have with written language. A large body of evidence shows what types of instruction struggling readers need to be successful (e.g., National Institute of Child Health and Human Development, 2000; Snow et al., 1998; Torgesen, 2000).

Now researchers can also "look" inside the brains of children before and after an intensive intervention and see for the first time the effects of the intervention on the brain activity of children with RD. The following are two such studies.

Aylward et al. (2003) imaged ten children with dyslexia and eleven average readers before and after a twenty-eight-hour intervention that only the students with dyslexia received. They compared the two groups of students on out-of-magnet reading tests as well as the level of activation during tasks of identifying letter sounds.

They found that while the control children showed no differences between the two imagings, the students who received the treatment showed a significant increase in activation in the areas important for reading and language during the phonological task. Before the intervention, the children with RD showed significant underactivation in these areas as compared to the control children, and after the treatment their profiles were very similar.

These results must be viewed with caution because of several limitations. One limitation is the lack of specificity about the intervention that was provided, another is the small sample size, and the last is the lack of an experimental control group (i.e., a group of children with RD who did not receive the treatment). Without an experimental control group, we cannot be certain that the intervention caused the changes found in the brain activation because of so many other possible explanations.

Shaywitz et al. (2004) addressed these limitations in their investigation of brain activation changes before and after an intervention. They studied seventy-eight second- and third-graders with reading disabilities who were randomly assigned to three groups:

- The experimental intervention

- School-based remedial programs

- Control

A summary of the instructional intervention is provided in Table 9.2 and a full and detailed description of the intervention and out-of-magnet reading assessments can be found in Blachman et al. (2004).

Before the intervention, all groups looked similar in their brain activity, but immediately after the intervention the experimental and

112

control groups had increased activation in the left hemispheric regions important for reading.

One year after intervention, the experimental group showed increased activity in the occipitotemporal region important for automatic, fluent reading, while at both time points the level of compensatory activation in the right hemisphere decreased.

Shaywitz et al. (2002) concluded, "These findings indicate that ... the use of an evidence-based phonologic reading intervention facilitates the development of those fast-paced neural systems that underlie skilled reading" (p. 931).

Table 9.2. Summary of intervention used in brain imaging study of students with RD

Duration

The individual tutoring intervention occurred daily for 50 minutes from September to June, which yielded an average of 126 sessions or 105 tutoring hours per student.

Instruction

Each session consisted of a framework of five steps that the tutors followed with each student. This framework was not scripted, but was individualized based on the student's progress.

Step 1: Brief and quick-paced review of sound-symbol relationships from previous lessons and introduction of new correspondences.

Step 2: Word work practice of phonemic segmentation and blending with letter cards or tiles, which occurred in a very systematic and explicit fashion.

Step 3: Fluency building with sight words and phonetically regular words made up of previously taught sound-symbol correspondences.

Step 4: Oral reading practice in phonetically controlled text, uncontrolled trade books, and nonfiction texts.

Step 5: Writing words with previously taught patterns from dictation.

Content

The intervention consisted of six levels that began with simple closed syllable words (e.g., cat) and ended with multisyllabic words consisting of all six syllable types.

For a complete description of the instructional intervention, see Blachman et al. (2004).

Important Considerations to Keep in Mind about the Brain Research

While research advances have allowed us to look more closely within the brain for the first time and revealed important information about how and where we think during reading, there are important considerations that must be remembered.

One is that with the exception of the research by B.E. Shaywitz, S. Shaywitz, and their colleagues, the sample sizes in each study are very small. The evidence from these small studies is converging into results that are reliable, but the results may change as more and more participants are included in the research base. This is especially true with children, where both the number of studies and the sample sizes are quite small.

Second, we must consider the type of task being used in the magnet. Because of the requirement that the person's head not move during the imaging, researchers are not able to study people actually reading aloud. Instead, they give tasks that require the person to read silently and then make a decision that he or she indicates with a push button (e.g., Do the letters t and v rhyme? Do leat and jete rhyme?).

Because the researchers have worked carefully on these tasks and have specified the particular process that is being measured, we can trust their conclusions about what the activation levels mean; however, the tasks are quite removed from natural classroom reading and should not be interpreted as if they were the same. The area of brain research is developing rapidly; technological advances are being made that will address these issues as time goes on.

Recommendations for Teachers

What does all of this information mean for school personnel and their students? Once teachers understand the underlying processes and causes of reading disabilities, they can use this information as they work with students and their families. The following are specific recommendations based on the neurological research.

Adequate assessment of language processing is important in determining why students struggle to learn to read. Dyslexia, or reading disability, is a disorder of the language processing systems in the brain. Specific information about exactly what sorts of weaknesses are present is needed in order to determine the appropriate instruction to meet each student's needs.

Imaging research confirms that simple tasks can more reliably be interpreted as "red flags" suggesting that a young child

114

may be at risk for dyslexia. It is vital to begin using screening and progress monitoring procedures early on to measure children's understanding of sounds in speech, letter sounds in words, and fluent word recognition. Using such assessment in an ongoing way throughout a child's school career can help teachers know what skills to teach and whether a child is developing these skills.

Explicit, intense, systematic instruction in the sound structure of language (phonemic awareness) and in how sounds relate to letters (phonics) is needed for readers with dyslexia. Imaging research confirmed that instruction in the alphabetic principle caused distinct differences in brain activation patterns in the students with RD (Shaywitz et al., 2004). Keep in mind that the intervention was explicit, intense, long term, and specifically focused on phonological processing, phonics, and fluency.

The roles of motivation and fear of failing are important when discussing reading problems. Students do not struggle simply because they are not trying hard enough. They may have a brain difference that requires them to be taught in a more intense fashion than their peers. Without intense intervention, low motivation may develop as students try to avoid a difficult and painful task.

School personnel can use their knowledge of the neurological characteristics and basis of dyslexia to help their students understand their strengths and weaknesses around reading and language. Understanding a possible reason why they find something difficult that no one else seems to struggle with may help relieve some of the mystery and negative feelings that many people with a disability feel. Sharing our knowledge of brain research may demystify dyslexia and help students and their parents realize that language processing is only one of many talents that they have and that they are not "stupid," they simply process language differently than their peers.

Recommendations for Parents

The identification of a child with dyslexia is a difficult time for parents and teachers. We suggest that teachers can help parents learn more about their child's difficulty in the following ways.

Teachers can share information about the student's specific areas of weakness and strength and help parents realize the underlying causes of their child's difficulty. This conversation can also include information about how to help their child use areas of strength to support areas of weakness.

It is critical to help parents get clear about what dyslexia is and is not. Sharing the common misconceptions and the correct information found in Table 9.1 with parents may help clear up any confusion that may exist.

Early intervention with intense, explicit instruction is critical for helping students avoid the lifelong consequences of poor reading. Engaging parents early in the process of identifying what programs and services are best for their child will ensure greater levels of success and cooperation between home and school.

There are many organizations devoted to supporting individuals with RD and their families. Accessing the knowledge, support, and advocacy of these organizations is critical for many families.

Finally, teachers can often best help families by simply listening to the parents and their concerns for their children. Understanding a disability label and what that means for the future of their child is a very emotional process for parents and many times teachers can help by providing a sympathetic ear as well as information.

Imaging research has demonstrated that the brains of people with dyslexia show different, less efficient, patterns of processing (including under and over activation) during tasks involving sounds in speech and letter sounds in words. Understanding this has the potential to increase the confidence teachers feel when designing and carrying out instruction for their students with dyslexia.

References

Adams, M.J. (1990). *Beginning to read: Thinking and learning about print.* Cambridge, MA: MIT Press.

American Optometric Association. (2004). The use of tinted lenses and colored overlays for the treatment of dyslexia and other related reading and learning disorders. St. Louis, MO: Author. Retrieved on June 12, 2005, from www.aoa.org/documents/TintedLenses.pdf

Aylward, E.H., Richards, T.L., Berninger, V.W., Nagy, W.E., Field, K.M., Grimme, A.C., et al. (2003). Instructional treatment associated with changes in brain activation in children with dyslexia. *Neurology*, 61, 212–19.

Blachman, B.A., Schatschneider, C., Fletcher, J.M., Francis, D.J., Clonan, S.M., Shaywitz, et al. (2004). Effects of intensive reading remediation for second and third graders and a 1-year follow-up. *Journal of Educational Psychology*, 96, 444–61.

Booth, J.R., and Burman, D.D. (2001). Development and disorders of neurocognitive systems for oral language and reading. *Learning Disability Quarterly*, 24, 205–15.

Catts, H.W., and Kamhi, A.G. (2005). *Language and reading disabilities (2nd ed.).* Boston: Pearson.

Deutsch, G.K., Dougherty, R.F., Bammer, R., Siok, W.T., Gabrieli, J.D., and Wandell, B. (2005). Children's reading performance is correlated with white matter structure measured by diffusion tensor imaging. *Cortex*, 41, 354–63.

Francis, D.J., Shaywitz, S.E., Stuebing, K.K., Shaywitz, B.A., and Fletcher, J.M. (1996). Developmental lag versus deficit models of reading disability: A longitudinal, individual growth curves analysis. *Journal of Educational Psychology*, 88, 3–17.

Heim, S., and Keil, A. (2004). Large-scale neural correlates of developmental dyslexia. *European Child & Adolescent Psychiatry*, 13, 125–40.

Iovino, I., Fletcher, J.M., Breitmeyer, B.G., and Foorman, B.R. (1998). Colored overlays for visual perceptual deficits in children with reading disability and attention deficit/hyperactivity disorder: Are they differentially effective? *Journal of Clinical & Experimental Neuropsychology*, 20, 791–806.

Joseph, J., Noble, K., and Eden, G. (2001). The neurobiological basis of reading. *Journal of Learning Disabilities*, 34, 566–79.

Lyon, G.R., Shaywitz, S.E., and Shaywitz, B.A. (2003). Defining dyslexia, comorbidity, teachers' knowledge of language and reading. *Annals of Dyslexia*, 53, 1–14.

Morris, R.D., Stuebing, K.K., Fletcher, J.M., Shaywitz, S.E., Shankweiler, D.P., Katz, L., et al. (1998). Subtypes of reading disability: Variability around a phonological core. *Journal of Educational Psychology*, 90, 347–73.

National Institute of Child Health and Human Development. (2000). Report of the National Reading Panel. Teaching children to read: An evidence-based assessment of the scientific research literature on reading and its implications for reading instruction (NIH Publication No. 00-4769). Washington, DC: U.S. Government Printing Office.

Papanicolaou, A.C., Pugh, K.R., Simos, P.G., and Mencl, W.E. (2004) Functional brain imaging: An introduction to concepts and applications. In P. McCardle & V. Chhabra (Eds.), *The voice of evidence in reading research*. Baltimore: Paul H. Brooks.

Rayner, K., Foorman, B.R., Perfetti, C.A., Pesetsky, D., and Seidenberg, M.S. (2001). How psychological science informs the teaching of reading. *Psychological Science in the Public Interest*, 2(2), 31–74.

Richards, T.L. (2001). Functional magnetic resonance imaging and spectroscopic imaging of the brain: Application of the fMRI and fMRS to reading disabilities and education. *Learning Disability Quarterly*, 24, 189–203.

Shaywitz, B.A., Shaywitz, S.E., Pugh, K.R., Mencl, W.E., Fulbright, R.K., Skudlarksi, P., et al. (2002). Disruption of posterior brain systems for reading in children with developmental dyslexia. *Biological Psychiatry*, 52, 101–10.

Shaywitz, S.E. (1996). Dyslexia. *Scientific American*, 275(5), 98–104.

Shaywitz, S.E., Fletcher, J.M., Holahan, J.M., Shneider, A.E., Marchione, K.E., Stuebing, K.K., et al. (1999). Persistence of dyslexia: The Connecticut Longitudinal Study at adolescence. *Pediatrics*, 104, 1351–59.

Shaywitz, B.A., Shaywitz, S.E., Blachman, B.A., Pugh, K.R., Fulbright, R.K., Skudlarski, P., et al. (2004). Development of left occipitotemporal systems for skilled reading in children after a phonologically-based intervention. *Biological Psychiatry*, 55, 926–33.

Shaywitz, S.E., Shaywitz, B.A., Fletcher, J.M., & Escobar, M.D. (1990). Prevalence of reading disability in boys and girls: Results of the Connecticut Longitudinal Study. *Journal of the American Medical Association*, 264, 998–1002.

Shaywitz, S.E., Shaywitz, B.A., Fulbright, R.K., Skudlarski, P., Mencl, W.E., Constable, R.T., et al. (2003). Neural systems for compensation and persistence: Young adult outcome of childhood reading disability. *Biological Psychiatry*, 54, 25–33.

Shaywitz, S.E., Shaywitz, B.A., Pugh, K.R., Fulbright, R.K., Constable, R.T., Mencl, W.E., et al. (1998). Functional disruption in the organization of the brain for reading in dyslexia. *Proceedings of the National Academy of Sciences*, 95, 2636–41.

Snow, C.E., Burns, M.S., and Griffin, P. (Eds.). (1998). *Preventing reading difficulties in young children*. Washington, DC: National Academy Press.

Torgesen, J.K. (2000). Individual differences in response to early interventions in reading: The lingering problem of treatment resisters. *Learning Disabilities Research & Practice*, 15, 55–64.

Torgesen, J.K. (2002). The prevention of reading difficulties. *Journal of School Psychology*, 40, 7–26.

Torgesen, J.K., Rashotte, C.A., and Alexander, A. (2001). Principles of fluency instruction in reading: Relationships with established empirical outcomes. In M. Wolf (Ed.), *Dyslexia, fluency, and the brain.* Timonium, MD: York.

Wagner, R.K., and Torgesen, J.K. (1987). The nature of phonological processing and its causal role in the acquisition of reading skills. *Psychological Bulletin*, 101, 192–212.

Ziegler, J.C., and Goswami, U. (2005). Reading acquisition, developmental dyslexia, and skilled reading across languages: A psycholinguistic grain size theory. *Psychological Bulletin*, 131, 3–29.

Chapter 10

Gifted but Learning Disabled

Who Are 2e Students?

Studies as early as the 1970s indicated that students from special populations could also be gifted. In 1981, a colloquium held at Johns Hopkins University convened experts from the fields of both learning disabilities and giftedness to consider this issue. At the time, interest in meeting the needs of gifted and talented students, as well as students with learning disabilities, was evident on many levels; but students who exhibited the characteristics of both exceptionalities, twice-exceptional (2e) students, had received little attention. The participants at the Johns Hopkins gathering concluded that 2e students do, in fact, exist but are often overlooked when assessed for either giftedness or learning disabilities (LDs). The colloquium did much toward establishing criteria for identifying 2e students as a population with special characteristics and needs (Fox, Brody, & Tobin, 1983).

In the intervening years, the concept of the 2e student has become commonly accepted among education researchers. Many books have been written on the subject, articles appear regularly in journals, and national education conferences focusing on either LDs or giftedness consistently include at least one session on the 2e student. Research has produced a generally accepted definition of the 2e student and the

---

"Twice-Exceptional Students: Who They Are and What They Need" by Micaela Bracamonte, © 2010 Micaela Bracamonte. Reprinted with permission. This article first appeared in the March 2010 issue of *2e: Twice-Exceptional Newsletter* (www.2enewsletter.com).

realization that 2e students require a unique combination of educational programs, enrichment, and counseling support.

How Many 2e Students Are There?

Since 2e students were first identified as a distinct group in 1977 with the publication of the book *Providing Programs for the Gifted Handicapped* (Maker 1977), their education has been of growing concern to an increasing number of researchers within both the realm of gifted/talented education and the field of special education. At the turn of the millennium, the U.S. Department of Education, Office of Civil Rights, began to collect data on the number of K–12 students identified as gifted/talented and receiving services for an LD. In the Individuals with Disabilities Educational Act (IDEA), these students are defined as having: "A disorder in one or more of the basic psychological processes involved in understanding or in using language, spoken or written, which may manifest itself in an imperfect ability to listen, speak, read, write, spell, or to do mathematical calculations."

In 2006, the most recent year for which these statistics are available, the number of K–12 students identified as 2e reached nearly seventy thousand among school districts that voluntarily tracked and reported this data. This number represents a percentage consistent with estimates that 2 to 5 percent of the gifted population have LDs and 2 to 5 percent of students with LDs are gifted. This number will continue to grow as more school districts become aware of twice exceptionality and as more districts participate in reporting this data.

However, despite a growing awareness of twice-exceptionality, 2e students are falling through the cracks of our educational system. With few exceptions, neither public nor private schools have kept pace with the research on who 2e students are and what they need to succeed. Furthermore, identifying students for gifted programs and identifying them for special education programs continue to be mutually exclusive activities (Boodoo et al. 1989).

2e Students in Profile

Who are 2e students? What are they like?

Julien: Typically 2e

At his third birthday party, Julien either ignored his guests or—using his vocabulary of twelve words—told them what to do. He ran around nonstop, touching everything and everybody, but made only fleeting eye contact with anyone. He also spent an hour by himself building an elaborate bridge system using Duplo® blocks. Earlier that year, during a state-mandated intelligence quotient (IQ) test, he largely ignored the tester and was determined to have an IQ of 84. But later that year, Julien learned to speak and read almost in tandem. A visit to one renowned psychiatrist yielded an Asperger syndrome diagnosis; a psychologist cited attention deficit hyperactivity disorder (ADHD) "tendencies"; and a neuropsychologist suggested Julien's hearing be tested. His pediatrician insisted Julien was a brilliant child on his own trajectory who just needed speech therapy.

Between the ages of three and nine, Julien attended four special education and three general education schools, none of them a good fit. He didn't score well on a kindergarten screening test for gifted programming because he couldn't stay in his seat during the test. He was removed from two general education kindergarten classrooms for calling out answers and asking off-topic questions, not sitting during circle time, and other "disruptive" and "noncompliant" behaviors.

Over the years, many teachers complained that Julien wasn't trying hard enough, that he didn't pay attention during group lessons (though he remembered everything that was said), that he refused to do worksheets in school, and that he would have a tantrum when asked to write. Julien complained that school was too hard and too easy. Because the special education schools he attended were so focused on controlling his classroom behavior, remediating his writing challenges and finding productive outlets for his talents were neglected.

Julien, now ten years old, is both "gifted"—with a full-scale IQ of 136—and "learning disabled," with diagnoses of ADHD (combined type), generalized anxiety disorder, and a disorder of written expression. He writes like a second-grader, but works on ninth-grade math, with college-level concepts thrown in "for fun." With his jigsaw collection of talents and relative deficits, Julien is a "typical" twice-exceptional child.

Simon: Why Don't I Fit In?

The first sign that Simon was out-of-sync with his age peers was when, at the age of two, he was kicked out of a playgroup. Parents complained that, though not aggressive, Simon was too physical with their children (e.g., grabbing and hugging too hard). Precociously verbal, Simon seemed to be trying to get and sustain his playmates' attention in a way he thought they'd understand.

In a Montessori preschool, Simon thrived at first; but as he sped ahead of classmates in reading, he became bored with the learning materials and increasingly disrupted the classroom routine. He narrowly missed score cutoffs for gifted kindergarten programs and was rejected by numerous private schools for being disrespectful at interviews and disobedient during group activities.

His public school kindergarten teacher tried engaging Simon by giving him extra homework, but Simon had trouble with everything from transitions, to standing in line, to the curriculum itself, which was several grades below his abilities. He got into trouble in class so that he'd be "punished" by having to sit outside the principal's office all day reading. On the playground, he was reprimanded for telling the other kids he was a monster. Later, Simon would tell his mother, "I wasn't pretending. I am a monster. I'm a freak."

First grade in a private school was similar—except that Simon had no problems whatsoever during his twice-weekly one-on-one periods with the school's learning specialist. He was asked to leave halfway during the school year.

Unfortunately, Simon's mixed bag of strengths—high creativity, precocious general knowledge, college-level reading skills—and his (relative) weaknesses—average processing, visual/spatial reasoning, and math skills, plus low frustration tolerance—make it hard to assess his abilities via formal testing. He frequently refuses to answer questions or complete tasks that are too repetitive, too simple, or too difficult. Also, despite his early advantage of being identified at the age of three both as gifted and as having ADHD (inattentive type), the absence of a school that could support both his exceptionalities has meant that, at the age of eight, he has four years' worth of negative school experiences under his belt. Simon fears that no schoolteacher will ever accept him for who he is.

Cameron: Passing as Average

Ten-year-old Cameron is a classic example of the child who falls through the cracks in school because his gifts and learning disabilities mask each other. Because he performs at or above grade level across the board and causes no disruptions in the classroom, Cameron's teachers see him as a model student. He's also very popular with his classmates. But Cameron dreads school and has been placed in five different schools in only four years.

In kindergarten, Cameron started begging his mother not to make him go to school. By second grade, he was getting sick to his stomach as he approached the school building. Cameron's undiagnosed dysgraphia made certain fine motor tasks laboriously difficult, causing him to work much harder than his classmates just to complete worksheets and writing assignments. His teachers suggested that he just wasn't trying hard enough. Though he wanted very much to please his teachers, Cameron's ADHD (hyperactive type) made it extremely difficult for him to sit still at a desk all day.

Despite his challenges, Cameron's superior-level intelligence, knack for higher-level science and abstract thinking, and high math aptitude helped him keep up and, at times, even exceed grade-level expectations. But because he was using all his mental and physical energy just to survive the school day, his gifts went unnoticed and unencouraged. When Cameron got home from school, he would fall apart, tell himself he was stupid, fear leaving home again, and cry himself to sleep. Although an enthusiastic learner, he became completely school avoidant at the age of eight, and his parents have home-schooled him for the last two years for lack of a better alternative.

Alex: A Gifted Dilemma

Alex has always been precocious as well as stubborn. At eighteen months, he would tell his parents the colors of passing cars; and, if he didn't get what he wanted, he would cry until he threw up. He was reading by three; by eight, diagnosed with diabetes; and by ten, enrolled in his third school in three years.

Alex has a superior-range IQ but is struggling to hang on in his gifted public education fourth-grade classroom, the last stop before his parents consider special education. His executive functioning challenges make it hard to organize his thoughts and work; and his diabetes makes him feel doubly different, physically and socially. What's hard for Alex academically is translating his ideas into something others can recognize and assess; so he struggles to write even a three-sentence essay (though he reads five-hundred-page books voraciously) or to show his work on a multi-step math problem he understands intuitively.

When faced with a task that comes easily to him, Alex doesn't read the directions; he rushes ahead and makes careless errors. When faced with a challenge, he either gives up quickly or refuses to try at all. Because of the vigilance and control his chronic illness requires, his parents feel Alex has a hard time accepting direction and control from authority figures in school. Because he's so empathetic and socially adept, he's well liked among classmates; but because he's so bright, perfectionistic, and self-directed, his teachers regard him as arrogant.

Ultimately, Alex's anxiety is his undoing, causing him to disengage from the education process altogether. He refuses to do his schoolwork, or he simply refuses to go to school at all.

Tying Together the Differences

As these profiles show, there are many expressions of twice exceptionality, even among children with identical diagnoses. It also merits mention that 2e girls, according to experts in the field, tend not to call attention to themselves with "disruptive behavior" until late middle school or high school, when their challenges start to exceed their ability to hide them. What binds these children together are their exceptional general intelligence, their asynchronous (unevenly developed) skills, their highly discrepant challenges, and the anxiety their differences cause socially and academically in typical classrooms. The challenges parents of 2e children face in finding appropriate, nurturing, and enriching environments are more than daunting. Specialized schools, both public and private, usually cater to children with learning disabilities or with gifts and talents, but not both.

How to Identify 2e Students

While 2e students have characteristics of both gifted and learning disabled students, they also have their own unique characteristics. Therefore, they need to be treated as a separate population. Unfortunately, although education researchers have known about 2e students for decades, most teachers and administrators are still largely unaware of these children, leaving them overlooked and underserved. An ongoing survey of school districts nationwide started in 2000 by Johns Hopkins University has indicated that the majority of school districts have no procedures in place for identifying or meeting the education needs of 2e children. At the same time, many of these same districts have indicated an interest in improving in this area.

By analyzing the records of students currently in 2e programs, researchers have developed a profile of twice exceptionality. 2e students typically perform at very high levels on some, but not all, of the gifted screening tests used by public schools. On the other hand, they tend to simultaneously perform very poorly on one or more of the local, state, or national standardized assessments used to measure individual student progress. One of the hallmarks of twice- exceptionality, then, is inconsistency in performance and, in particular, in test results.

Because 2e children are inconsistent performers with uneven skills and asynchronous development, it's critical to separate out their test scores on IQ tests, education experts suggest. The commonly used Wechsler Intelligence Scales for Children (WISC) includes a series of subtests, and a review of these subtest IQ scores can help identify 2e students (Bannatyne 1974; Baum et al. 1991; Coleman 1997, Kaufman 2002).

Most 2e students tend to do well on the WISC's spatial, pattern recognition, verbal comprehension, and abstract conceptualization measures; there's a strong tendency for these children to be creative problem solvers. On the other hand, most 2e students tend to do less well on measures of processing details and rote memorization (Baum 2004).

Researchers have worked to shed light on the pattern of abilities and relative deficits displayed by 2e students in order to simplify their identification by teachers and administrators. These students are a diverse group, however, embracing a wide variety of gifts and talents in combination with multifarious learning challenges that often resist categorization. There is, in fact, no single defining pattern of characteristics or test scores. Nevertheless, it can be safely said that hallmarks include:

- evidence of a discrepancy between expected and actual achievement;

- evidence of an outstanding talent or ability;

- coincident evidence of a processing deficit (with processing defined broadly as the ability to interpret higher-order perceptions, as in auditory processing).

A multidimensional approach to identifying twice-exceptionality should include not only written assessments such as the WISC, but behavioral checklists completed by parents, teachers, and students alike, as well as portfolio reviews and interviews (Krochak and Ryan 2007). Only through a combination of formal and informal assessments can a full picture of an individual 2e student emerge.

What Works (and What Doesn't) for 2e Students

The goal of education is to provide opportunities for students to build knowledge, skills, and attitudes so that they can become successful, contributing members of a global society. 2e students need not be excluded from this vision. In fact, according to Thomas West in his 1997 book, *In the Mind's Eye*, these very individuals have made and will make some of the most extraordinary contributions to our world.

The needs of 2e students can be met through appropriate identification and an individualized approach to education. However, the classroom teacher must have support from both gifted educators and special educators to implement effective strategies. The best results are achieved where there is collaboration between the classroom teacher, gifted educator, special educator, parents, and the student.

Programming for 2e students must include strategies to:

- nurture the student's strengths and interests;

- foster their social/emotional development;

- enhance their capacity to cope with mixed abilities;

- identify learning gaps and provide explicit, remediative instruction;

- support the development of compensatory strategies. (Reis and McCoach 2000, and Smutny 2001).

Clearly, 2e students have needs that differ considerably from those of gifted students without LDs, students without exceptional abilities who have LDs, and average students whose abilities are more evenly distributed. Individualized instruction is, of course, optimal for all students, so that pace, level, and content can be geared to ability, interests, and learning style. However, it is essential for students whose abilities are clearly discrepant. Ideally, a continuum of placement options should be available so that teachers can develop a plan that builds heavily on students' strengths but also provides academic and cognitive remediation as well as support for social and emotional needs.

A study of 2e students found that those receiving either a combination of both gifted and LD services or only gifted programming reported higher self-concept than did those students receiving intensive or exclusive LD services (Nielsen and Morton-Albert 1989). Thus, there may be positive social and emotional effects, as well as positive academic effects, of making accelerated or enriched academic experiences available to those identified as 2e. Given the strong concern among educators that 2e students be challenged in their areas of strength, placement in a gifted program for at least part of the day is advisable.

There are a number of helpful classroom strategies for 2e students on which education researchers agree. They include the following five strategies.

Strategy 1: Playing to their Strengths

An encouraging and exciting learning environment for 2e students is one in which their giftedness is recognized first, not their disability. Despite their difficulties in reading, writing, math, or attending to the task at hand, these learners must be allowed to engage in a challenging curriculum tailored to their strengths (Baum 2004). Strength-based instruction is one of the most effective strategies for 2e students, emphasizing talent development over remediation of deficiencies. In "playing to strengths," the teacher provides opportunities for high-level abstract thinking, creativity, and problem solving. Strength-based interventions are often more successful because they engage students' interests and abilities, enhancing motivation and increasing frustration tolerance.

2e students are most likely to accept academic challenge when instruction plays to their strengths. In creating individualized learning programs, teachers will find their 2e students far more motivated to work when given options based on their interests and talents, as well as on their learning style. For example, as gifted education author Lisa Rivero explains: "Visual learners prefer to use their eyes to learn and auditory learners their ears. Kinesthetic learners prefer to use their bodies to learn [through movement], while tactile learners prefer to use their sense of touch. Allowing students to use their preferred learning style results in deeper, more meaningful learning. Being prohibited from using it often leads to frustration, decreased learning, underachievement, and lowered self-concept" (Rivero 2002).

Research shows that 2e children are quite capable of high-level abstract thinking, demonstrate significant creativity, and are able to take unique problem-solving approaches to tasks (Trail 2000). Offering learning opportunities that draw on these abilities is likely to engage these students and give them opportunities for success. At the same time, caution is essential when setting the level of challenge for 2e students. It needs to be appropriate—high enough so that they must stretch to meet the challenge, but not so high that they will fail. Here is where supports in the learning environment come into play.

Strategy 2: Addressing Social and Emotional Needs

2e students need a nurturing environment that supports the development of their potential. An encouraging approach is recommended over implementing measures from a punitive perspective (Strop and Goldman 2002). Teachers provide a nurturing environment when:

- they value individual differences and learning styles;
- student readiness, interests, and learning profile shape instruction;
- instruction includes activities for multiple intelligences;
- flexible grouping is used for instruction;
- the development of student potential is encouraged;
- students are assessed in accordance with their abilities;
- excellence is defined by individual growth.

Strategy 3: Incorporating Counseling Support

The drive to achieve perfection, common in many gifted children, generates much psychological conflict in academically talented children who have difficulty achieving (Olenchak 1994). One survey of gifted students with LDs found them to be emotionally upset and generally unhappy because of their frustrations; in particular, "virtually all had some idea that they could not make their brain, body, or both do what they wanted" (Schiff et al. 1981). Furthermore, 2e students can be very self-critical, which can lead to a particularly dysfunctional form of perfectionism. Counseling is recommended to address their unique needs and should be available on an as-needed basis.

The importance of providing counseling for these students has been noted in many studies from the time 2e children were first identified (Brown-Mizuno 1990; Hishinuma 1993; Mendaglio 1993; Olenchak 1994; Suter and Wolf 1987). The benefits of both group and individual counseling have been identified by numerous researchers (Baum 1994; Mendaglio 1993; Olenchak 1994). Group counseling can, for example, help students see that others' experiences are similar to their own. Learning in a classroom with other 2e students, in itself, can go a long way towards providing this support. The counseling role can sometimes be undertaken by teachers who understand well the needs of 2e students (Baum et al. 1991; Daniels 1983; Hishinuma 1993). However, some students may require individual counseling. Parents also need information and, in cases, counseling to help them understand the characteristics and needs of their gifted children with learning challenges (Bricklin 1983; Brown-Mizuno 1990; Daniels 1983).

Strategy 4: Providing Organizational Guidance and One-on-one Tutoring Opportunities

A lack of organizational, time management, and study skills can have a negative impact on both the emotional well-being and school performance of twice-exceptional students. Many in the 2e research community agree that it is critical that students receive explicit instruction and support to develop this battery of skills. These students also need prescriptive, individualized intervention services related to their areas of academic challenge, such as reading, writing, or math. This focus on relative weaknesses should, as much as possible, be woven into projects in areas of student strengths, with accommodations and adaptations in place as long as students need them (and no longer). Long-term, project-based learning affords ample opportunities for teachers to naturalistically scaffold acquisition of these skills in both group learning and one-on-one mentored situations.

Strategy 5: Integrating Technology

Accommodations, particularly the use of assistive technology, are highly recommended to help these academically talented students compensate for their learning challenges (Baum et al. 1991; Howard 1994; Suter and Wolf 1987; Torgesen 1986). Such techniques may be helpful to many LD students, but they are especially beneficial to those who are also gifted and in need of moving ahead in their areas of strength. For example, students who are capable of a high level of mathematical problem solving, but who have difficulty with simple computations, could be given a calculator so that they won't be held back. A laptop computer loaded with voice-recognition software, word prediction, brainstorming/planning software, and a spell checker can be enormously helpful to a student whose problems lie in writing and/ or spelling, but whose ideas are complex and sophisticated. Students who have difficulty taking notes in class can be allowed to record lectures. Recorded books and other information sources not dependent on reading (such as films) might also help students who have reading challenges but strong auditory processing skills.

What's Needed

The ideal classroom environment for the twice-exceptional student is very far from what exists. No Child Left Behind legislation has failed to provide services for 2e students, much less offer a framework for identifying them on a large scale. With a handful of exceptions, highly promising, creative students with learning differences continue to be systematically denied what they need in school—a flexible combination of acceleration, remediation, and social/emotional supports—whether the context is general, gifted, or special education.

To meet the needs of these children, there must be a paradigm shift from a remediation or deficit model to a strength-based model of education. This is particularly true as a growing body of research demonstrates that learning disabilities also appear to afford and co-exist with unique learning strengths. These children need programs and schools that transform the research on twice exceptionality into a daily commitment to combine academic rigor with individualized accommodations and adaptations.

One million of our nation's most promising, most innovative thinkers—bright children who learn differently, not "deficiently"—constitute a neglected national resource. Twice-exceptional children need an education that fits, and it's in all of our interests to give it to them.

References

Bannatyne, A. (1974). Diagnosis: A note on recategorization of the WISC scaled scores. *Journal of Learning Disabilities*, 7, 272–73.

Baum, S. (1994). Meeting the needs of gifted/learning disabled students. *The Journal of Secondary Gifted Education*, 5(3), 6–16.

Baum, S., Owen, S. V., & Dixon, J. (1991). *To be gifted and learning disabled: From identification to practical intervention strategies.* Mansfield Center, CT: Creative Learning Press.

Baum, S. and Owen, S. V. (2004). *To be gifted and learning disabled: Strategies for helping bright students with LD, ADHD, and more.* Mansfield Center, CT: Creative Learning Press.

Boodoo, G. M., Bradley, C. L., Frontera, R. L., Pitts, J. R., and Wright, L. B. (1989). A survey of procedures used for identifying gifted learning disabled children. *Gifted Child Quarterly*, 33(3), 110–14.

Bricklin, P. M. (1983). Working with parents of learning disabled/gifted children. In L. H. Fox, L. Brody, and D. Tobin (Eds.), *Learning disabled / gifted children: Identification and programming* (pp. 243–60). Baltimore: University Park Press.

Brown-Mizuno, C. (1990). Success strategies for learners who are learning disabled as well as gifted. *Teaching Exceptional Children*, 23(1), 10–12.

Coleman, M. R., Gallagher, J. J. and Foster, A. (1998). *Updated report on state policies related to the identification of gifted students.* Chapel Hill, NC: University of North Carolina Press.

Daniels, P. R. (1983). *Teaching the gifted / learning disabled child.* Rockville, MD: Aspen.

Fox, L. H., Brody, L., and Tobin, D. (Eds.). (1983*). Learning disabled / gifted children: Identification and programming.* Baltimore: University Park Press.

Hishinuma, E. S. (1993). Counseling gifted/at risk and gifted/dyslexic youngsters. *Gifted Child Today*, 16(1), 30–33.

Howard, J. B. (1994). Addressing needs through strengths. *The Journal of Secondary Gifted Education*, 5(3), 23–34.

Kaufman, A. S. and Lichtenberger, E. O. (2002). *Assessing adolescent and adult intelligence (2nd ed.).* Boston, MA: Allyn and Bacon.

Krochak, L. A. and Ryan, T. G. (2007). The challenge of identifying gifted/learning disabled students. *International Journal of Special Education*, 22(3), 44–53.

Maker, C. (1977). *Providing programs for the gifted handicapped.* Reston, VA: Council for Exceptional Children.

Mendaglio, S. (1993). Counseling gifted learning disabled: Individual and group counseling techniques. In L. K. Silverman (Ed.), *Counseling the gifted and talented* (pp. 131–49). Denver: Love Publishing.

Nielsen, M. E. and Morton-Albert, S. (1989). The effects of special education on the self-concept and school attitude of learning-disabled/gifted students. *Roeper Review*, 12, 29–26.

Olenchak, F. R. (1994). Talent development. *The Journal of Secondary Gifted Education*, 5(3), 40–52.

Reis, S. and McCoach, D. B. (2000). The underachievement of gifted students: What do we know and where do we go? *Gifted Child Quarterly*, 44, 152–70.

Rivero, L. (2002). *Creative homeschooling for gifted children: A resource guide for smart families.* Scottsdale, AZ: Great Potential Press.

Schiff, M., Kaufman, N. and Kaufman, A. (1981). Scatter analysis of WISC-R profiles for LD children with superior intelligence. *Journal of Learning Disabilities*, 14(7), 400–404.

Smutny, J. F. (2001). Meeting the needs of gifted underachievers—Individually! *Gifted Education Communicator*, 32(3).

Strop, J. and Goldman, D. (2002). The affective side: Emotional issues of twice-exceptional students. From *Understanding Our Gifted*, Winter, 28–29.

Suter, D. P., and Wolf, J. S. (1987). Issues in the identification and programming of the gifted/learning disabled child. *Journal for the Education of the Gifted*, 10, 227–37.

Torgesen, J. K. (1986). Computer assisted instruction with learning disabled children. In J. K. Torgesen and B. Y. L. Wong (Eds.), *Psychological and educational perspectives on learning disabilities* (pp. 417–35). Orlando, FL: Academic Press.

Trail, B. (2000). A collaborative approach to meeting the needs of twice-exceptional students. In K. Kay (Ed.), *Uniquely gifted: Identifying and meeting the needs of the twice-exceptional student*. Gilsum, NH: Avocus Publishing.

West, T. G. (1991). *In the mind's eye: Visual thinkers, gifted people with learning difficulties, computer images, and the ironies of creativity*. Buffalo, NY: Prometheus Books.

Chapter 11

Nonverbal Learning Disability

What is non-verbal learning disability (NLD or NVLD)?

Kids with NLD are very verbal, and may not have academic problems until they get into the upper grades in school. Often their biggest problem is with social skills.

NLD is very like Asperger syndrome. It may be that the diagnoses of Asperger syndrome (AS) and NLD simply "provide different perspectives on a heterogeneous, yet overlapping, group of individuals sharing at least some common aspects."[1] AS and NLD are generally thought to describe pretty much the same kind of disorder, but to differ in severity—with AS describing more severe symptoms.

What are the signs of NLD?

- Great vocabulary and verbal expression

- Excellent memory skills

- Attention to detail, but misses the big picture

- Trouble understanding reading

- Difficulty with math, especially word problems

- Poor abstract reasoning
- Physically awkward; poor coordination
- Messy and laborious handwriting
- Concrete thinking; taking things very literally
- Trouble with nonverbal communication, like body language, facial expression, and tone of voice
- Poor social skills; difficulty making and keeping friends
- Fear of new situations
- Trouble adjusting to changes
- May be very naïve and lack common sense
- Anxiety, depression, low self-esteem
- May withdraw, becoming agoraphobic (abnormal fear of open spaces)

What are some parenting tips for kids with NLD?

- Keep the environment predictable and familiar.
- Provide structure and routine.
- Prepare your child for changes, giving logical explanations.
- Pay attention to sensory input from the environment, like noise, temperature, smells, many people around, etc. Help your child learn coping skills for dealing with anxiety and sensory difficulties.
- Be logical, organized, clear, concise, and concrete. Avoid jargon, double meanings, sarcasm, nicknames, and teasing.
- State your expectations clearly.
- Be very specific about cause and effect relationships.
- Work with your child's school to modify homework assignments, testing (time and content), grading, art, and physical education.
- Have your child use the computer at school and at home for schoolwork.
- Help your child learn organizational and time management skills.
- Make use of your child's verbal skills to help with social interactions and nonverbal experiences. For example, giving a verbal explanation of visual material.

- Teach your child about nonverbal communication (facial expressions, gestures, etc.). Help them learn how to tell from others' reactions whether they are communicating well.
- Learn about social competence and how to teach it.
- Help your child out in group activities.
- Get your child into the therapies they need, such as: occupational and physical therapy, psychological, or speech and language (to address social issues).

How can parents help kids with poor social skills?

According to Mel Levine, in a book chapter titled "Unpopular Children"[2] there are many ways parents can help kids with social skills problems. Here are some ways parents can help their kids:

- Steer your child toward a playmate they have something in common with and set up a play date. This is a way to get some social skills experience in a small, controlled, less-threatening way.
- See if you can find a small-group social skills training program in your school system, medical system, or community. This kind of program will probably not be available in smaller communities.
- Encourage your child to develop interests that will build their self-esteem and help them relate to other kids. For example, if your child is interested in Pokémon, pursuing this interest may open social doors for them with schoolmates.
- Talk to your child in private after you have gone with them to a group activity. You can discuss with them how they could improve the way they interact with other kids. For example, you might point out that other kids don't feel comfortable when your child stands so close to them. Help them practice the social skills you explain to them through role-playing.
- Bullying is unacceptable. Your child's school must make every effort to prevent it. If talking to your child's teachers and principal does not put an end to the victimization, ask your child's doctor to write a letter to the school, and pursue the issue up to higher channels in the school district if necessary.
- These kids need as few handicaps as possible, so make sure your child is getting the counseling, therapies, and/or medication they need to treat any other problems or medical conditions they might have.

- Reassure your child that you value them for who they are. It's a little tricky to help your child improve social skills, and at the same time nurture their confidence to hold on to their unique individuality.

Notes

1. Klin, A., Volkmar, FR. Asperger's syndrome: guidelines for assessment and diagnosis. Yale Child Study Center. Developmental Disabilities Clinic. Available from: URL: http://info.med.yale.edu/chldstdy/autism/asdiagnosis.html.

2. Levine, MD. Unpopular Children. In: Parker, S., Zuckerman, B., editors. *Behavioral and developmental pediatrics: a handbook for primary care*. Boston: Little, Brown and Company; 1995, p. 327.

Chapter 12

Speech, Language, and Communication Disorders

Chapter Contents

Section 12.1

What Is a Communication Disorder?

"Speech and Language Impairments," National Dissemination
Center for Children with Disabilities, January 2011.

Definition

There are many kinds of speech and language disorders that can
affect children. In this section, we'll talk about four major areas in
which these impairments occur. These are the areas of:

- **articulation:** speech impairments where the child produces
  sounds incorrectly (e.g., lisp, difficulty articulating certain
  sounds, such as "l" or "r");

- **fluency:** speech impairments where a child's flow of speech is
  disrupted by sounds, syllables, and words that are repeated, prolonged, or avoided and where there may be silent blocks or inappropriate inhalation, exhalation, or phonation patterns;

- **voice:** speech impairments where the child's voice has an abnormal quality to its pitch, resonance, or loudness; and

- **language:** language impairments where the child has problems
  expressing needs, ideas, or information, and/or in understanding
  what others say.[1]

These areas are reflected in how "speech or language impairment" is
defined by the nation's special education law, the Individuals with Disabilities Education Act, given below. IDEA is the law that makes early intervention services available to infants and toddlers with disabilities, and
special education available to school-aged children with disabilities.

Definition of "Speech or Language Impairment" under IDEA

The Individuals with Disabilities Education Act, or IDEA, defines the term "speech or language impairment" as follows: "Speech

or language impairment means a communication disorder, such as stuttering, impaired articulation, a language impairment, or a voice impairment, that adversely affects a child's educational performance."

Development of Speech and Language Skills in Childhood

Speech and language skills develop in childhood according to fairly well defined milestones. Parents and other caregivers may become concerned if a child's language seems noticeably behind (or different from) the language of same-aged peers. This may motivate parents to investigate further and, eventually, to have the child evaluated by a professional.

Having the child's hearing checked is a critical first step. The child may not have a speech or language impairment at all but, rather, a hearing impairment that is interfering with his or her development of language.

It's important to realize that a language delay isn't the same thing as a speech or language impairment. Language delay is a very common developmental problem—in fact, the most common, affecting 5 to 10 percent of children in preschool.[2] With language delay, children's language is developing in the expected sequence, only at a slower rate. In contrast, speech and language disorder refers to abnormal language development.[3] Distinguishing between the two is most reliably done by a certified speech-language pathologist.

Characteristics of Speech or Language Impairments

The characteristics of speech or language impairments will vary depending upon the type of impairment involved. There may also be a combination of several problems.

When a child has an articulation disorder, he or she has difficulty making certain sounds. These sounds may be left off, added, changed, or distorted, which makes it hard for people to understand the child.

Leaving out or changing certain sounds is common when young children are learning to talk, of course. A good example of this is saying "wabbit" for "rabbit." The incorrect articulation isn't necessarily a cause for concern unless it continues past the age where children are expected to produce such sounds correctly.[4]

Fluency refers to the flow of speech. A fluency disorder means that something is disrupting the rhythmic and forward flow of speech—

usually, a stutter. As a result, the child's speech contains an "abnormal number of repetitions, hesitations, prolongations, or disturbances. Tension may also be seen in the face, neck, shoulders, or fists."[5]

Voice is the sound that's produced when air from the lungs pushes through the voice box in the throat (also called the larynx), making the vocal folds within vibrate. From there, the sound generated travels up through the spaces of the throat, nose, and mouth, and emerges as our "voice."

A voice disorder involves problems with the pitch, loudness, resonance, or quality of the voice.[6] The voice may be hoarse, raspy, or harsh. For some, it may sound quite nasal; others might seem as if they are "stuffed up." People with voice problems often notice changes in pitch, loss of voice, loss of endurance, and sometimes a sharp or dull pain associated with voice use.[7]

Language has to do with meanings, rather than sounds.[8] A language disorder refers to an impaired ability to understand and/or use words in context.[9] A child may have an expressive language disorder (difficulty in expressing ideas or needs), a receptive language disorder (difficulty in understanding what others are saying), or a mixed language disorder (which involves both).

Some characteristics of language disorders include:

• improper use of words and their meanings;

• inability to express ideas;

• inappropriate grammatical patterns;

• reduced vocabulary; and

• inability to follow directions.[10]

Children may hear or see a word but not be able to understand its meaning. They may have trouble getting others to understand what they are trying to communicate. These symptoms can easily be mistaken for other disabilities such as autism or learning disabilities, so it's very important to ensure that the child receives a thorough evaluation by a certified speech-language pathologist.

What Causes Speech and Language Disorders?

Some causes of speech and language disorders include hearing loss, neurological disorders, brain injury, intellectual disabilities, drug abuse, physical impairments such as cleft lip or palate, and vocal abuse or misuse. Frequently, however, the cause is unknown.

Incidence

Of the 6.1 million children with disabilities who received special education under IDEA in public schools in the 2005–2006 school year, more than 1.1 million were served under the category of speech or language impairment.[11] This estimate does not include children who have speech/language problems secondary to other conditions such as deafness, intellectual disability, autism, or cerebral palsy. Because many disabilities do impact the individual's ability to communicate, the actual incidence of children with speech-language impairment is undoubtedly much higher.

Finding Help

Because all communication disorders carry the potential to isolate individuals from their social and educational surroundings, it is essential to provide help and support as soon as a problem is identified. While many speech and language patterns can be called "baby talk" and are part of children's normal development, they can become problems if they are not outgrown as expected.

Therefore, it's important to take action if you suspect that your child has a speech or language impairment (or other disability or delay).

References

1.   Minnesota Department of Education. (2010). Speech or language impairments. Online at: http://education.state.mn.us/MDE/EdExc/SpecEdClass/DisabCateg/SpeechLangImpair/index.html

2.   Boyse, K. (2008). Speech and language delay and disorder. Retrieved from the University of Michigan Health System website: http://www.med.umich.edu/yourchild/topics/speech.htm

3.   Ibid.

4.   American Speech-Language-Hearing Association. (n.d.). Speech sound disorders: Articulation and phonological processes. Online at: http://www.asha.org/public/speech/disorders/speechsounddisorders.htm

5.   Cincinnati Children's Hospital. (n.d.). Speech conditions and diagnoses. Online at: http://www.cincinnatichildrens.org/health/info/speech/diagnose/speech-disorder.htm

6. National Institute on Deafness and Other Communication Disorders. (2002). What is voice? What is speech? What is language? Online at: http://www.nidcd.nih.gov/health/voice/pages/whatis_vsl.aspx

7. American Academy of Otolaryngology—Head and Neck Surgery. (n.d.). Fact sheet: About your voice. Online at: http://www.entnet.org/HealthInformation/aboutVoice.cfm

8. Boyse, K. (2008). Speech and language delay and disorder. Retrieved from the University of Michigan Health System website: http://www.med.umich.edu/yourchild/topics/speech.htm

9. Encyclopedia of Nursing & Allied Health. (n.d.). Language disorders. Online at: http://www.enotes.com/nursing-encyclopedia/language-disorders

10. Ibid.

11. U.S. Department of Education. (2010, December). Twenty-ninth annual report to Congress on the Implementation of the Individuals with Disabilities Education Act: 2007. Online at: http://www2.ed.gov/about/reports/annual/osep/2007/parts-b-c/index.html

Section 12.2

Apraxia of Speech

Reprinted from the National Institute on Deafness and Other
Communication Disorders, National Institutes of Health, June 7, 2010.

What is apraxia of speech?

Apraxia of speech, also known as verbal apraxia or dyspraxia, is a
speech disorder in which a person has trouble saying what he or she
wants to say correctly and consistently. It is not due to weakness or paralysis of the speech muscles (the muscles of the face, tongue, and lips).
The severity of apraxia of speech can range from mild to severe.

What are the types and causes of apraxia?

There are two main types of speech apraxia: acquired apraxia of
speech and developmental apraxia of speech. Acquired apraxia of
speech can affect a person at any age, although it most typically occurs in adults. It is caused by damage to the parts of the brain that are
involved in speaking, and involves the loss or impairment of existing
speech abilities. The disorder may result from a stroke, head injury,
tumor, or other illness affecting the brain. Acquired apraxia of speech
may occur together with muscle weakness affecting speech production
(dysarthria) or language difficulties caused by damage to the nervous
system (aphasia).

Developmental apraxia of speech (DAS) occurs in children and is
present from birth. It appears to affect more boys than girls. This speech
disorder goes by several other names, including developmental verbal
apraxia, developmental verbal dyspraxia, articulatory apraxia, and
childhood apraxia of speech. DAS is different from what is known as
a developmental delay of speech, in which a child follows the "typical"
path of speech development but does so more slowly than normal.

The cause or causes of DAS are not yet known. Some scientists
believe that DAS is a disorder related to a child's overall language development. Others believe it is a neurological disorder that affects the
brain's ability to send the proper signals to move the muscles involved

145

in speech. However, brain imaging and other studies have not found evidence of specific brain lesions or differences in brain structure in children with DAS. Children with DAS often have family members who have a history of communication disorders or learning disabilities. This observation and recent research findings suggest that genetic factors may play a role in the disorder.

What are the symptoms?

People with either form of apraxia of speech may have a number of different speech characteristics, or symptoms. One of the most notable symptoms is difficulty putting sounds and syllables together in the correct order to form words. Longer or more complex words are usually harder to say than shorter or simpler words. People with apraxia of speech also tend to make inconsistent mistakes when speaking. For example, they may say a difficult word correctly but then have trouble repeating it, or they may be able to say a particular sound one day and have trouble with the same sound the next day. People with apraxia of speech often appear to be groping for the right sound or word, and may try saying a word several times before they say it correctly. Another common characteristic of apraxia of speech is the incorrect use of "prosody"—that is, the varying rhythms, stresses, and inflections of speech that are used to help express meaning.

Children with developmental apraxia of speech generally can understand language much better than they are able to use language to express themselves. Some children with the disorder may also have other problems. These can include other speech problems, such as dysarthria; language problems such as poor vocabulary, incorrect grammar, and difficulty in clearly organizing spoken information; problems with reading, writing, spelling, or math; coordination or "motor-skill" problems; and chewing and swallowing difficulties.

The severity of both acquired and developmental apraxia of speech varies from person to person. Apraxia can be so mild that a person has trouble with very few speech sounds or only has occasional problems pronouncing words with many syllables. In the most severe cases, a person may not be able to communicate effectively with speech, and may need the help of alternative or additional communication methods.

How is it diagnosed?

Professionals known as speech-language pathologists play a key role in diagnosing and treating apraxia of speech. There is no single factor or test that can be used to diagnose apraxia. In addition, speech-language experts do not agree about which specific symptoms are part of developmental apraxia. The person making the diagnosis generally looks for the presence of some, or many, of a group of symptoms, including those described above. Ruling out other contributing factors, such as muscle weakness or language-comprehension problems, can also help with the diagnosis.

To diagnose developmental apraxia of speech, parents and professionals may need to observe a child's speech over a period of time. In formal testing for both acquired and developmental apraxia, the speech-language pathologist may ask the person to perform speech tasks such as repeating a particular word several times or repeating a list of words of increasing length (for example, love, loving, lovingly). For acquired apraxia of speech, a speech-language pathologist may also examine a person's ability to converse, read, write, and perform nonspeech movements. Brain-imaging tests such as magnetic resonance imaging (MRI) may also be used to help distinguish acquired apraxia of speech from other communication disorders in people who have experienced brain damage.

How is it treated?

In some cases, people with acquired apraxia of speech recover some or all of their speech abilities on their own. This is called spontaneous recovery. Children with developmental apraxia of speech will not outgrow the problem on their own. Speech-language therapy is often helpful for these children and for people with acquired apraxia who do not spontaneously recover all of their speech abilities.

Speech-language pathologists use different approaches to treat apraxia of speech, and no single approach has been proven to be the most effective. Therapy is tailored to the individual and is designed to treat other speech or language problems that may occur together with apraxia. Each person responds differently to therapy, and some people will make more progress than others. People with apraxia of speech usually need frequent and intensive one-on-one therapy. Support and encouragement from family members and friends are also important.

In severe cases, people with acquired or developmental apraxia of speech may need to use other ways to express themselves. These might include formal or informal sign language, a language notebook with pictures or written words that the person can show to other people, or an electronic communication device such as a portable computer that writes and produces speech.

What research is being done?

Researchers are searching for the causes of developmental apraxia of speech, including the possible role of abnormalities in the brain or other parts of the nervous system. They are also looking for genetic factors that may play a role in DAS. Other research on DAS is aimed at identifying more specific criteria and new techniques that can be used to diagnose the disorder and distinguish it from other communication disorders. Research on acquired apraxia of speech includes studies to pinpoint the specific areas of the brain that are involved in the disorder. In addition, researchers are studying the effectiveness of various treatment approaches for acquired and developmental apraxia of speech.

Section 12.3

The Impact of Language Difficulties on Learning Ability

"Language Abilities and the Impact of Language Difficulties," *The Parent Letter*, March 2005, updated January 2012. Written and developed by the staff of the Institute for Learning and Academic Achievement at the NYU Child Study Center. © NYU Child Study Center (www.aboutourkids.org). All rights reserved. Reprinted with permission.

When does language start?

Think of your child when she was an infant and recall the way that she cooed, warbled, and gurgled, even before she said her first word. Your child was practicing for later communication but neither her brain nor her vocal apparatus were developed enough for her to use words to communicate her needs. As children grow, however, they come to recognize that sets of particular sounds, when organized in a certain way, have meaning. Children also gradually learn that words go together in many different ways and that they can communicate their ideas to other people. These language abilities develop automatically for most children because they regularly listen to and talk with members of their families.

Indeed, studies have shown that talking to young children is important, and that families differ in how much they talk to their infants. Even before children turn twelve to fifteen months old (a milestone around which most children will utter their first words), parents may have exposed them to thousands of new words, and millions of words may have been spoken in their presence. Studies of how families communicate before the age of eighteen months show that children whose parents talked to them a lot had stronger skills when they began school than children whose parents had spoken to them less. For the average child, the best foundation for academic success is increased exposure to language.

What are the basic building blocks of language?

By the age of four or five, children typically have the ability to name many objects, understand straightforward communications, follow two- and three-step instructions, and listen to and comprehend short stories. These skills are called receptive language abilities because they involve the understanding of information spoken by others. Most children at that age also have the capacity to repeat information told to them and to express their ideas according to specific rules, called syntax, which is equivalent to the rules of grammar. These are called expressive language skills. As children develop, they demonstrate greater abilities to listen to and understand lengthier communications, they can remember and retain more verbal information, and they also add skills involved in understanding figurative communications and pragmatic language rules, like turn taking in dialogues and the methods of practical and social language use.

How much learning is based on these language skills?

Many aspects of school instruction involve language skills. For example, a teacher may deliver a brief lecture as a form of teaching, and classroom discussions often serve as an opportunity to learn new information. Children are also expected to remember what was said to them for later use.

Children with receptive and/or expressive language difficulties will likely struggle in school because they cannot easily learn in these conditions. These children cannot always keep up with the pace of verbal instruction. They may not consistently understand the content of ideas being discussed, and they may not have strong skills for communicating what they do or do not know. As a result, they may become withdrawn in school or appear inattentive because they lose their focus when they do not understand what is being discussed. For these children, language skills need to be evaluated and, when necessary, speech and language therapy should be instituted. As language skills improve, they feel more productive in the classroom.

How do language abilities influence a child's performance in reading, math, and writing?

Some language skills play a significant role in academic development. Young children should be able to rhyme, to understand that letters stand for specific sounds, and to detect individual speech sounds, called phonemes, in words. They can then recognize and manipulate speech sounds. This skill, which is the foundation of learning to read, has been labeled "phonological awareness" or "phonological decoding."

As an example, when a child learns to read he must sound out each letter before he recognizes the word. Children with difficulties in phonological awareness will not consistently recognize the sounds associated with each letter and will struggle to learn to read fluently. Research studies have shown that these problems in phonological decoding are evident in almost all cases of developmental dyslexia or reading disorder.

Difficulties manipulating speech sounds for the purposes of reading and writing are called "language-based," but they are not the same difficulties seen in children with receptive and expressive language difficulties; dyslexic children often understand other people's oral communication and verbally express their ideas with ease.

What can be done to help children with language-based learning difficulties?

If you suspect your child has a learning disability, a psychoeducational evaluation is recommended in order to identify the cause and severity of his or her difficulties. The Committee for Special Education through the Department or Board of Education in your school district can complete these assessments, or a local psychologist may be able to evaluate your child for the presence of these problems. These difficulties do not resolve by themselves as your child grows older, so if a disorder is diagnosed, specialized interventions are necessary. Early intervention is crucial so that the child does not fall further and further behind her peers.

What is the emotional impact of language difficulties or learning disorders?

Children who are diagnosed with a language-based learning disability or a language disorder can feel demoralized and defeated by their struggles. Many children with these difficulties become aware that they are not performing as well as other children and they may withdraw or avoid academic challenges. Helping these children overcome these weaknesses is imperative so that they can experience more success when approaching academic challenges.

Section 12.4

Long-Term Impacts of Early Speech, Language, and Communication Disorders

Speech, language, and communication difficulties can have a profound and lasting effect on children's lives. For a small percentage of children their disability cannot be prevented, but early intervention is just as vital as for those with less severe difficulties to help give a child the best possible support that they need. The impact of these difficulties will vary according to the severity of the problem, the support the child receives, the child's confidence, and the demands of the child's environment. This section pulls together research findings on the consequences of speech and language impairment for children and young people in order to highlight the seriousness of the issue overall. References are listed at the end.

General

- Young children with speech and language impairments are at risk for continued communication problems, as well as for associated cognitive, academic, behavioral, social, and psychiatric difficulties (Bashir and Scavuzzo 1992).

- The initial pattern of speech and/or language deficits is related to overall prognosis. Children whose impairments involve only articulation/phonology generally fare better than those whose impairments involve language [processing] (Beitchman et al. 1994).

Social and Behavioral Problems

- Children with specific language impairment (SLI) have been reported to experience concurrent difficulties in the area of social and behavioral development (Redmond and Rice 1998). This has often been thought to arise from such factors as frustration, peer rejection, and lack of confidence in the face of poor linguistic skills.

- Studies have shown that substantial proportions of children with SLI experience social and behavioral problems as they reach high school age and that these problems increase over time (Redmond and Rice 2002).

Withdrawn Behavior

- Many children with SLI appear to show withdrawn social interaction styles. This may include being less likely to initiate conversation, playing alone, and being liked less by others in the class (Coster, Goorhuis-Brouwer, Nakken, and Spelberg 1999).

- Paul and Kellogg (1997) found that children with slow expressive development at two years of age were rated as shyer and less outgoing than peers when followed up at six years of age.

- Poor interaction and increased withdrawal may also lead to poor self-esteem, as some studies have found this to be a feature of older but not younger children with language difficulties (Jerome, Fujiki, Brinton, and James 2002).

- Children with early language impairment have significantly higher rates of anxiety disorder in young adulthood compared with nonimpaired children. The majority of participants with anxiety disorders had a diagnosis of social phobia (Beitchman et al 2001).

Aggressive Behavior

- Behavioral difficulties of an aggressive nature have been reported as showing increased prevalence in young children with speech and language impairment (Carson, Klee, Perry, Muskina, and Donaghy 1998).

- In the epidemiological study by Beitchman and colleagues (1996), nearly half of the five-year-old speech-language-impaired group was found to have behavioral disorders, of which attention hyperactivity difficulties were the main source.

Difficulty Relating to Others

- Even in a preschool setting, children with language difficulties are less likely than peers to be chosen as friendship partners (Gertner, Rice, and Hadley 1994).

- Language impaired children are at risk of being the target of bullies at school (Conti-Ramsden and Botting 2004).

Learning Difficulties

- Comprehension difficulties make children very vulnerable in relation to education (Hooper et al. 2003).

- Early language impairment (rather than speech impairment) is clearly associated with continued academic difficulties into adulthood. (Young et al. 2002)

- Tomblin, Zhang, Buckwalter, and Catts (2000) found that children with language impairment were at risk of both reading and behavioral problems and, furthermore, that the behavioral difficulties were associated with the reading impairments. Levels of frustration, misunderstanding, and inability to access the curriculum could result in subsequent aggressive behavior, as could failure to understand other children and adults.

Crime

- High levels of speech, language, and communication difficulties are found among the young offender population (Bryan 2004).

- Low education and speech and literacy difficulties are risk factors for offending (Tomblin 2000).

Lasting Impact

- Speech and language impairment identified at age five has long-lasting effects. In one study more than 72 percent of children who had SLI at age five remained impaired at age twelve (Beitchman et al. 1994).

- Social and behavioral difficulties are not a short-term problem for children with speech and language impairment. To the contrary, social difficulties appear to increase. A large cohort of 242 children who had been attending infant language units at seven years of age was followed up when the children were in their final year of primary school (aged eleven). More than half of the children were showing clinical-level difficulties (Conti-Ramsden and Botting 2004).

- A study of young adults who were initially identified as having SLI at age five and subsequently followed at ages twelve and nineteen found: (a) high rates of continued communication difficulties in those with a history of impairment; (b) considerable stability in language performance over time; (c) better long-term outcomes for those with initial speech impairments than for those with language impairments; and (d) more favorable prognoses for those with specific language impairments than for those with impairments secondary to sensory, structural, neurological, or cognitive deficits (Johnson et al. 1999).

References

Bashir, Anthony S., and Scavuzzo, Annebelle. (1992). Children with language disorders: Natural history and academic success. *Journal of Learning Disabilities*, 25 (1), 53–65.

Beitchman, J. H., Brownlie, E. B., Inglis, A., Wild, J., Matthews, R., Schachter, D., et al. (1994). Seven-year follow-up of speech/language impaired and control children: Speech/language stability and outcome. *Journal of the American Academy of Child and Adolescent Psychiatry*, 33, 1322–30.

Beitchman, J. H., Wilson, B., Brownlie, E. B., Walters, H., Inglis, A., and Lancee, W. (1996). Long-term consistency in speech/language profiles: II. behavioural, emotional and social outcomes. *Journal of the American Academy of Child and Adolescent Psychiatry*, 35(6), 815–25.

Beitchman, J. H., Wilson, B., Johnson, C. J., Atkinson, L., Young, A., Adlaf, E., et al. (2001). Fourteen-year follow-up of speech/language impaired children and control children: psychiatric outcome. *Journal of the American Academy of Child and Adolescent Psychiatry*, 40(1), 75–82.

Bryan, K. (2004) Preliminary study of the prelance of speech and language difficulties in young offenders. *International Journal of Language and Communication Disorders*; 39:3, 391–400.

Carson, D. K., Klee, T., Perry, C. K., Muskina, G., and Donaghy, T. (1998). Comparisons of children with delayed and normal language at 24 months of age on measures of behavioural difficulties, social and cognitive development. *Infant Mental Health Journal*, 19, 59–75.

Conti-Ramsden, G., and Botting, N. (2004). Social difficulties and victimisation in children with SLI at 11 years of age. *Journal of Speech, Language and Hearing Research*, 47(1), 145–72.

Coster, F.W, Goorhuis-Brouwer, S.M, Nakken, H, Lutje Spelberg H.C. (1999). Specific Language Impairments and Behavioural Problems. *Folia Phoniatrica et Logopaedica*, 51:99–107.

Gertner, B.L., Rice, M.L., and Hadley, P.A. (1994). Influence of communicative competence on peer preferences in a preschool classroom. *Journal of Speech and Hearing Research*, 37, 913–23.

Hooper, S J, Roberts J E, Zeisel, SA, and Poe, M. (2003). Core language predictors of behavioural functioning in early elementary school children: Concurrent and longitudinal findings. *Behavioral Disorders*, 29(1), 10–21.

Jerome AC, Fujiki M, Brinton B, James SL. (2002). Self-esteem in children with specific language impairment, *Journal of Speech Language and Hearing Research* Aug; 45(4): 700–14.

Johnson, C., Beitchman, J. H., Young, A. R., Escobar, M., Atkinson, L., Wilson, B., et al. (1999). Fourteen-year follow-up of children with and without speech/language impairments: Speech/language stability and outcomes. *Journal of Speech, Language and Hearing Research*, 42, 744–60.

Paul, R. and Kellogg, L. Temperament in late talkers. *Journal of Child Psychology and Psychiatry*, 38, (1997): 803–10.

Redmond, S.M. and Rice M.L. (1998) The socio-emotional behaviours of children with Speech and Language Impairment: Social adaptation or social deviance? *Journal of Speech, Language and Hearing Research*, 41, 688–700.

Redmond, S.M. and Rice, M.L. (2002). Stability of behavioral ratings of children with specific language impairment. *Journal of Speech, Language, and Hearing Research*, 45, 190–201.

Tomblin, J. B., Zhang, X., Buckwalter, P., and Catts, H. (2000). The association of reading disability, behavioural disorders and language impairment among second-grade children. *Journal of Child Psychology and Psychiatry*, 41(4), 473–82.

Young, A. R., Beitchman, J. H., Johnson, C., Douglas, L., Atkinson, L., Escobar, M., et al. (2002). Young adult academic outcomes in a longitudinal sample of early identified language impaired and control children. *Journal of Child Psychology and Psychiatry*, 43(5), 635–45.

Chapter 13

Visual Processing Disorders

There are lots of ways the brain processes visual information. Weaknesses in a particular kind of visual processing can often be seen in specific difficulties with practical, everyday tasks.

Below is an explanation of each of the types of visual processing. Each category also includes:

- possible difficulties that can occur if there is a weakness in that area;

- possible strategies that may help overcome the difficulties.

Be aware that weakness can occur in one or more category at the same time.

It is also important to note that many people without any kind of visual processing disorder experience problems with learning and behavior from time to time. However, if a person consistently displays difficulties with these tasks over time, testing for visual processing disorders by trained professionals should be considered.

Visual Discrimination
The Skill

Using the sense of sight to notice and compare the features of different items to distinguish one item from another.

Difficulties Observed

- Seeing the difference between two similar letters, shapes, or objects
- Noticing the similarities and differences between certain colors, shapes, and patterns

Types of Helpful Strategies

- Clearly space words/problems on a page.
- Anticipate confusions and point out examples of correct responses.

Visual Figure-Ground Discrimination

The Skill

Discriminating a shape or printed character from its background.

Difficulties Observed

- Finding a specific bit of information on a printed page full of words and numbers
- Seeing an image within a competing background

Types of Helpful Strategies

- Practice with "find the item" challenges, such as "Where's Waldo?"
- Use an index card or marker when reading to blot out distraction of other words.
- Highlight useful information while reading.

Visual Sequencing

The Skill

The ability to see and distinguish the order of symbols, words or images.

Difficulties Observed

- Using a separate answer sheet
- Staying in the right place while reading a paragraph (example: skipping lines, reading the same line over and over)

- Reversing or misreading letters, numbers, and words
- Understanding math equations

Types of Helpful Strategies

- Combine reading with oral presentation.
- Color code written instruction.

Visual Motor Processing

The Skill

Using feedback from the eyes to coordinate the movement of other parts of the body.

Difficulties Observed

- Writing within lines or margins of a piece of paper
- Copying from a board or book
- Moving around without bumping into things
- Participating in sports that require well-timed and precise movements in space

Types of Helpful Strategies

- Allow use of a computer.
- Allow use of a tape recorder for lectures.
- Substitute oral reports for written ones.
- Provide a "note buddy" to check that topic notes are clear and well organized.

Visual Memory

The Skill

There are two kinds of visual memory:

- Long-term visual memory is the ability to recall something seen some time ago.
- Short-term visual memory is the ability to remember something seen very recently.

Difficulties Observed

- Remembering the spelling of familiar words with irregular spelling
- Reading comprehension
- Using a calculator or keyboard with speed and accuracy
- Remembering phone numbers

Types of Helpful Strategies

- Provide handouts that are clearly written.
- Provide oral instruction to reinforce written directions.

Visual Closure

The Skill

The ability to know what an object is when only parts of it are visible.

Difficulties Observed

- Recognizing a picture of a familiar object from a partial image (example: a truck without its wheels)
- Identifying a word with a letter missing
- Recognizing a face when one feature (such as the nose) is missing

Types of Helpful Strategies

- Practice with jigsaw puzzles and rebus-type games.

Spatial Relationships

The Skill

The ability to understand how objects are positioned in space in relation to oneself. This involves the understanding of distance (near or far), as well as the relationship of objects and characters described on paper or in a spoken narrative.

Difficulties Observed

- Getting from one place to another
- Spacing letters and words on paper

- Judging time
- Reading maps

Types of Helpful Strategies

- Practice estimating distance with ball games and using a tape measure.
- Create maps and travel logs.
- Practice social skills that focus on judging appropriate physical proximity to others.

Part Three

Other Disorders that
Make Learning Difficult

Chapter 14

Aphasia

What is aphasia?

Aphasia is a disorder that results from damage to portions of the brain that are responsible for language. For most people, these are areas on the left side (hemisphere) of the brain. Aphasia usually occurs suddenly, often as the result of a stroke or head injury, but it may also develop slowly, as in the case of a brain tumor, an infection, or dementia. The disorder impairs the expression and understanding of language as well as reading and writing. Aphasia may co-occur with speech disorders such as dysarthria or apraxia of speech, which also result from brain damage.

Who has aphasia?

Anyone can acquire aphasia, including children, but most people who have aphasia are middle-aged or older. Men and women are equally affected. According to the National Aphasia Association, approximately eighty thousand individuals acquire aphasia each year from strokes. About one million people in the United States currently have aphasia.

What causes aphasia?

Aphasia is caused by damage to one or more of the language areas of the brain. Many times, the cause of the brain injury is a stroke. A

Excerpted from the National Institute on Deafness and Other Communication Disorders, National Institutes of Health, NIH Publication No. 97-4257, October 2008.

stroke occurs when blood is unable to reach a part of the brain. Brain cells die when they do not receive their normal supply of blood, which carries oxygen and important nutrients. Other causes of brain injury are severe blows to the head, brain tumors, brain infections, and other conditions that affect the brain.

What types of aphasia are there?

There are two broad categories of aphasia: fluent and nonfluent.

Damage to the temporal lobe (the side portion) of the brain may result in a fluent aphasia called Wernicke aphasia. In most people, the damage occurs in the left temporal lobe, although it can result from damage to the right lobe as well. People with Wernicke aphasia may speak in long sentences that have no meaning, add unnecessary words, and even create made-up words. For example, someone with Wernicke aphasia may say, "You know that smoodle pinkered and that I want to get him round and take care of him like you want before." As a result, it is often difficult to follow what the person is trying to say. People with Wernicke aphasia usually have great difficulty understanding speech, and they are often unaware of their mistakes. These individuals usually have no body weakness because their brain injury is not near the parts of the brain that control movement.

A type of nonfluent aphasia is Broca aphasia. People with Broca aphasia have damage to the frontal lobe of the brain. They frequently speak in short phrases that make sense but are produced with great effort. They often omit small words such as "is," "and," and "the." For example, a person with Broca aphasia may say, "Walk dog," meaning, "I will take the dog for a walk," or "book book two table," for "There are two books on the table." People with Broca aphasia typically understand the speech of others fairly well. Because of this, they are often aware of their difficulties and can become easily frustrated. People with Broca aphasia often have right-sided weakness or paralysis of the arm and leg because the frontal lobe is also important for motor movements.

Another type of nonfluent aphasia, global aphasia, results from damage to extensive portions of the language areas of the brain. Individuals with global aphasia have severe communication difficulties and may be extremely limited in their ability to speak or comprehend language.

There are other types of aphasia, each of which results from damage to different language areas in the brain. Some people may have difficulty repeating words and sentences even though they can speak and they understand the meaning of the word or sentence. Others may have difficulty naming objects even though they know what the object is and what it may be used for.

How is aphasia diagnosed?

Aphasia is usually first recognized by the physician who treats the person for his or her brain injury. Frequently this is a neurologist. The physician typically performs tests that require the person to follow commands, answer questions, name objects, and carry on a conversation. If the physician suspects aphasia, the patient is often referred to a speech-language pathologist, who performs a comprehensive examination of the person's communication abilities. The examination includes the person's ability to speak, express ideas, converse socially, understand language, read, and write, as well as the ability to swallow and to use alternative and augmentative communication.

How is aphasia treated?

In some cases, a person will completely recover from aphasia without treatment. This type of spontaneous recovery usually occurs following a type of stroke in which blood flow to the brain is temporarily interrupted but quickly restored, called a transient ischemic attack. In these circumstances, language abilities may return in a few hours or a few days.

For most cases, however, language recovery is not as quick or as complete. While many people with aphasia experience partial spontaneous recovery, in which some language abilities return a few days to a month after the brain injury, some amount of aphasia typically remains. In these instances, speech-language therapy is often helpful. Recovery usually continues over a two-year period. Many health professionals believe that the most effective treatment begins early in the recovery process. Some of the factors that influence the amount of improvement include the cause of the brain damage, the area of the brain that was damaged, the extent of the brain injury, and the age and health of the individual. Additional factors include motivation, handedness, and educational level.

Aphasia therapy aims to improve a person's ability to communicate by helping him or her to use remaining language abilities, restore language abilities as much as possible, compensate for language problems, and learn other methods of communicating. Individual therapy focuses on the specific needs of the person, while group therapy offers the opportunity to use new communication skills in a small-group setting. Stroke clubs, regional support groups formed by people who have had a stroke, are available in most major cities. These clubs also offer the opportunity for people with aphasia to try new communication skills. In addition, stroke clubs can help a person and his or her family adjust to the life changes that accompany stroke and aphasia.

Family involvement is often a crucial component of aphasia treatment so that family members can learn the best way to communicate with their loved one.

Family members are encouraged to do the following:

- Simplify language by using short, uncomplicated sentences.

- Repeat the content words or write down key words to clarify meaning as needed.

- Maintain a natural conversational manner appropriate for an adult.

- Minimize distractions, such as a loud radio or TV, whenever possible.

- Include the person with aphasia in conversations.

- Ask for and value the opinion of the person with aphasia, especially regarding family matters.

- Encourage any type of communication, whether it is speech, gesture, pointing, or drawing.

- Avoid correcting the person's speech.

- Allow the person plenty of time to talk.

- Help the person become involved outside the home. Seek out support groups such as stroke clubs.

Other treatment approaches involve the use of computers to improve the language abilities of people with aphasia. Studies have shown that computer-assisted therapy can help people with aphasia retrieve certain parts of speech, such as the use of verbs. Computers can also provide an alternative system of communication for people with difficulty expressing language.

Chapter 15

Attention Deficit Hyperactivity Disorder

Chapter Contents

Section 15.1

ADHD in Children

Lisa's son Jack had always been a handful. Even as a preschooler, he would tear through the house like a tornado, shouting, roughhousing, and climbing the furniture. No toy or activity ever held his interest for more than a few minutes and he would often dart off without warning, seemingly unaware of the dangers of a busy street or a crowded mall.

It was exhausting to parent Jack, but Lisa hadn't been too concerned back then. Boys will be boys, she figured. But at age eight, he was no easier to handle. It was a struggle to get Jack to settle down long enough to complete even the simplest tasks, from chores to homework. When his teacher's comments about his inattention and disruptive behavior in class became too frequent to ignore, Lisa took Jack to the doctor, who recommended an evaluation for attention deficit hyperactivity disorder (ADHD).

ADHD is a common behavioral disorder that affects an estimated 8 to 10 percent of school-age children. Boys are about three times more likely than girls to be diagnosed with it, though it's not yet understood why.

Kids with ADHD act without thinking, are hyperactive, and have trouble focusing. They may understand what's expected of them but have trouble following through because they can't sit still, pay attention, or attend to details.

Of course, all kids (especially younger ones) act this way at times, particularly when they're anxious or excited. But the difference with ADHD is that symptoms are present over a longer period of time and occur in different settings. They impair a child's ability to function socially, academically, and at home.

The good news is that with proper treatment, kids with ADHD can learn to successfully live with and manage their symptoms.

Symptoms

ADHD used to be known as attention deficit disorder, or ADD. In 1994, it was renamed ADHD and broken down into three subtypes, each with its own pattern of behaviors:

1. An inattentive type, with signs that include:

    - inability to pay attention to details or a tendency to make careless errors in schoolwork or other activities;

    - difficulty with sustained attention in tasks or play activities;

    - apparent listening problems;

    - difficulty following instructions;

    - problems with organization;

    - avoidance or dislike of tasks that require mental effort;

    - tendency to lose things like toys, notebooks, or homework;

    - distractibility;

    - forgetfulness in daily activities.

2. A hyperactive-impulsive type, with signs that include:

    - fidgeting or squirming;

    - difficulty remaining seated;

    - excessive running or climbing;

    - difficulty playing quietly;

    - always seeming to be "on the go";

    - excessive talking;

    - blurting out answers before hearing the full question;

    - difficulty waiting for a turn or in line;

    - problems with interrupting or intruding.

3. A combined type, which involves a combination of the other two types and is the most common.

Although it can be challenging to raise kids with ADHD, it's important to remember they aren't "bad," "acting out," or being difficult on purpose. And they have difficulty controlling their behavior without medication or behavioral therapy.

Diagnosis

Because there's no test that can determine the presence of ADHD, a diagnosis depends on a complete evaluation. Many children and adolescents diagnosed with ADHD are evaluated and treated by primary care doctors, including pediatricians and family practitioners, but your child may also be referred to one of several different specialists (psychiatrists, psychologists, neurologists), especially when the diagnosis is in doubt, or if there are other concerns, such as Tourette syndrome, a learning disability, anxiety, or depression.

To be considered for a diagnosis of ADHD:

- a child must display behaviors from one of the three subtypes before age seven;

- these behaviors must be more severe than in other kids the same age;

- the behaviors must last for at least six months;

- the behaviors must occur in and negatively affect at least two areas of a child's life (such as school, home, daycare settings, or friendships).

The behaviors must also not only be linked to stress at home. Kids who have experienced a divorce, a move, an illness, a change in school, or other significant life event may suddenly begin to act out or become forgetful. To avoid a misdiagnosis, it's important to consider whether these factors played a role in the onset of symptoms.

First, your child's doctor may perform a physical examination and take a medical history that includes questions about any concerns and symptoms, your child's past health, your family's health, any medications your child is taking, any allergies your child may have, and other issues.

The doctor may also check hearing and vision so other medical conditions can be ruled out. Because some emotional conditions, such as extreme stress, depression, and anxiety, can also look like ADHD, you'll likely be asked to fill out questionnaires to help rule them out.

You'll be asked many questions about your child's development and behaviors at home, school, and among friends. Other adults who see your child regularly (like teachers, who are often the first to notice ADHD symptoms) probably will be consulted, too. An educational evaluation, which usually includes a school psychologist, may also be done. It's important for everyone involved to be as honest and thorough as possible about your child's strengths and weaknesses.

Causes of ADHD

ADHD is not caused by poor parenting, too much sugar, or vaccines.

ADHD has biological origins that aren't yet clearly understood. No single cause has been identified, but researchers are exploring a number of possible genetic and environmental links. Studies have shown that many kids with ADHD have a close relative who also has the disorder.

Although experts are unsure whether this is a cause of the disorder, they have found that certain areas of the brain are about 5 to 10 percent smaller in size and activity in kids with ADHD. Chemical changes in the brain also have been found.

Research also links smoking during pregnancy to later ADHD in a child. Other risk factors may include premature delivery, very low birth weight, and injuries to the brain at birth.

Some studies have even suggested a link between excessive early television watching and future attention problems. Parents should follow the American Academy of Pediatrics' (AAP) guidelines, which say that children under two years old should not have any "screen time" (TV, DVDs or videotapes, computers, or video games) and that kids two years and older should be limited to one to two hours per day, or less, of quality television programming.

Related Problems

One of the difficulties in diagnosing ADHD is that it's often found in conjunction with other problems. These are called coexisting conditions, and about two-thirds of kids with ADHD have one. The most common coexisting conditions are:

- **Oppositional defiant disorder (ODD) and conduct disorder (CD):** At least 35 percent of kids with ADHD also have oppositional defiant disorder, which is characterized by stubbornness, outbursts of temper, and acts of defiance and rule breaking. Conduct disorder is similar but features more severe hostility and aggression. Kids who have conduct disorder are more likely to get in trouble with authority figures and, later, possibly with the law. Oppositional defiant disorder and conduct disorder are seen most commonly with the hyperactive and combined subtypes of ADHD.

- **Mood disorders:** About 18 percent of kids with ADHD, particularly the inattentive subtype, also experience depression. They may feel inadequate, isolated, frustrated by school failures and social problems, and have low self-esteem.

• **Anxiety disorders:** Anxiety disorders affect about 25 percent of kids with ADHD. Symptoms include excessive worry, fear, or panic, which can also lead to physical symptoms such as a racing heart, sweating, stomach pains, and diarrhea. Other forms of anxiety that can accompany ADHD are obsessive-compulsive disorder and Tourette syndrome, as well as motor or vocal tics (movements or sounds that are repeated over and over). A child who has symptoms of these other conditions should be evaluated by a specialist.

• **Learning disabilities:** About half of all kids with ADHD also have a specific learning disability. The most common learning problems are with reading (dyslexia) and handwriting. Although ADHD isn't categorized as a learning disability, its interference with concentration and attention can make it even more difficult for a child to perform well in school.

If your child has ADHD and a coexisting condition, the doctor will carefully consider that when developing a treatment plan. Some treatments are better than others at addressing specific combinations of symptoms.

Treating ADHD

ADHD can't be cured, but it can be successfully managed. Your child's doctor will work with you to develop an individualized, long-term plan. The goal is to help a child learn to control his or her own behavior and to help families create an atmosphere in which this is most likely to happen.

In most cases, ADHD is best treated with a combination of medication and behavior therapy. Any good treatment plan will require close follow-up and monitoring, and your doctor may make adjustments along the way. Because it's important for parents to actively participate in their child's treatment plan, parent education is also considered an important part of ADHD management.

Medications

Several different types of medications may be used to treat ADHD:

• Stimulants are the best-known treatments—they've been used for more than fifty years in the treatment of ADHD. Some require several doses per day, each lasting about four hours; some last up to twelve hours. Possible side effects include decreased appetite, stomachache, irritability, and insomnia. There's currently no evidence of long-term side effects.

- Nonstimulants represent a good alternative to stimulants or are sometimes used along with a stimulant to treat ADHD. The first nonstimulant was approved for treating ADHD in 2003. They may have fewer side effects than stimulants and can last up to twenty-four hours.

- Antidepressants are sometimes a treatment option; however, in 2004 the U.S. Food and Drug Administration (FDA) issued a warning that these drugs may lead to a rare increased risk of suicide in children and teens. If an antidepressant is recommended for your child, be sure to discuss these risks with your doctor.

Medications can affect kids differently, and a child may respond well to one but not another. When determining the correct treatment, the doctor might try various medications in various doses, especially if your child is being treated for ADHD along with another disorder.

Behavioral Therapy

Research has shown that medications used to help curb impulsive behavior and attention difficulties are more effective when combined with behavioral therapy.

Behavioral therapy attempts to change behavior patterns by:

- reorganizing a child's home and school environment;

- giving clear directions and commands;

- setting up a system of consistent rewards for appropriate behaviors and negative consequences for inappropriate ones.

Here are examples of behavioral strategies that may help a child with ADHD:

- Create a routine. Try to follow the same schedule every day, from wake-up time to bedtime. Post the schedule in a prominent place, so your child can see what's expected throughout the day and when it's time for homework, play, and chores.

- Get organized. Put schoolbags, clothing, and toys in the same place every day so your child will be less likely to lose them.

- Avoid distractions. Turn off the TV, radio, and computer games, especially when your child is doing homework.

- Limit choices. Offer a choice between two things (this outfit, meal, toy, etc., or that one) so that your child isn't overwhelmed and overstimulated.

- Change your interactions with your child. Instead of long-winded explanations and cajoling, use clear, brief directions to remind your child of responsibilities.

- Use goals and rewards. Use a chart to list goals and track positive behaviors, then reward your child's efforts. Be sure the goals are realistic (think baby steps rather than overnight success).

- Discipline effectively. Instead of yelling or spanking, use time-outs or removal of privileges as consequences for inappropriate behavior. Younger kids may simply need to be distracted or ignored until they display better behavior.

- Help your child discover a talent. All kids need to experience success to feel good about themselves. Finding out what your child does well—whether it's sports, art, or music—can boost social skills and self-esteem.

Alternative Treatments

Currently, the only ADHD therapies that have been proven effective in scientific studies are medications and behavioral therapy. But your doctor may recommend additional treatments and interventions depending on your child's symptoms and needs. Some kids with ADHD, for example, may also need special educational interventions such as tutoring, occupational therapy, etc. Every child's needs are different.

A number of other alternative therapies are promoted and tried by parents, including: megavitamins, body treatments, diet manipulation, allergy treatment, chiropractic treatment, attention training, visual training, and traditional one-on-one "talking" psychotherapy. However, scientific research has not found them to be effective, and most have not been studied carefully, if at all.

Parents should always be wary of any therapy that promises an ADHD "cure." If you're interested in trying something new, speak with your doctor first.

Parent Training

Parenting a child with ADHD often brings special challenges. Kids with ADHD may not respond well to typical parenting practices. Also, because ADHD tends to run in families, parents may also have some problems with organization and consistency themselves and need active coaching to help learn these skills.

Experts recommend parent education and support groups to help family members accept the diagnosis and to teach them how to help kids organize their environment, develop problem-solving skills, and cope with frustrations. Training can also teach parents to respond appropriately to a child's most trying behaviors with calm disciplining techniques. Individual or family counseling can also be helpful.

ADHD in the Classroom

As your child's most important advocate, you should become familiar with your child's medical, legal, and educational rights.

Kids with ADHD are eligible for special services or accommodations at school under the Individuals with Disabilities in Education Act (IDEA) and an anti-discrimination law known as Section 504. Keep in touch with teachers and school officials to monitor your child's progress.

In addition to using routines and a clear system of rewards, here are some other tips to share with teachers for classroom success:

- Reduce seating distractions. Lessening distractions might be as simple as seating your child near the teacher instead of near the window.

- Use a homework folder for parent-teacher communications. The teacher can include assignments and progress notes, and you can check to make sure all work is completed on time.

- Break down assignments. Keep instructions clear and brief, breaking down larger tasks into smaller, more manageable pieces.

- Give positive reinforcement. Always be on the lookout for positive behaviors. Ask the teacher to offer praise when your child stays seated, doesn't call out, or waits his or her turn instead of criticizing when he or she doesn't.

- Teach good study skills. Underlining, note taking, and reading out loud can help your child stay focused and retain information.

- Supervise. Check that your child goes and comes from school with the correct books and materials. Sometimes kids are paired with a buddy to can help them stay on track.

- Be sensitive to self-esteem issues. Ask the teacher to provide feedback to your child in private, and avoid asking your child to perform a task in public that might be too difficult.

- Involve the school counselor or psychologist. He or she can help design behavioral programs to address specific problems in the classroom.

Helping Your Child

You're a stronger advocate for your child when you foster good partnerships with everyone involved in your child's treatment—that includes teachers, doctors, therapists, and even other family members. Take advantage of all the support and education that's available, and you'll help your child navigate toward success.

Section 15.2

ADHD in Adults

"Can Adults Have ADHD?" National
Institute of Mental Health, January 23, 2009.

Some children with attention deficit hyperactivity disorder (ADHD) continue to have it as adults. And many adults who have the disorder don't know it. They may feel that it is impossible to get organized, stick to a job, or remember and keep appointments. Daily tasks such as getting up in the morning, preparing to leave the house for work, arriving at work on time, and being productive on the job can be especially challenging for adults with ADHD.

These adults may have a history of failure at school, problems at work, or difficult or failed relationships. Many have had multiple traffic accidents. Like teens, adults with ADHD may seem restless and may try to do several things at once, most of them unsuccessfully. They also tend to prefer "quick fixes," rather than taking the steps needed to achieve greater rewards.

How is ADHD diagnosed in adults?

Like children, adults who suspect they have ADHD should be evaluated by a licensed mental health professional. But the professional may need to consider a wider range of symptoms when assessing adults for ADHD because their symptoms tend to be more varied and possibly not as clear cut as symptoms seen in children.

To be diagnosed with the condition, an adult must have ADHD symptoms that began in childhood and continued throughout adulthood. Health professionals use certain rating scales to determine if an adult meets the diagnostic criteria for ADHD. The mental health professional also will look at the person's history of childhood behavior and school experiences, and will interview spouses or partners, parents, close friends, and other associates. The person will also undergo a physical exam and various psychological tests.

For some adults, a diagnosis of ADHD can bring a sense of relief. Adults who have had the disorder since childhood, but who have not been diagnosed, may have developed negative feelings about themselves over the years. Receiving a diagnosis allows them to understand the reasons for their problems, and treatment will allow them to deal with their problems more effectively.

How is ADHD treated in adults?

Much like children with the disorder, adults with ADHD are treated with medication, psychotherapy, or a combination of treatments.

Medications: ADHD medications, including extended-release forms, often are prescribed for adults with ADHD, but not all of these medications are approved for adults. However, those not approved for adults still may be prescribed by a doctor on an "off-label" basis.

Although not approved by the U.S. Food and Drug Association (FDA) specifically for the treatment of ADHD, antidepressants are sometimes used to treat adults with ADHD. Older antidepressants, called tricyclics, sometimes are used because they, like stimulants, affect the brain chemicals norepinephrine and dopamine. A newer antidepressant, venlafaxine (Effexor), also may be prescribed for its effect on the brain chemical norepinephrine. And in recent clinical trials, the antidepressant bupropion (Wellbutrin), which affects the brain chemical dopamine, showed benefits for adults with ADHD.

Adult prescriptions for stimulants and other medications require special considerations. For example, adults often require other medications for physical problems, such as diabetes or high blood pressure, or for anxiety and depression. Some of these medications may interact badly with stimulants. An adult with ADHD should discuss potential medication options with his or her doctor. These and other issues must be taken into account when a medication is prescribed.

Education and psychotherapy: A professional counselor or therapist can help an adult with ADHD learn how to organize his or her life with tools such as a large calendar or date book, lists, reminder notes, and by assigning a special place for keys, bills, and paperwork. Large tasks can be broken down into more manageable, smaller steps so that completing each part of the task provides a sense of accomplishment.

Psychotherapy, including cognitive behavioral therapy, also can help change one's poor self-image by examining the experiences that produced it. The therapist encourages the adult with ADHD to adjust to the life changes that come with treatment, such as thinking before acting, or resisting the urge to take unnecessary risks.

Chapter 16

Cerebral Palsy

What is CP?

Cerebral palsy—also known as CP—is a condition caused by injury to the parts of the brain that control our ability to use our muscles and bodies. Cerebral means having to do with the brain. Palsy means weakness or problems with using the muscles. Often the injury happens before birth, sometimes during delivery, or soon after being born.

CP can be mild, moderate, or severe. Mild CP may mean a child is clumsy. Moderate CP may mean the child walks with a limp. He or she may need a special leg brace or a cane. More severe CP can affect all parts of a child's physical abilities. A child with moderate or severe CP may have to use a wheelchair and other special equipment.

Sometimes children with CP can also have learning problems, problems with hearing or seeing (called sensory problems), or intellectual disabilities. Usually, the greater the injury to the brain, the more severe the CP. However, CP doesn't get worse over time, and most children with CP have a normal life span.

What are the signs of CP?

There are four main types of CP:

- Spastic CP is where there is too much muscle tone or tightness. Movements are stiff, especially in the legs, arms, and/or back.

Excerpted from "Cerebral Palsy," National Dissemination Center for Children with Disabilities, June 2010.

Children with this form of CP move their legs awkwardly, turning in or scissoring their legs as they try to walk. This form of CP occurs in 50 to 75 percent of all cases.

- Athetoid CP (also called dyskinetic CP) can affect movements of the entire body. Typically, this form of CP involves slow, uncontrolled body movements and low muscle tone that makes it hard for the person to sit straight and walk. This form occurs in 10 to 20 percent of all cases.

- Ataxic CP involves poor coordination, balance, and depth perception and occurs in approximately 5 to 10 percent of all cases.

- Mixed CP is a combination of the symptoms listed above. A child with mixed CP has both high- and low-tone muscle. Some muscles are too tight, and others are too loose, creating a mix of stiffness and involuntary movements. (United Cerebral Palsy 2001)

Is there help available?

Yes, there's a lot of help available, beginning with the free evaluation of the child. The nation's special education law, the Individuals with Disabilities Education Act (IDEA), requires that all children suspected of having a disability be evaluated without cost to their parents to determine if they do have a disability and, because of the disability, need special services under IDEA. Those special services are:

- **Early intervention:** A system of services to support infants and toddlers with disabilities (before their third birthday) and their families.

- **Special education and related services:** Services available through the public school system for school-aged children, including preschoolers (ages three to twenty-one).

Under IDEA, children with CP are usually found eligible for services under the category of "orthopedic impairment." IDEA's definition of orthopedic impairment reads as follows:

> . . . a severe orthopedic impairment that adversely affects a child's educational performance. The term includes impairments caused by a congenital anomaly, impairments caused by disease (e.g., poliomyelitis, bone tuberculosis), and impairments from other causes (e.g., cerebral palsy, amputations, and fractures or burns that cause contractures). [34 CFR §300.8(c)(9)]

What about Treatment?

With early and ongoing treatment the effects of CP can be reduced. Many children learn how to get their bodies to work for them in other ways. For example, one infant whose CP keeps him from crawling may be able to get around by rolling from place to place.

Typically, children with CP may need different kinds of therapy, including:

- Physical therapy (PT), which helps the child develop stronger muscles such as those in the legs and trunk. Through PT, the child works on skills such as walking, sitting, and keeping his or her balance.

- Occupational therapy (OT), which helps the child develop fine motor skills such as dressing, feeding, writing, and other daily living tasks.

- Speech-language pathology (S/L), which helps the child develop his or her communication skills. The child may work in particular on speaking, which may be difficult due to problems with muscle tone of the tongue and throat.

All of these are available as related services in both early intervention programs (for very young children) and special education (for school-aged children).

Children with CP may also find a variety of special equipment helpful. For example, braces (also called ankle-foot orthoses, or AFOs) may be used to hold the foot in place when the child stands or walks. Custom splints can provide support to help a child use his or her hands. A variety of therapy equipment and adapted toys are available to help children play and have fun while they are working their bodies. Activities such as swimming or horseback riding can help strengthen weaker muscles and relax the tighter ones.

What about school?

A child with CP can face many challenges in school and is likely to need individualized help. Fortunately, states are responsible for meeting the educational needs of children with disabilities.

As we've said, for children up to the third birthday, services are provided through an early intervention system. Staff work with the child's family to develop what is known as an Individualized Family Services Plan, or IFSP. The IFSP will describe the child's unique needs as well as the services the child will receive to address those needs. The IFSP will also emphasize the unique needs of the family, so that parents and other family members will know how to help their young child with CP. Early intervention services may be provided on a sliding-fee basis, meaning that the costs to the family will depend upon their income.

For school-aged children, including preschoolers, special education and related services will be provided through the school system. School staff will work with the child's parents to develop an Individualized Education Program, or IEP. The IEP is similar to an IFSP in that it describes the child's unique needs and the services that have been designed to meet those needs. Special education and related services, which can include PT, OT, and speech-language pathology, are provided at no cost to parents.

In addition to therapy services and special equipment, children with CP may need what is known as assistive technology. Examples of assistive technology include:

- Communication devices, which can range from the simple to the sophisticated. Communication boards, for example, have pictures, symbols, letters, or words attached. The child communicates by pointing to or gazing at the pictures or symbols. Augmentative communication devices are more sophisticated and include voice synthesizers that enable the child to "talk" with others.

- Computer technology, which can range from electronic toys with special switches to sophisticated computer programs operated by simple switch pads or keyboard adaptations.

The ability of the brain to find new ways of working after an injury is remarkable. Even so, it can be difficult for parents to imagine what their child's future will be like. Good therapy and handling can help, but the most important "treatment" the child can receive is love and encouragement, with lots of typical childhood experiences, family, and friends. With the right mix of support, equipment, extra time, and accommodations, all children with CP can be successful learners and full participants in life.

What can parents do?

- Learn about CP. The more you know, the more you can help yourself and your child.

- Love and play with your child. Treat your son or daughter as you would a child without disabilities. Take your child places, read together, have fun.

- Learn from professionals and other parents how to meet your child's special needs, but try not to turn your lives into one round of therapy after another.

- Ask for help from family and friends. Caring for a child with CP is hard work. Teach others what to do and give them plenty of opportunities to practice while you take a break.

- Keep informed about new treatments and technologies that may help. New approaches are constantly being worked on and can make a huge difference to the quality of your child's life. However, be careful about unproven new "fads."

- Learn about assistive technology that can help your child. This may include a simple communication board to help your child express needs and desires, or may be as sophisticated as a computer with special software.

- Be patient, keep up your hope for improvement. Your child, like every child, has a whole lifetime to learn and grow.

- Work with professionals in early intervention or in your school to develop an IFSP or an IEP that reflects your child's needs and abilities. Be sure to include related services such as speech-language pathology, physical therapy, and occupational therapy if your child needs these. Don't forget about assistive technology either!

What can teachers do?

- Learn more about CP.

- This may seem obvious, but sometimes the "look" of CP can give the mistaken impression that a child who has CP cannot learn as much as others. Focus on the individual child and learn firsthand what needs and capabilities he or she has.

- Tap into the strategies that teachers of students with learning disabilities use for their students. Become knowledgeable about different learning styles. Then you can use the approach best suited for a particular child, based upon that child's learning abilities as well as physical abilities.

- Be inventive. Ask yourself (and others), "How can I adapt this lesson for this child to maximize active, hands-on learning?"

- Learn to love assistive technology. Find experts within and outside your school to help you. Assistive technology can mean the difference between independence for your student or not.

- Always remember, parents are experts, too. Talk candidly with your student's parents. They can tell you a great deal about their daughter or son's special needs and abilities.

- Effective teamwork for the child with CP needs to bring together professionals with diverse backgrounds and expertise. The team must combine the knowledge of its members to plan, implement, and coordinate the child's services.

Chapter 17

Chromosomal Disorders

Chapter Contents

Section 17.1

47,XYY Syndrome

Excerpted from Genetics Home Reference, July 25, 2011.

What is 47,XYY syndrome?

47,XYY syndrome is characterized by an extra copy of the Y chromosome in each of a male's cells. Although males with this condition may be taller than average, this chromosomal change typically causes no unusual physical features. Most males with 47,XYY syndrome have normal sexual development and are able to father children.

47,XYY syndrome is associated with an increased risk of learning disabilities and delayed development of speech and language skills. Delayed development of motor skills (such as sitting and walking), weak muscle tone (hypotonia), hand tremors or other involuntary movements (motor tics), and behavioral and emotional difficulties are also possible. These characteristics vary widely among affected boys and men.

A small percentage of males with 47,XYY syndrome are diagnosed with autistic spectrum disorders, which are developmental conditions that affect communication and social interaction.

How common is 47,XYY syndrome?

This condition occurs in about one in one thousand newborn boys. Five to ten boys with 47,XYY syndrome are born in the United States each day.

What are the genetic changes related to 47,XYY syndrome?

People normally have forty-six chromosomes in each cell. Two of the forty-six chromosomes, known as X and Y, are called sex chromosomes because they help determine whether a person will develop male or female sex characteristics. Females typically have two X chromosomes (46,XX), and males have one X chromosome and one Y chromosome (46,XY).

47,XYY syndrome is caused by the presence of an extra copy of the Y chromosome in each of a male's cells. As a result of the extra Y chromosome, each cell has a total of forty-seven chromosomes instead of the usual forty-six. It is unclear why an extra copy of the Y chromosome is associated with tall stature, learning problems, and other features in some boys and men.

Some males with 47,XYY syndrome have an extra Y chromosome in only some of their cells. This phenomenon is called 46,XY/47,XYY mosaicism.

Can 47,XYY syndrome be inherited?

Most cases of 47,XYY syndrome are not inherited. The chromosomal change usually occurs as a random event during the formation of sperm cells. An error in cell division called nondisjunction can result in sperm cells with an extra copy of the Y chromosome. If one of these atypical reproductive cells contributes to the genetic makeup of a child, the child will have an extra Y chromosome in each of the body's cells.

46,XY/47,XYY mosaicism is also not inherited. It occurs as a random event during cell division in early embryonic development. As a result, some of an affected person's cells have one X chromosome and one Y chromosome (46,XY), and other cells have one X chromosome and two Y chromosomes (47,XYY).

What other names do people use for 47,XYY syndrome?

- Jacob syndrome
- XYY karyotype
- XYY syndrome
- YY syndrome

Section 17.2

Down Syndrome

Excerpted from "Down Syndrome," National Dissemination
Center for Children with Disabilities, June 2010.

Down syndrome is the most common and readily identifiable chromosomal condition associated with intellectual disabilities. It is caused by a chromosomal abnormality: for some unknown reason, an accident in cell development results in forty-seven instead of the usual forty-six chromosomes. This extra chromosome changes the orderly development of the body and brain. In most cases, the diagnosis of Down syndrome is made according to results from a chromosome test administered shortly after birth.

Just as in the normal population, there is a wide variation in mental abilities, behavior, and developmental progress in individuals with Down syndrome. Their level of intellectual disability may range from mild to severe, with the majority functioning in the mild to moderate range.

Because children with Down syndrome differ in ability, it's important that families and members of the intervention team place few limitations on potential capabilities and possible achievements. Each child with Down syndrome has his or her own talents and unique capacities, and it's important to recognize these and reinforce them.

Incidence of Down Syndrome

Nearly five thousand babies are born with Down syndrome in the United States each year. This means that 1 in every 733 babies is born with this condition. Although parents of any age may have a child with Down syndrome, 80 percent are born to women under the age of thirty-five.

Down syndrome is not a disease, nor is it contagious. Its most common forms usually do not occur more than once in a family.

Characteristics of Down Syndrome

There are over fifty clinical signs of Down syndrome, but it is rare to find all or even most of them in one person. Every child with Down syndrome is different. Some common characteristics include the following:

- Poor muscle tone

- Slanting eyes with folds of skin at the inner corners (called epicanthal folds)

- Hyperflexibility (excessive ability to extend the joints)

- Short, broad hands with a single crease across the palm on one or both hands

- Broad feet with short toes

- Flat bridge of the nose

- Short, low-set ears

- Short neck and small head

- Small oral cavity

- Short, high-pitched cries in infancy

Individuals with Down syndrome are usually smaller than their nondisabled peers, and their physical as well as intellectual development is slower.

Help for Babies and Toddlers

When a baby is born with Down syndrome, his or her parents should know that there's a lot of help available—and immediately. Shortly after the diagnosis of Down syndrome is confirmed, parents will want to get in touch with the early intervention system in their community.

Early intervention is a system of services designed to help infants and toddlers with disabilities (before their third birthday) and their families. It's mandated by federal law—the Individuals with Disabilities Education Act (IDEA), the nation's special education law. Staff work with the child's family to develop what is known as an Individualized Family Services Plan, or IFSP. The IFSP will describe the child's unique needs as well as the services he or she will receive to address those needs. The IFSP will also emphasize the unique needs of the family, so that parents and other family members will know how to help their young child with Down syndrome. Early intervention services may be provided on a sliding-fee basis, meaning that the costs to the family will depend upon their income.

Help for School-Aged Children

Just as IDEA requires that early intervention be made available to babies and toddlers with disabilities, it requires that special education and related services be made available free of charge to every eligible child with a disability, including preschoolers (ages three to twenty-one). These services are specially designed to address the child's individual needs associated with the disability—in this case, Down syndrome.

There is a lot to know about the special education process. To begin, however, and access special education services for a school-aged child in your area, get in touch with your local public school system. Calling the elementary school in your neighborhood is an excellent place to start.

Health Considerations

Besides having a distinct physical appearance, children with Down syndrome frequently have specific health-related problems. A lowered resistance to infection makes these children more prone to respiratory problems. Visual problems such as crossed eyes and far- or nearsightedness are common in individuals with Down syndrome, as are mild to moderate hearing loss and speech difficulty. Approximately one-third of babies born with Down syndrome have heart defects, most of which are now successfully correctable. Some individuals are born with gastrointestinal tract problems that can be surgically corrected.

Some people with Down syndrome also may have a condition known as atlantoaxial instability, a misalignment of the top two vertebrae of the neck. This condition makes these individuals more prone to injury if they participate in activities that overextend or flex the neck. Parents are urged to have their child examined by a physician to determine whether or not their child should be restricted from sports and activities that place stress on the neck. Although this misalignment is a potentially serious condition, proper diagnosis can help prevent serious injury.

Children with Down syndrome may have a tendency to become obese as they grow older. Besides having negative social implications, this weight gain threatens these individuals' health and longevity. A supervised diet and exercise program may help reduce this problem.

Educating Children with Down Syndrome

When a child with Down syndrome reaches school age (after the third birthday), the public school system becomes responsible for educating the child and for addressing the child's unique needs related to his or her disability. Parents and school personnel will work together to develop what is known as an Individualized Education Program (IEP) for the child. The IEP is similar to an IFSP in that it describes the child's unique needs and the services that will be provided to meet those needs. The IEP will include annual goals for learning and much more.

Much information is available for teachers to learn more about effective teaching practices for children with Down syndrome. It's important for teachers to take into consideration the degree of intellectual disability involved, the child's talents and interests, and the supports and services he or she needs, as specified in the IEP. Generally speaking, teachers will find it more effective to emphasize concrete concepts with a student who has Down syndrome, instead of abstract ideas. Teaching skills in a step-by-step fashion with frequent reinforcement and consistent feedback has proven successful. Other suggestions for teachers are given at the end of this section.

Today, the majority of children with Down syndrome are educated in the regular classroom, alongside their peers without disabilities. This is in keeping with the inclusion movement of the last decade and the requirements of IDEA, which states that each school system must ensure that:

Special classes, separate schooling, or other removal of children with disabilities from the regular educational environment occurs only if the nature or severity of the disability is such that education in regular classes with the use of supplementary aids and services cannot be achieved satisfactorily.

Equally clear is this requirement of IDEA:

A child with a disability [may not be] removed from education in age-appropriate regular classrooms solely because of needed modifications in the general education curriculum.

For High School Students with Down Syndrome

While the student is still in secondary school, parents, the IEP team, and the student himself (or herself!) will need to plan for the future and the student's life as an adult. This involves considering, for example, issues such as employment (with or without supports), independent living and self-care skills, the possibility of higher education or vocational training, and how to connect with adult service systems. Under IDEA, the process of planning for transition to adulthood should begin no later than the student's sixteenth birthday. For adolescents with Down syndrome, it's usually important to begin earlier than that.

Adult life for individuals with Down syndrome has changed noticeably from just two decades ago. Opportunities to live and work independently in the community have greatly expanded for those with Down syndrome. This owes much to the more inclusive and comprehensive education IDEA promotes and to improved public attitudes towards disability. Today, there's a nationwide network of independent living centers, as well as apartments that are group-shared and supervised for those who need this level of support. Training, education, and assistance are also available to eligible adults with Down syndrome through service systems such as Vocational Rehabilitation and Social Security. Adult life holds many opportunities for those with Down syndrome, so it's important to plan ahead with optimism and vigor.

Tips for Parents

- Learn about Down syndrome. The more you know, the more you can help yourself and your child.

- Love and play with your child. Treat your son or daughter as you would a child without disabilities. Take your child places, read together, have fun.

- Encourage your child to be independent. For example, help your son or daughter learn self-care skills such as getting dressed, grooming, and doing laundry.

- Give your child chores. Keep in mind his or her age, mental capacity, attention span, and abilities. Divide tasks into small steps. Explain what your child is supposed to do, step by step, until the chore is done. Demonstrate. Offer help when it's needed and praise when things go well.

- Work with the professionals who are working with your child. Participate in team meetings where your child's education or program is being planned, share your unique knowledge of who your son or daughter is, advocate that the program address your child's needs.

- Find out what your child is learning at school. Look for ways to apply it at home. For example, if the teacher is reviewing concepts of money, take your child to the supermarket with you to help keep track of what money you're spending.

- Look for social opportunities in the community (such as Scouts) or activities offered through the department of sports and leisure. Joining in and taking part will help your child develop social skills and have fun.

- Talk with other parents whose children have Down syndrome. They can be a fountain of practical advice and emotional support.

- Be patient, be hopeful. Your child, like every child, has a whole lifetime to learn and grow.

- Take pleasure in your beautiful one. He—she—is a treasure. Learn from your child, too. Those with Down syndrome have a special light within—let it shine.

Tips for Teachers

- Learn as much as possible about Down syndrome.

- This may seem obvious, but sometimes the appearance of Down syndrome can give the mistaken impression that the child cannot learn. Focus on the individual child and learn firsthand what needs and capabilities he or she has.

- Realize that you can make a big difference in this student's life! Use the student's abilities and interests to involve and motivate. Give lots of opportunities for the student to be successful.

- Talk candidly with your student's parents. They're experts and can tell you a great deal about their daughter's or son's special needs and abilities.

- Work with the student's parents and other school personnel to develop and implement a special educational plan (IEP) that addresses the individual needs of the student. Share information on a regular basis with parents about how things are going for the student at home and in school.

- If you're not part of the student's IEP team, ask for a copy of this important document. The student's educational goals will be listed there, as will the services and accommodations that he or she is supposed to receive, including in your class.

- Talk to specialists in your school (for example, special educators), as necessary. They can help you identify methods that are effective for teaching a student with disabilities, ways to adapt the curriculum, and how to address the student's IEP goals in the classroom.

- Be as concrete as possible with the student. Demonstrate what you want to see happen instead of giving only verbal instructions. When you share concrete information verbally, also show a photograph. Give the student practical materials and experiences and the opportunity to touch and examine objects.

- Divide new tasks and large tasks into smaller steps. Demonstrate the steps. Have the student do the steps, one by one. Offer help when necessary.

- Give the student immediate, concrete feedback.

Section 17.3

Fragile X Syndrome

"Learning about Fragile X Syndrome," National Human Genome Research Institute, National Institutes of Health, June 24, 2010.

What is fragile X syndrome?

Fragile X syndrome is the most common form of inherited mental retardation in males and is also a significant cause of mental retardation in females. It affects about one in four thousand males and one in eight thousand females and occurs in all racial and ethnic groups.

Nearly all cases of fragile X syndrome are caused by an alteration (mutation) in the FMR1 gene where a deoxyribonucleic acid (DNA) segment, known as the CGG triplet repeat, is expanded. Normally, this DNA segment is repeated from five to about forty times. In people with fragile X syndrome, however, the CGG segment is repeated more than two hundred times. The abnormally expanded CGG segment inactivates (silences) the FMR1 gene, which prevents the gene from producing a protein called fragile X mental retardation protein. Loss of this protein leads to the signs and symptoms of fragile X syndrome. Both boys and girls can be affected, but because boys have only one X chromosome, a single fragile X is likely to affect them more severely.

What are the symptoms of fragile X syndrome?

A boy who has the full FMR1 mutation has fragile X syndrome and will have moderate mental retardation. They have a particular facial appearance, characterized by a large head size, a long face, prominent forehead and chin, and protruding ears. In addition males who have fragile X syndrome have loose joints (joint laxity), and large testes (after puberty).

Affected boys may have behavioral problems such as hyperactivity, hand flapping, hand biting, temper tantrums, and autism. Other behaviors in boys after they have reached puberty include poor eye contact, perseverative speech, problems in impulse control, and distractibility. Physical problems that have been seen include eye, orthopedic, heart, and skin problems.

Girls who have the full FMR1 mutation have mild mental retardation.

Family members who have fewer repeats in the FMR1 gene may not have mental retardation, but may have other problems. Women with less severe changes may have premature menopause or difficulty becoming pregnant.

Both men and women may have problems with tremors and poor coordination.

What does it mean to have a fragile X premutation?

People with about fifty-five to two hundred repeats of the CGG segment are said to have an FMR1 premutation (an intermediate variation of the gene). In women, the premutation is liable to expand to more than two hundred repeats in cells that develop into eggs. This means that women with the FMR1 premutation have an increased risk of having a child with fragile X syndrome. By contrast, the premutation CGG repeat in men remains at the same size or shortens as it is passed to the next generation.

Males and females who have a fragile X premutation have normal intellect and appearance. A few individuals with a premutation have subtle intellectual or behavioral symptoms, such as learning difficulties or social anxiety. The difficulties are usually not socially debilitating, and these individuals may still marry and have children.

Males who have a premutation with fifty-nine to two hundred CGG trinucleotide repeats are usually unaffected and are at risk for fragile X–associated tremor/ataxia syndrome (FXTAS). The fragile X–associated tremor/ataxia syndrome (FXTAS) is characterized by late-onset, progressive cerebellar ataxia and intention tremor in males who have a premutation. Other neurologic findings include short-term memory loss, executive function deficits, cognitive decline, parkinsonism, peripheral neuropathy, lower-limb proximal muscle weakness, and autonomic dysfunction.

The degree to which clinical symptoms of fragile X are present (penetrance) is age related; symptoms are seen in 17 percent of males aged fifty to fifty-nine years, in 38 percent of males aged sixty to sixty-nine years, in 47 percent of males aged seventy to seventy-nine years, and in 75 percent of males aged eighty years or older. Some female premutation carriers may also develop tremor and ataxia.

Females who have a premutation usually are unaffected, but may be at risk for premature ovarian failure and FXTAS. Premature ovarian failure (POF) is defined as cessation of menses before age forty years, has been observed in carriers of premutation alleles. A review by Sherman (2005) concluded that the risk for POF was 21 percent in premutation carriers compared to 1 percent for the general population.

How is fragile X syndrome diagnosed?

There are very few outward signs of fragile X syndrome in babies, but one is a tendency to have a large head circumference. An experienced geneticist may note subtle differences in facial characteristics. Mental retardation is the hallmark of this condition and, in females, this may be the only sign of the problem.

A specific genetic test (polymerase chain reaction [PCR]) can now be performed to diagnose fragile X syndrome. This test looks for an expanded mutation (called a triplet repeat) in the FMR1 gene.

How is fragile X syndrome treated?

There is no specific treatment available for fragile X syndrome. Supportive therapy for children who have fragile X syndrome includes the following:

- Special education and anticipatory management including avoidance of excessive stimulation to decrease behavioral problems

- Medication to manage behavioral issues, although no specific medication has been shown to be beneficial

- Early intervention, special education, and vocational training

Vision, hearing, connective tissue problems, and heart problems when present are treated in the usual manner.

Is fragile X syndrome inherited?

This condition is inherited in an X-linked dominant pattern. A condition is considered X-linked if the mutated gene that causes the disorder is located on the X chromosome, one of the two sex chromosomes. The inheritance is dominant if one copy of the altered gene in each cell is sufficient to cause the condition. In most cases, males experience more severe symptoms of the disorder than females. A striking characteristic of X-linked inheritance is that fathers cannot pass X-linked traits to their sons.

Section 17.4

Klinefelter Syndrome

"Learning about Klinefelter Syndrome," National Human Genome Research Institute, National Institutes of Health, July 20, 2010.

What is Klinefelter syndrome?

Klinefelter syndrome is a condition that occurs in men as a result of an extra X chromosome. The most common symptom is infertility.

Humans have forty-six chromosomes, which contain all of a person's genes and deoxyribonucleic acid (DNA). Two of these chromosomes, the sex chromosomes, determine a person's gender. Both of the sex chromosomes in females are called X chromosomes. (This is written as XX.) Males have an X and a Y chromosome (written as XY). The two sex chromosomes help a person develop fertility and the sexual characteristics of their gender.

Most often, Klinefelter syndrome is the result of one extra X (written as XXY). Occasionally, variations of the XXY chromosome count may occur, the most common being the XY/XXY mosaic. In this variation, some of the cells in the male's body have an additional X chromosome, and the rest have the normal XY chromosome count. The percentage of cells containing the extra chromosome varies from case to case. In some instances, XY/XXY mosaics may have enough normally functioning cells in the testes to allow them to father children.

Klinefelter syndrome is found in about one out of every five hundred to one thousand newborn males. The additional sex chromosome results from a random error during the formation of the egg or sperm. About half of the time the error occurs in the formation of sperm, while the remainder are due to errors in egg development. Women who have pregnancies after age thirty-five have a slightly increased chance of having a boy with this syndrome.

What are the symptoms of Klinefelter syndrome?

Males who have Klinefelter syndrome may have the following symptoms: small, firm testes, a small penis, sparse pubic, armpit, and facial hair, enlarged breasts (called gynecomastia), tall stature, and abnormal body proportions (long legs, short trunk).

School-age children may be diagnosed if they are referred to a doctor to evaluate learning disabilities. The diagnosis may also be considered in the adolescent male when puberty is not progressing as expected. Adult males may come to the doctor because of infertility.

Klinefelter syndrome is associated with an increased risk for breast cancer, a rare tumor called extragonadal germ cell tumor, lung disease, varicose veins, and osteoporosis. Men who have Klinefelter syndrome also have an increased risk for autoimmune disorders such as lupus, rheumatoid arthritis, and Sjögren syndrome.

How is Klinefelter syndrome diagnosed?

A chromosomal analysis (karyotype) is used to confirm the diagnosis. In this procedure, a small blood sample is drawn. White blood cells are then separated from the sample, mixed with tissue culture medium, incubated, and checked for chromosomal abnormalities, such as an extra X chromosome.

The chromosome analysis looks at a number of cells, usually at least twenty, which allows for the diagnosis of genetic conditions in both the full and mosaic state. In some cases, low-level mosaicism may be missed. However, if mosaicism is suspected (based on hormone levels, sperm counts, or physical characteristics), additional cells can be analyzed from within the same blood draw.

How is Klinefelter syndrome treated?

Testosterone therapy is used to increase strength, promote muscular development, grow body hair, improve mood and self-esteem, increase energy, and improve concentration.

Most men who have Klinefelter syndrome are not able to father children. However, some men with an extra X chromosome have fathered healthy offspring, sometimes with the help of infertility specialists.

Most men who have Klinefelter syndrome can expect to have a normal and productive life. Early diagnosis, in conjunction with educational interventions, medical management, and strong social support will optimize each individual's potential in adulthood.

Section 17.5

Prader-Willi Syndrome

Reprinted from the National Institute of Child Health and Human Development, National Institutes of Health, March 24, 2010.

What is Prader-Willi syndrome?

Prader-Willi Syndrome is the most common genetic cause of life-threatening obesity in children.

People with Prader-Willi syndrome have a problem in their hypothalamus, a part of the brain that normally controls feelings of fullness or hunger. As a result, they never feel full and have a constant urge to eat that they cannot control.

Most cases of Prader-Willi syndrome result from a spontaneous genetic error in genes on chromosome 15 that occurs at conception. In very rare cases, the mutation is inherited.

What are the symptoms of Prader-Willi syndrome?

There are generally two stages of symptoms for people with Prader-Willi syndrome:

- **Stage 1:** As newborns, babies with Prader-Willi can have low muscle tone, which can affect their ability to suck properly. As a result, babies may need special feeding techniques to help them eat, and infants may have problems gaining weight. As these babies grow older, their strength and muscle tone usually get better. They meet motor milestones, but are usually slower in doing so.

- **Stage 2:** Between the ages of one and six years old, the disorder changes to one of constant hunger and food seeking. Most people with Prader-Willi syndrome have an insatiable appetite, meaning they never feel full. In fact, their brains are telling them they are starving. They may have trouble regulating their own eating and may need external restrictions on food, including locked kitchen and food storage areas.

This problem is made worse because people with Prader-Willi syndrome use fewer calories than those without the syndrome because they have less muscle mass. The combination of eating massive amounts of food and not burning enough calories can lead to life-threatening obesity if the diet is not kept under strict control.

There are other symptoms that may affect people with Prader-Willi, including the following:

- Behavioral problems, usually during transitions and unanticipated changes, such as stubbornness or temper tantrums

- Delayed motor skills and speech due to low muscle tone

- Cognitive problems, ranging from near normal intelligence to mild intellectual and developmental disabilities; learning disabilities are common

- Repetitive thoughts and verbalizations

- Collecting and hoarding of possessions

- Picking at skin

- Low sex hormone levels

Prader-Willi syndrome is considered a spectrum disorder, meaning not all symptoms will occur in everyone affected and the symptoms may range from mild to severe.

People with Prader-Willi often have some mental strengths as well, such as skills in jigsaw puzzles. If obesity is prevented, people with the syndrome can live a normal lifespan.

What are the treatments for Prader-Willi syndrome?

Prader-Willi syndrome cannot be cured, but early intervention can help people build skills for adapting to the disorder. Early diagnosis can also help parents learn about the condition and prepare for future challenges. A healthcare provider can do a blood test to check for Prader-Willi syndrome.

Exercise and physical activity can help control weight and help with motor skills. Speech therapy may be needed to help with oral skills.

Human growth hormone has been found to be helpful in treating Prader-Willi syndrome. It can help to increase height, decrease body fat, and increase muscle mass. However, no medications have yet been found to control appetite in those with Prader-Willi.

Section 17.6

Triple X Syndrome

Excerpted from "XXX Syndrome (Trisomy X)," http://www.med.umich.edu/ yourchild/topics/xxxsyn.htm, written and compiled by Kyla Boyse, R.N., reviewed by Autumn Tansky, MS, updated July 2010. Content provided by the University of Michigan Health System, © 2010. All rights reserved. Reprinted with permission.

What is XXX or triple X syndrome?

XXX syndrome (also called trisomy X or triple X) is caused by the presence of an extra "X" chromosome in every cell. Typically, a female has two X chromosomes in every cell of their body, so the extra "X" is unusual. The extra "X" chromosome is typically inherited from the mother, but is a random event—not caused by anything she did or could prevent. Trisomy X is often not diagnosed until later in life, if ever. The risk of having a second child with an extra chromosome is approximately 1 percent, until mom is older than thirty-eight years of age, as it is thought that this random event becomes more common as a woman ages. Prenatal testing is available in future pregnancies.

How common is trisomy X?

The extra "X" chromosome occurs in about one in every one thousand newborn girls.

What are the features of triple X syndrome?

Many girls and women with triple X have no signs or symptoms. Signs and symptoms vary a lot between individuals, but can include:

- Physical:
  - Tall stature (height)
  - Possible mild facial characteristics: increased width between eyes, skin fold at inner eyelid (epicanthal fold), proportionately smaller head size
- Developmental:
  - Learning disabilities (70 percent): Normal IQ, but may be ten to fifteen points below siblings
  - Speech and language delays (50 percent)
  - Delayed motor skills: Poor coordination, awkwardness, clumsiness
- Behavioral:
  - Introverted, difficulty with interpersonal relationships

How is triple X diagnosed and treated?

XXX syndrome is diagnosed prenatally, through CVS or amniocentesis, or after the child is born by a blood test. These tests are all able to look at a person's chromosomes (karyotype.) There is no way to remove the extra X chromosome. Treatment depends on what needs the child has. Girls with XXX syndrome may need to be seen by physical, developmental, occupational, or speech therapists if they have developmental or speech problems. Additionally, a pediatric psychologist or group therapy may be helpful if they have social troubles. Girls with trisomy X are treated as any other child with a developmental or psychological concern would be treated.

What is 46,XX/47,XXX mosaicism?

This describes a chromosome study that shows a mixture of normal cells and cells with an extra X chromosome. A girl with mosaicism will usually have fewer effects of the extra chromosome, because not all of her cells have this extra genetic material. She will probably not be much different than she would be if her chromosome study showed all normal cells.

Section 17.7

Turner Syndrome

"Learning about Turner Syndrome," National Human Genome
Research Institute, National Institutes of Health, June 28, 2010.

What is Turner syndrome?

Turner syndrome is a chromosomal condition that alters development
in females. Women with this condition tend to be shorter than average
and are usually unable to conceive a child (infertile) because of an absence of ovarian function. Other features of this condition that can vary
among women who have Turner syndrome include: extra skin on the
neck (webbed neck), puffiness or swelling (lymphedema) of the hands
and feet, skeletal abnormalities, heart defects, and kidney problems.

This condition occurs in about 1 in 2,500 female births worldwide,
but is much more common among pregnancies that do not survive to
term (miscarriages and stillbirths).

Turner syndrome is a chromosomal condition related to the X chromosome.

Researchers have not yet determined which genes on the X chromosome are responsible for most signs and symptoms of Turner syndrome. They have, however, identified one gene called SHOX that is
important for bone development and growth. Missing one copy of this
gene likely causes short stature and skeletal abnormalities in women
with Turner syndrome.

What are the symptoms of Turner syndrome?

Girls who have Turner syndrome are shorter than average. They
often have normal height for the first three years of life, but then
have a slow growth rate. At puberty they do not have the usual
growth spurt.

Nonfunctioning ovaries are another symptom of Turner syndrome.
Normally a girl's ovaries begin to produce sex hormones (estrogen and
progesterone) at puberty. This does not happen in most girls who have
Turner syndrome. They do not start their periods or develop breasts
without hormone treatment at the age of puberty.

Even though many women who have Turner have nonfunctioning ovaries and are infertile, their vagina and womb are totally normal.

In early childhood, girls who have Turner syndrome may have frequent middle ear infections. Recurrent infections can lead to hearing loss in some cases.

Girls with Turner syndrome are usually of normal intelligence with good verbal skills and reading skills. Some girls, however, have problems with math, memory skills, and fine-finger movements.

Additional symptoms of Turner syndrome include the following:

- An especially wide neck (webbed neck) and a low or indistinct hairline.

- A broad chest and widely spaced nipples.

- Arms that turn out slightly at the elbow.

- A heart murmur, sometimes associated with narrowing of the aorta (blood vessel exiting the heart).

- A tendency to develop high blood pressure (so this should be checked regularly).

- Minor eye problems that are corrected by glasses.

- Scoliosis (deformity of the spine) occurs in 10 percent of adolescent girls who have Turner syndrome.

- The thyroid gland becomes underactive in about 10 percent of women who have Turner syndrome. Regular blood tests are necessary to detect it early and if necessary treat with thyroid replacement.

- Older or overweight women with Turner syndrome are slightly more at risk of developing diabetes.

- Osteoporosis can develop because of a lack of estrogen, but this can largely be prevented by taking hormone replacement therapy.

How is Turner syndrome diagnosed?

A diagnosis of Turner syndrome may be suspected when there are a number of typical physical features observed such as webbed neck, a broad chest, and widely spaced nipples. Sometimes diagnosis is made at birth because of heart problems, an unusually wide neck, or swelling of the hands and feet.

The two main clinical features of Turner syndrome are short stature and the lack of the development of the ovaries.

Many girls are diagnosed in early childhood when a slow growth rate and other features are identified. Diagnosis sometimes takes place later when puberty does not occur.

Turner syndrome may be suspected in pregnancy during an ultrasound test. This can be confirmed by prenatal testing—chorionic villous sampling or amniocentesis—to obtain cells from the unborn baby for chromosomal analysis. If a diagnosis is confirmed prenatally, the baby may be under the care of a specialist pediatrician immediately after birth.

Diagnosis is confirmed by a blood test, called a karyotype. This is used to analyze the chromosomal composition of the female.

What is the treatment for Turner syndrome?

During childhood and adolescence, girls may be under the care of a pediatric endocrinologist, who is a specialist in childhood conditions of the hormones and metabolism.

Growth hormone injections are beneficial in some individuals with Turner syndrome. Injections often begin in early childhood and may increase final adult height by a few inches.

Estrogen replacement therapy is usually started at the time of normal puberty, around twelve years, to start breast development. Estrogen and progesterone are given a little later to begin a monthly "period," which is necessary to keep the womb healthy. Estrogen is also given to prevent osteoporosis.

Babies born with a heart murmur or narrowing of the aorta may need surgery to correct the problem. A heart expert (cardiologist) will assess and follow up any treatment necessary.

Girls who have Turner syndrome are more likely to get middle ear infections. Repeated infections may lead to hearing loss and should be evaluated by the pediatrician. An ear, nose, and throat specialist (ENT) may be involved in caring for this health issue.

High blood pressure is quite common in women who have Turner syndrome. In some cases, the elevated blood pressure is due to narrowing of the aorta or a kidney abnormality. However, most of the time, no specific cause for the elevation is identified. Blood pressure should be checked routinely and, if necessary, treated with medication. Women who have Turner syndrome have a slightly higher risk of having an underactive thyroid or developing diabetes. This should also be monitored during routine health maintenance visits and treated if necessary.

Regular health checks are very important. Special clinics for the care of girls and women who have Turner syndrome are available in some areas, with access to a variety of specialists. Early preventive care and treatment is very important.

Almost all women with Turner Syndrome are infertile, but pregnancy with donor embryos may be possible.

Having appropriate medical treatment and support allows a woman with Turner syndrome to lead a normal, healthy and happy life.

Is Turner syndrome inherited?

Turner syndrome is not usually inherited in families. Turner syndrome occurs when one of the two X chromosomes normally found in women is missing or incomplete. Although the exact cause of Turner syndrome is not known, it appears to occur as a result of a random error during the formation of either the eggs or sperm.

Humans have forty-six chromosomes, which contain all of a person's genes and deoxyribonucleic acid (DNA). Two of these chromosomes, the sex chromosomes, determine a person's gender. Both of the sex chromosomes in females are called X chromosomes. (This is written as XX.) Males have an X and a Y chromosome (written as XY). The two sex chromosomes help a person develop fertility and the sexual characteristics of their gender.

In Turner syndrome, the girl does not have the usual pair of two complete X chromosomes. The most common scenario is that the girl has only one X chromosome in her cells. Some girls with Turner syndrome do have two X chromosomes, but one of the X chromosomes is incomplete. In another scenario, the girl has some cells in her body with two X chromosomes, but other cells have only one. This is called mosaicism.

Section 17.8

Velocardiofacial Syndrome

"Learning about Velocardiofacial Syndrome," National Human Genome
Research Institute, National Institutes of Health, June 28, 2010.

What is velocardiofacial syndrome?

Velocardiofacial syndrome (VCFS) is a genetic condition that is
sometimes hereditary. VCFS is characterized by a combination of medical problems that vary from child to child. These medical problems
include: cleft palate, or an opening in the roof of the mouth, and other
differences in the palate; heart defects; problems fighting infection; low
calcium levels; differences in the way the kidneys are formed or work;
a characteristic facial appearance; learning problems; and speech and
feeding problems.

The name velocardiofacial syndrome comes from the Latin words
"velum," meaning palate, "cardia," meaning heart, and "facies," having to do with the face. Not all of these identifying features are found
in each child who is born with VCFS. The most common features are
palatal differences (~75 percent), heart defects (75 percent), problems
fighting infection (77 percent), low calcium levels (50 percent), differences in the kidney (35 percent), characteristic facial appearance
(numbers vary depending on the individual's ethnic and racial background), learning problems (~90 percent), and speech (~75 percent)
and feeding problems (35 percent).

Two genes—COMT and TBX1—are associated with VCFS. However, not all of the genes that cause VCFS have been identified. Most
children who have been diagnosed with this syndrome are missing a
small part of chromosome 22. Chromosomes are threadlike structures
found in every cell of the body. Each chromosome contains hundreds
of genes. A human cell normally contains 46 chromosomes (23 from
each parent). The specific location or address of the missing segment
in individuals with VCFS is 22q11.2.

VCFS is also called the 22q11.2 deletion syndrome. It also has other
clinical names such as DiGeorge syndrome, conotruncal anomaly face
syndrome (CTAF), autosomal dominant Opitz G/BBB syndrome or

Cayler cardiofacial syndrome. As a result of this deletion, about thirty genes are generally absent from this chromosome.

VCFS affects about one in four thousand newborns. VCFS may affect more individuals, however, because some people who have the 22q11.2 deletion may not be diagnosed, as they have very few signs and symptoms.

What are the symptoms of VCFS?

Despite the involvement of a very specific portion of chromosome 22, there is great variation in the symptoms of this syndrome. At least thirty different symptoms have been associated with the 22q11 deletion. Most of these symptoms are not present in all individuals who have VCFS.

Symptoms include: cleft palate, usually of the soft palate (the roof of the mouth nearest the throat, which is behind the bony palate); heart problems; similar faces (elongated face, almond-shaped eyes, wide nose, small ears); eye problems; feeding problems that include food coming through the nose (nasal regurgitation) because of the palatal differences; middle-ear infections (otitis media); low calcium due to hypoparathyroidism (low levels of the parathyroid hormone that can result in seizures); immune system problems which make it difficult for the body to fight infections; differences in the way the kidneys are formed or how they work; weak muscles; differences in the spine such as curvature of the spine (scoliosis) or bony abnormalities in the neck or upper back; and tapered fingers. Children are born with these features.

Children who have VCFS also often have learning difficulties and developmental delays. About 65 percent of individuals with the 22q11.2 deletion are found to have a nonverbal learning disability. When tested, their verbal intelligence quotient (IQ) scores are greater than ten points higher than their performance IQ scores. This combination of test scores brings down the full-scale IQ scores but they won't represent the abilities of the individual accurately. As a result of this type of learning disability, students will have relative strengths in reading and rote memorization but will struggle with math and abstract reasoning. These individuals may also have communication and social interaction problems such as autism. As adults, these individuals have an increased risk for developing mental illness such as depression, anxiety, and schizophrenia.

How is VCFS diagnosed?

VCFS is suspected as a diagnosis based on clinical examination and the presence of the signs and symptoms of the syndrome.

A special blood test called FISH (fluorescence in situ hybridization) is then done to look for the deletion in chromosome 22q11.2. More than 95 percent of individuals who have VCFS have a deletion in chromosome 22q11.2.

Those individuals who do not have the 22q11.2 deletion by standard FISH testing may have a smaller deletion that may only be found using more sophisticated lab studies such as comparative genomic hybridization, multiplex ligation-dependent probe amplification (MLPA), additional FISH studies performed in a research laboratory, or using specific gene studies to look for mutations in the genes known to be in this region. Again, these studies may only be available through a research lab.

What is the treatment for VCFS?

Treatment is based on the type of symptoms that are present. For example, heart defects are treated as they would normally be via surgical interventions in the newborn period. Individuals who have low calcium levels are given calcium supplements and frequently vitamin D to help them absorb the calcium. Palate problems are treated by a team of specialists called a cleft palate or craniofacial team and again often require surgical interventions and intensive speech therapy. Infections are generally treated aggressively with antibiotics in infants and children with immune problems.

Early intervention and speech therapies are started when possible at one year of age to assess and treat developmental delays.

Is VCFS inherited?

VCFS is due to a 22q11.2 deletion. Most often neither parent has the deletion and so it is new in the child (93 percent) and the chance for the couple to have another child with VCFS is quite low (close to zero). However, once the deletion is present in a person he or she has a 50 percent chance for having children who also have the deletion. The 22q11 deletion happens as an accident when either the egg or sperm are being formed or early in fetal development.

In less than 10 percent of cases, a person with VCFS inherits the deletion in chromosome 22 from a parent. When VCFS is inherited in families, this means that other family members may be affected as well.

Since some people with the 22q11.2 deletion are very mildly affected, it is suggested that all parents of children with the deletion have testing. Furthermore, some people with the deletion have no symptoms but they have the deletion in some of their cells but not all. This is called mosaicism. Even other people have the deletion only in their egg cells or sperm cells but not in their blood cells. It is recommended that all parents of a child with a 22q11.2 deletion seek genetic counseling before or during a subsequent pregnancy to learn more about their chances of having another child with VCFS.

Section 17.9

Williams Syndrome

"Williams Syndrome Information Page," National Institute of Neurological Disorders and Stroke, National Institutes of Health, September 9, 2008.

What is Williams syndrome?

Williams syndrome (WS) is a rare genetic disorder characterized by mild to moderate mental retardation or learning difficulties, a distinctive facial appearance, and a unique personality that combines overfriendliness and high levels of empathy with anxiety. The most significant medical problem associated with WS is cardiovascular disease caused by narrowed arteries. WS is also associated with elevated blood calcium levels in infancy. A random genetic mutation (deletion of a small piece of chromosome 7), rather than inheritance, most often causes the disorder. However, individuals who have WS have a 50 percent chance of passing it on if they decide to have children. The characteristic facial features of WS include puffiness around the eyes, a short nose with a broad nasal tip, wide mouth, full cheeks, full lips, and a small chin. People with WS are also likely to have a long neck, sloping shoulders, short stature, limited mobility in their joints, and curvature of the spine. Some individuals with WS have a starlike pattern in the iris of their eyes. Infants with WS are often irritable and colicky, with feeding problems that keep them from gaining weight. Chronic abdominal pain is common in adolescents and adults. By age thirty, the majority of individuals with WS have diabetes or pre-diabetes and mild to moderate sensorineural hearing loss (a form of deafness due to disturbed function of the auditory nerve). For some people, hearing loss may begin as early as late childhood. WS also is associated with a characteristic "cognitive profile" of mental strengths and weaknesses composed of strengths in verbal short-term memory and language, combined with severe weakness in visuospatial construction (the skills used to copy patterns, draw, or write). Within language, the strongest skills are typically in concrete, practical vocabulary, which in many cases is in the low average to average range for the general population. Abstract or conceptual-relational vocabulary is much more limited. Most older children and adults with WS speak fluently and use good grammar. More than 50 percent of children with WS have attention deficit disorders (attention deficit disorder [ADD] or attention deficit hyperactivity disorder [ADHD]), and about 50 percent have specific phobias, such as a fear of loud noises. The majority of individuals with WS worry excessively.

Is there any treatment?

There is no cure for Williams syndrome, nor is there a standard course of treatment. Because WS is an uncommon and complex disorder, multidisciplinary clinics have been established at several centers in the United States. Treatments are based on an individual's particular symptoms. People with WS require regular cardiovascular monitoring for potential medical problems, such as symptomatic narrowing of the blood vessels, high blood pressure, and heart failure.

What is the prognosis?

The prognosis for individuals with WS varies. Some degree of mental retardation is found in most people with the disorder. Some adults are able to function independently, complete academic or vocational school, and live in supervised homes or on their own; most live with a caregiver. Parents can increase the likelihood that their child will be able to live semi-independently by teaching self-help skills early. Early intervention and individualized educational programs designed with the distinct cognitive and personality profiles of WS in mind also help individuals maximize their potential. Medical complications associated with the disorder may shorten the life spans of some individuals with WS.

What research is being done?

The National Institutes of Health (NIH), and the National Institute of Neurological Disorders and Stroke (NINDS), have funded many of the research studies exploring the genetic and neurobiological origins of WS. In the early 1990s, researchers located and identified the genetic mutation responsible for the disorder: the deletion of a small section of chromosome 7 that contains approximately twenty-five genes. NINDS continues to support WS researchers including, for example, groups that are attempting to link specific genes with the corresponding facial, cognitive, personality, and neurological characteristics of WS.

Chapter 18

Emotional Disturbance

The mental health of our children is a natural and important concern for us all. The fact is, many mental disorders have their beginnings in childhood or adolescence, yet may go undiagnosed and untreated for years.[1]

We refer to mental disorders using different "umbrella" terms such as emotional disturbance, behavioral disorders, or mental illness. Beneath these umbrella terms, there is actually a wide range of specific conditions that differ from one another in their characteristics and treatment. These include (but are not limited to) the following:

- Anxiety disorders
- Bipolar disorder (sometimes called manic-depression)
- Conduct disorders
- Eating disorders
- Obsessive-compulsive disorder (OCD)
- Psychotic disorders

Definition

We've chosen to use the term "emotional disturbance" in this chapter because that is the term used in the nation's special education law,

Excerpted from "Emotional Disturbance," National Dissemination Center for Children with Disabilities, June 2010.

the Individuals with Disabilities Education Act (IDEA). IDEA defines emotional disturbance as follows:

> . . . a condition exhibiting one or more of the following characteristics over a long period of time and to a marked degree that adversely affects a child's educational performance:
>
> (A) An inability to learn that cannot be explained by intellectual, sensory, or health factors.
>
> (B) An inability to build or maintain satisfactory interpersonal relationships with peers and teachers.
>
> (C) Inappropriate types of behavior or feelings under normal circumstances.
>
> (D) A general pervasive mood of unhappiness or depression.
>
> (E) A tendency to develop physical symptoms or fears associated with personal or school problems.[2]

As defined by IDEA, emotional disturbance includes schizophrenia but does not apply to children who are socially maladjusted, unless it is determined that they have an emotional disturbance.[3]

Characteristics

As is evident in IDEA's definition, emotional disturbances can affect an individual in areas beyond the emotional. Depending on the specific mental disorder involved, a person's physical, social, or cognitive skills may also be affected. The National Alliance on Mental Illness (NAMI) puts this very well:

> Mental illnesses are medical conditions that disrupt a person's thinking, feeling, mood, ability to relate to others and daily functioning. Just as diabetes is a disorder of the pancreas, mental illnesses are medical conditions that often result in a diminished capacity for coping with the ordinary demands of life.[4]

Some of the characteristics and behaviors seen in children who have an emotional disturbance include the following:

- Hyperactivity (short attention span, impulsiveness)
- Aggression or self-injurious behavior (acting out, fighting)
- Withdrawal (not interacting socially with others, excessive fear or anxiety)

- Immaturity (inappropriate crying, temper tantrums, poor coping skills)

- Learning difficulties (academically performing below grade level)

Children with the most serious emotional disturbances may exhibit distorted thinking, excessive anxiety, bizarre motor acts, and abnormal mood swings.

Many children who do not have emotional disturbance may display some of these same behaviors at various times during their development. However, when children have an emotional disturbance, these behaviors continue over long periods of time. Their behavior signals that they are not coping with their environment or peers.

Causes

No one knows the actual cause or causes of emotional disturbance, although several factors—heredity, brain disorder, diet, stress, and family functioning—have been suggested and vigorously researched. A great deal of research goes on every day, but to date, researchers have not found that any of these factors are the direct cause of behavioral or emotional problems.

According to NAMI, mental illnesses can affect persons of any age, race, religion, or income. Further:

Mental illnesses are not the result of personal weakness, lack of character, or poor upbringing. Mental illnesses are treatable. Most people diagnosed with a serious mental illness can experience relief from their symptoms by actively participating in an individual treatment plan.[5]

Frequency

According to the Centers for Disease Control and Prevention (CDC), approximately 8.3 million children (14.5 percent) aged four to seventeen years have parents who've talked with a healthcare provider or school staff about the child's emotional or behavioral difficulties.[6] Nearly 2.9 million children have been prescribed medication for these difficulties.[7]

Help for School-Aged Children

IDEA requires that special education and related services be made available free of charge to every eligible child with a disability, including

217

preschoolers (ages three to twenty-one). These services are specially designed to address the child's individual needs associated with the disability—in this case, emotional disturbance, as defined by IDEA (and further specified by states). In the 2003–2004 school year, more than 484,000 children and youth with emotional disturbance received these services to address their individual needs related to emotional disturbance.[8]

Determining a child's eligibility for special education and related services begins with a full and individual evaluation of the child. Under IDEA, this evaluation is provided free of charge in public schools.

A Look at Specific Emotional Disturbances

As we mentioned, emotional disturbance is a commonly used umbrella term for a number of different mental disorders. Let's take a brief look at some of the most common of these.

Anxiety Disorders

We all experience anxiety from time to time, but for many people, including children, anxiety can be excessive, persistent, seemingly uncontrollable, and overwhelming. An irrational fear of everyday situations may be involved. This high level of anxiety is a definite warning sign that a person may have an anxiety disorder.

As with the term emotional disturbance, "anxiety disorder" is an umbrella term that actually refers to several distinct disabilities that share the core characteristic of irrational fear: generalized anxiety disorder (GAD), obsessive-compulsive disorder (OCD), panic disorder, posttraumatic stress disorder (PTSD), social anxiety disorder (also called social phobia), and specific phobias.[9]

According to the Anxiety Disorders Association of America, anxiety disorders are the most common psychiatric illnesses affecting children and adults.[10] They are also highly treatable. Unfortunately, only about one-third of those affected receive treatment.[11]

Bipolar Disorder

Also known as manic-depressive illness, bipolar disorder is a serious medical condition that causes dramatic mood swings from overly "high" and/or irritable to sad and hopeless, and then back again, often with periods of normal mood in between. Severe changes in energy and behavior go along with these changes in mood.[12]

For most people with bipolar disorder, these mood swings and related symptoms can be stabilized over time using an approach that combines medication and psychosocial treatment.[13]

Conduct Disorder

Conduct disorder refers to a group of behavioral and emotional problems in youngsters. Children and adolescents with this disorder have great difficulty following rules and behaving in a socially acceptable way.[14] This may include some of the following behaviors:

- Aggression to people and animals

- Destruction of property

- Deceitfulness, lying, or stealing

- Truancy or other serious violations of rules.[15]

Although conduct disorder is one of the most difficult behavior disorders to treat, young people often benefit from a range of services that include the following:

- Training for parents on how to handle child or adolescent behavior

- Family therapy

- Training in problem-solving skills for children or adolescents

- Community-based services that focus on the young person within the context of family and community influences[16]

Eating Disorders

Eating disorders are characterized by extremes in eating behavior—either too much or too little—or feelings of extreme distress or concern about body weight or shape. Females are much more likely than males to develop an eating disorder.[17]

Anorexia nervosa and bulimia nervosa are the two most common types of eating disorders. Anorexia nervosa is characterized by self-starvation and dramatic loss of weight. Bulimia nervosa involves a cycle of binge eating, then self-induced vomiting or purging. Both of these disorders are potentially life threatening.[18]

Binge eating is also considered an eating disorder. It's characterized by eating excessive amounts of food, while feeling unable to control how much or what is eaten. Unlike with bulimia, people who binge eat usually do not purge afterward by vomiting or using laxatives.[19]

According to the National Eating Disorders Association:

The most effective and long-lasting treatment for an eating disorder is some form of psychotherapy or counseling, coupled with careful attention to medical and nutritional needs. Some medications have been shown to be helpful. Ideally, whatever treatment is offered should be tailored to the individual, and this will vary according to both the severity of the disorder and the patient's individual problems, needs, and strengths.[20]

Obsessive-Compulsive Disorder

Often referred to as OCD, obsessive-compulsive disorder is actually considered an anxiety disorder (which was discussed earlier in this chapter). OCD is characterized by recurrent, unwanted thoughts (obsessions) and/or repetitive behaviors (compulsions). Repetitive behaviors (hand washing, counting, checking, or cleaning) are often performed with the hope of preventing obsessive thoughts or making them go away. Performing these so-called rituals, however, provides only temporary relief, and not performing them markedly increases anxiety.[21]

A large body of scientific evidence suggests that OCD results from a chemical imbalance in the brain.[22] Treatment for most people with OCD should include one or more of the following:

- Therapist trained in behavior therapy

- Cognitive behavior therapy (CBT)

- Medication (usually an antidepressant)[23]

Psychotic Disorders

"Psychotic disorders" is another umbrella term used to refer to severe mental disorders that cause abnormal thinking and perceptions. Two of the main symptoms are delusions and hallucinations. Delusions are false beliefs, such as thinking that someone is plotting against you. Hallucinations are false perceptions, such as hearing, seeing, or feeling something that is not there. Schizophrenia is one type of psychotic disorder.[24] There are others as well.

Treatment for psychotic disorders will differ from person to person, depending on the specific disorder involved. Most are treated with a combination of medications and psychotherapy (a type of counseling).[25]

More about School

As mentioned, emotional disturbance is one of the categories of disability specified in IDEA. This means that a child with an emotional disturbance may be eligible for special education and related services in public school. These services can be of tremendous help to students who have an emotional disturbance.

Typically, educational programs for children with an emotional disturbance need to include attention to providing emotional and behavioral support as well as helping them to master academics, develop social skills, and increase self-awareness, self-control, and self-esteem. A large body of research exists regarding methods of providing students with positive behavioral support (PBS) in the school environment, so that problem behaviors are minimized and positive, appropriate behaviors are fostered. It is also important to know that, within the school setting, the following is true:

- For a child whose behavior impedes learning (including the learning of others), the team developing the child's Individualized Education Program (IEP) needs to consider, if appropriate, strategies to address that behavior, including positive behavioral interventions, strategies, and supports.

- Students eligible for special education services under the category of emotional disturbance may have IEPs that include psychological or counseling services. These are important related services available under IDEA and are to be provided by a qualified social worker, psychologist, guidance counselor, or other qualified personnel.

Other Considerations

Children and adolescents with an emotional disturbance should receive services based on their individual needs, and everyone involved in their education or care needs to be well informed about the care that they are receiving. It's important to coordinate services between home, school, and community, keeping the communication channels open between all parties involved.

The Importance of Support

Families often need help in understanding their child's disability and how to address the needs that arise from the disability. Help is available from psychiatrists, psychologists, and other mental health professionals that work in the public or private sector. There is also a network of mental health support operating in every state as well as locally.

References

1. National Institute of Mental Health (NIMH). (2010). Child and adolescent mental health. Available online at: http://www.nimh.nih.gov/health/topics/child-and-adolescent-mental-health/index.shtml.

2. Code of Federal Regulations, Title 34, §300.8(c)(4)(i).

3. Code of Federal Regulations, Title 34, §300.8(c)(4)(ii).

4. National Alliance on Mental Illness. (2010). What is mental illness: Mental illness facts. Available online at: http://tinyurl.com/3ew3d.

5. Ibid.

6. Simpson, G.A., Cohen, R.A., Pastor, P.N., and Reuben, C.A. (2008, September). Use of mental health services in the past 12 months by children aged 4–17 years: United States, 2005–2006. NCHS Data Brief, No. 8, 1–8. Available online at: http://www.cdc.gov/nchs/data/databriefs/db08.pdf.

7. Ibid.

8. U.S. Department of Education. (2007). 27th annual report to Congress on the implementation of the Individuals with Disabilities Education Act, 2005 (Vol. 2). Washington, DC: Author.

9. NIMH. (2010, March). Anxiety disorders. Available online at: www.nimh.nih.gov/health/publications/anxiety-disorders/complete-index.shtml

10. Anxiety Disorders Association of America. (2010). Understanding anxiety. Available online at: http://www.adaa.org/understanding-anxiety.

11. Ibid.

12. NIMH. (2010, May). Bipolar disorder. Available online at: http://www.nimh.nih.gov/health/topics/bipolar-disorder/index.shtml.

13. Ibid.

14. American Academy of Adolescent and Child Psychiatry. (2004, July). Conduct disorder: Facts for families. Available online at: http://www.aacap.org/cs/root/facts_for_families/conduct_disorder.

15. Ibid.

16. National Mental Health Information Center. (2003). Children's mental health facts: Children and adolescents with conduct disorder. Available online at: http://mentalhealth.samhsa.gov/publications/allpubs/ca-0010/default.asp.

17. NIMH. (2009). Eating disorders. Available online at: http://www.nimh.nih.gov/health/publications/eating-disorders/complete-index.shtml.

18. National Eating Disorders Association. (2010). Terms and definitions. Available online at: http://www.nationaleatingdisorders.org/information-resources/general-information.php.

19. Weight-control Information Network. (2008, June). Binge eating disorder. Available online at: http://www.win.niddk.nih.gov/publications/binge.htm.

20. National Eating Disorders Association. (2010). Treatment of eating disorders. Available online at: http://tinyurl.com/25f6v76.

21. NIMH. (2010, May). Obsessive-compulsive disorder, OCD. Available online at: http://www.nimh.nih.gov/health/topics/obsessive-compulsive-disorder-ocd/index.shtml.

22. National Alliance for Mental Illness. (2003). Mental illnesses: Obsessive-compulsive disorder. Available online at: http://tinyurl.com/2h2xne.

23. International OCD Foundation. (n.d.). Treatment of OCD. Available online at: www.ocfoundation.org/treatment.aspx.

24. Medline Plus. (2010, April). Psychotic disorders. Available online at: http://www.nlm.nih.gov/medlineplus/psychotic disorders.html.

25. MedicineNet.com. (n.d.). Psychotic disorders (cont.). Available online at: http://www.medicinenet.com/psychotic_disorders/page2.htm.

Chapter 19

Epilepsy

Jeremy's Story

When Jeremy was four months old, he had his first seizure. His mother Caroline knew at once that something was wrong, because she'd never seen him so stiff and pale, with his eyes rolling back.

The seizure passed quickly, although, to Caroline, it seemed to last forever. Then Jeremy took a deep breath, opened his eyes, and looked at her. Soon afterward, the baby fell into a deep sleep.

That was fifteen years ago. Jeremy's a teenager now, and you wouldn't guess from his alert eyes, quick smile, or quirky sense of humor that his brain is subject sometimes to brief, strong surges of electrical activity that dramatically affect his cognition and physical functioning. It's taken a lot of doctor visits, different medications, and one brain surgery to get his epilepsy under control. He still has seizures, but they don't happen very often now, much to everyone's relief, especially his mom and dad.

This year, for the first time, Jeremy and Caroline took part in the National Walk for Epilepsy, where they joined with thousands of others to raise funds for research, education, advocacy, and services for people with epilepsy and their caregivers. The best part of the day for Jeremy and Caroline was meeting so many other people who live with epilepsy every day, just like they do themselves.

Reprinted from "Epilepsy," National Dissemination Center for Children with Disabilities, June 2010.

Definition

Epilepsy is a seizure disorder. According to the Epilepsy Foundation of America, a seizure happens when a brief, strong surge of electrical activity affects part or all of the brain.[1] Seizures can last from a few seconds to a few minutes. They can have different symptoms, too, from convulsions and loss of consciousness, to signs such as blank staring, lip smacking, or jerking movements of arms and legs.[2]

Some people can have a seizure and yet not have epilepsy. For example, many young children have convulsions from fevers. Other types of seizures not classified as epilepsy include those caused by an imbalance of body fluids or chemicals or by alcohol or drug withdrawal. Thus, a single seizure does not mean that the person has epilepsy. Generally speaking, the diagnosis of epilepsy is made when a person has two or more unprovoked seizures.[3]

Incidence

About three million Americans have epilepsy. Of the two hundred thousand new cases diagnosed each year, nearly forty-five thousand are children and adolescents.[4] Epilepsy affects people in all nations and of all races. Its incidence is greater in African American and socially disadvantaged populations.[5]

Characteristics

Although the symptoms listed below do not necessarily mean that a person has epilepsy, it is wise to consult a doctor if you or a member of your family experiences one or more of them:

- "Blackouts" or periods of confused memory

- Episodes of staring or unexplained periods of unresponsiveness

- Involuntary movement of arms and legs

- "Fainting spells" with incontinence or followed by excessive fatigue

- Odd sounds, distorted perceptions, or episodic feelings of fear that cannot be explained.

Doctors have described more than thirty different types of seizures.[6] These are divided into two major categories—generalized seizures and partial seizures (also known as focal seizures).

Generalized seizures: This type of seizure involves both sides of the brain from the beginning of the seizure. The best-known subtype of generalized seizures is the grand mal seizure. In a grand mal seizure, the person's arms and legs stiffen (the tonic phase), and then begin to jerk (the clonic phase). That's why the grand mal seizure is also known as a generalized tonic clonic seizure.

Grand mal seizures typically last one to two minutes and are followed by a period of confusion and then deep sleep. The person will not remember what happened during the seizure.

You may also have heard of the petit mal seizure, which is an older term for another type of generalized seizure. It's now called an absence seizure, because during the seizure, the person stares blankly off into space and doesn't seem to be aware of his or her surroundings. The person may also blink rapidly and seem to chew. Absence seizures typically last from two to fifteen seconds and may not be noticed by others. Afterwards, the person will resume whatever he or she was doing at the time of the seizure, without any memory of the event.

Partial seizures: Partial seizures are so named because they involve only one hemisphere of the brain. They may be simple partial seizures (in which the person jerks and may have odd sensations and perceptions, but doesn't lose consciousness) or complex partial seizures (in which consciousness is impaired or lost). Complex partial seizures often involve periods of "automatic behavior" and altered consciousness. This is typified by purposeful-looking behavior, such as buttoning or unbuttoning a shirt. Such behavior, however, is unconscious, may be repetitive, and is usually not remembered afterwards.

Diagnosis

Diagnosing epilepsy is a multistep process. According to the Epilepsy Foundation of America: "... the doctor's main tool ... is a careful medical history with as much information as possible about what the seizures looked like and what happened just before they began. The doctor will also perform a thorough physical examination, especially of the nervous system, as well as analysis of blood and other bodily fluids."[7]

The doctor may also order an electroencephalograph (EEG) of the patient's brain activity, which may show patterns that help the doctor decide whether or not someone has epilepsy. Other tests may also be used—such as the CT (computerized tomography) or MRI (magnetic resonance imaging)—in order to look for any growths, scars, or other physical conditions in the brain that may be causing the seizures.

Which tests and how many of them are ordered may vary, depending on how much each test reveals.[8]

Treatment

Anti-epileptic medication is the most common treatment for epilepsy. It's effective in stopping seizures in 70 percent of patients.[9] Interestingly, it's not uncommon for doctors to wait a while before prescribing an anti-seizure medication, especially if the patient is a young child. Unless the EEG of the patient's brain is clearly abnormal, doctors may suggest waiting until a second or even third seizure occurs. Why? Because studies show that an otherwise normal child who has had a single seizure has a relatively low 15 percent risk of a second one.[10]

When anti-epileptic medications are not effective in stopping a person's seizures, other treatment options may be discussed. These include the following:

- Surgery to remove the areas of the brain that are producing the seizures

- Stimulation of the vagus nerve (a large nerve in the neck), where short bursts of electrical energy are directed into the brain via the vagus nerve

- A ketogenic diet (one that is very high in fats and low in carbohydrates), which makes the body burn fat for energy instead of glucose.

According to the Epilepsy Foundation of America, 10 percent of new patients cannot bring their seizures disorder under control despite optimal medical management.[11]

Educational and Developmental Considerations

It's not unusual for seizures to interfere with a child's development and learning. For example, if a student has the type of seizure characterized by periods of fixed staring, he or she is likely to miss parts of what the teacher is saying. If teachers—or other caregivers such as babysitters, daycare providers, preschool teachers, K–12 personnel—observe such an episode, it's important that they document and report it promptly to parents (and the school nurse, if appropriate).

Because epilepsy can affect a child's learning and development (even babies), families will want to learn more about the systems of help that are available. Much of that help comes from the nation's special education law, the Individuals with Disabilities Education Act (IDEA), which makes available these two sets of services:

- **Early intervention:** A system of services to help infants and toddlers with disabilities (before their third birthday) and their families.

- **Special education and related services:** Services available through the public school system for school-aged children, including preschoolers (ages three to twenty-one).

In both of these systems, eligible children receive special services designed to address the developmental, functional, and educational needs resulting from their disability.

More about Services under IDEA

The process of finding a child eligible for early intervention or special education and related services under IDEA begins with a comprehensive and individual evaluation of the child in order to:

- establish that the child does, indeed, have a disability;

- get a detailed picture of how the disability affects the child functionally, developmentally, and academically; and

- document the child's special needs related to the disability.

This evaluation is provided free of charge through either the early intervention system (for infants and toddlers under the age of three) or through the local school system (for children ages three to twenty-one). Under IDEA, children with epilepsy are usually found eligible for services under the category of "Other Health Impairment" (OHI). We've included IDEA's definition of OHI below.

IDEA's Definition of "Other Health Impairment"

The nation's special education law specifically mentions epilepsy in its definition of "Other Health Impairment," a category under which children may be found eligible for special education and related services. Here's IDEA's definition:

> (9) Other health impairment means having limited strength, vitality, or alertness, including a heightened alertness to environmental stimuli, that results in limited alertness with respect to the educational environment, that—

(i) Is due to chronic or acute health problems such as asthma, attention deficit disorder or attention deficit hyperactivity disorder, diabetes, epilepsy, a heart condition, hemophilia, lead poisoning, leukemia, nephritis, rheumatic fever, sickle cell anemia, and Tourette syndrome; and

(ii) Adversely affects a child's educational performance. [34 CFR §300.8(c)(9)]

When a baby or toddler is found eligible for early intervention, parents meet with the early intervention staff, and together they develop what is known as an Individualized Family Service Plan, or IFSP. The IFSP will describe the child's unique needs as well as the services the child will receive to address those needs. The IFSP will also emphasize the unique needs of the family, so that parents and other family members will know how to help their young child with epilepsy. Early intervention services may be provided on a sliding-fee basis, meaning that the costs to the family will depend upon their income.

When a child is found eligible for special education and related services, school staff and parents meet and develop what is known as an Individualized Education Program, or IEP. This document is very important in the educational life of a child with epilepsy, because it details the nature of the child's needs and the services that the public school system will provide free of charge to address those needs.

Succeeding at School

Special education and related services can be very helpful to children with epilepsy attending public school. Because the disorder affects memory and concentration, accommodations in the classroom and during testing are key to students' academic success.

Related services may be every bit as important for children with epilepsy, especially school health services and school nurse services—which can provide the child's medication during school hours or give first aid instruction on seizure management to the student's teachers, for example.

Depending on the child's unique needs, other related services may also be necessary so that the student benefits from his or her special education program—for example, counseling services. Children and youth with epilepsy must deal with the psychological and social aspects of the condition. These include public misperceptions and fear of seizures, loss of self-control during the seizure episode, and compliance with medications. Counseling services may help students with epilepsy address the complexities of living with this disorder. The school can also help by providing epilepsy education programs for staff and students, including information on how to recognize a seizure and what to do if a seizure occurs.

It is important that the teachers and school staff are informed about the child's condition, possible effects of medication, and what to do in case a seizure occurs at school. Most parents find that a friendly conversation with the teacher(s) at the beginning of the school year is the best way to handle the situation. Even if a child has seizures that are largely controlled by medication, it is still best to notify the school staff about the condition.

School personnel and the family should work together to monitor the effectiveness of medication as well as any side effects. If a child's physical or intellectual skills seem to change, it is important to tell the doctor. There may also be hearing or perception problems caused by changes in the brain. Written observations of both the family and school staff will be helpful in discussions with the child's doctor.

Accommodations in the Classroom

The accommodations that a child with epilepsy receives are determined by his or her IEP team (which includes the parents). Here are some possibilities to consider.[12]

To address memory deficits, do the following:

- Provide written or pictorial instructions.

- Use voice recordings of verbal instructions.

- Have a peer buddy take notes for the student or permit tape recording.

- Divide large tasks into smaller steps.

- Provide a checklist of assignments and a calendar with due dates.

- Decrease memory demands during class work and testing (e.g., use recognition rather than recall tasks).

To address health concerns, do the following:

- Be flexible about time missed from school to seek treatment or adjust to new medications.

- Provide extra time for assignments and a modified workload (fatigue is a common side effect of seizures and medications).

- Replace fluorescent lighting with full-spectrum lighting.
- Provide private area to rest or recover from a seizure.

References

1. Epilepsy Foundation of America. (n.d.). What is epilepsy? Available online at: http://www.epilepsyfoundation.org/about/.

2. Ibid.

3. National Institute of Neurological Disorders and Stroke. (2010, May). NINDS epilepsy information page. Available online at: http://www.ninds.nih.gov/disorders/epilepsy/epilepsy.htm.

4. Epilepsy Foundation of America. (n.d.). Epilepsy and seizure statistics. Available online at: www.epilepsyfoundation.org/about/statistics.cfm.

5. Ibid.

6. National Institute of Neurological Disorders and Stroke. (2010, May). Seizures and epilepsy: Hope through research. Available online at: http://www.ninds.nih.gov/disorders/epilepsy/detail_epilepsy.htm.

7. Epilepsy Foundation of America. (n.d.). Epilepsy and seizure statistics. Available online at: http://www.epilepsyfoundation.org/about/diagnosis/.

8. Ibid.

9. Epilepsy Foundation of America. (n.d.). Epilepsy and seizure statistics. Available online at: www.epilepsyfoundation.org/about/statistics.cfm.

10. Epilepsy Foundation of America. (n.d.). The decision to treat. Available online at: http://www.epilepsyfoundation.org/about/treatment/.

11. Epilepsy Foundation of America. (n.d.). Epilepsy and seizure statistics. Available online at: www.epilepsyfoundation.org/about/statistics.cfm.

12. Kitchen, S.G. (2010). Accommodation and compliance series: Employees with epilepsy. Available online at the Job Accommodations Network website: http://askjan.org/media/epilepsy.html.

Chapter 20

Fetal Alcohol Spectrum Disorders

Chapter Contents

Section 20.1

Facts about Fetal Alcohol Spectrum Disorders

Reprinted from "Facts about FASDs," Centers for Disease Control and Prevention, October 6, 2010.

Fetal alcohol spectrum disorders (FASDs) are a group of conditions that can occur in a person whose mother drank alcohol during pregnancy. These effects can include physical problems and problems with behavior and learning. Often, a person with an FASD has a mix of these problems.

Cause and Prevention

FASDs are caused by a woman drinking alcohol during pregnancy. There is no known amount of alcohol that is safe to drink while pregnant. There is also no safe time to drink during pregnancy and no safe kind of alcohol to drink while pregnant.

To prevent FASDs, a woman should not drink alcohol while she is pregnant, or even when she might get pregnant. This is because a woman could get pregnant and not know for several weeks or more. In the United States, half of pregnancies are unplanned.

Signs and Symptoms

FASDs refer to the whole range of effects that can happen to a person whose mother drank alcohol during pregnancy. These conditions can affect each person in different ways, and can range from mild to severe.

A person with an FASD might have the following:

- Abnormal facial features, such as a smooth ridge between the nose and upper lip (this ridge is called the philtrum)

- Small head size

- Shorter-than-average height

- Low body weight

- Poor coordination

- Hyperactive behavior

- Difficulty paying attention

- Poor memory

- Difficulty in school (especially with math)

- Learning disabilities

- Speech and language delays

- Intellectual disability or low intelligence quotient (IQ)

- Poor reasoning and judgment skills

- Sleep and sucking problems as a baby

- Vision or hearing problems

- Problems with the heart, kidneys, or bones

Types of FASDs

Different terms are used to describe FASDs, depending on the type of symptoms:

- **Fetal alcohol syndrome (FAS):** FAS represents the severe end of the FASD spectrum. Fetal death is the most extreme outcome from drinking alcohol during pregnancy. People with FAS might have abnormal facial features, growth problems, and central nervous system (CNS) problems. People with FAS can have problems with learning, memory, attention span, communication, vision, or hearing. They might have a mix of these problems. People with FAS often have a hard time in school and trouble getting along with others.

- **Alcohol-related neurodevelopmental disorder (ARND):** People with ARND might have intellectual disabilities and problems with behavior and learning. They might do poorly in school and have difficulties with math, memory, attention, judgment, and poor impulse control.

- **Alcohol-related birth defects (ARBD):** People with ARBD might have problems with the heart, kidneys, or bones or with hearing. They might have a mix of these.

The term "fetal alcohol effects" (FAE) was previously used to describe intellectual disabilities and problems with behavior and learning in a person whose mother drank alcohol during pregnancy. In 1996, the Institute of Medicine (IOM) replaced FAE with the terms "alcohol-related neurodevelopmental disorder" (ARND) and "alcohol-related birth defects" (ARBD).

Diagnosis

The term "FASDs" is not meant for use as a clinical diagnosis. The Centers for Disease Control and Prevention (CDC) worked with a group of experts and organizations to review the research and develop guidelines for diagnosing FAS. The guidelines were developed for FAS only. CDC and its partners are working to put together diagnostic criteria for other FASDs, such as ARND. Clinical and scientific research on these conditions is going on now.

Diagnosing FAS can be hard because there is no medical test, like a blood test, for it. And other disorders, such as ADHD (attention deficit hyperactivity disorder) and Williams syndrome, have some symptoms like FAS.

To diagnose FAS, doctors look for the following things:

- Abnormal facial features (e.g., smooth ridge between nose and upper lip)

- Lower-than-average height, weight, or both

- Central nervous system problems (e.g., small head size, problems with attention and hyperactivity, poor coordination)

- Prenatal alcohol exposure, although confirmation is not required to make a diagnosis

Treatment

FASDs last a lifetime. There is no cure for FASDs, but research shows that early intervention treatment services can improve a child's development.

There are many types of treatment options, including medication to help with some symptoms, behavior and education therapy, parent training, and other alternative approaches. No one treatment is right for every child. Good treatment plans will include close monitoring, follow-ups, and changes as needed along the way.

Also, "protective factors" can help reduce the effects of FASDs and help people with these conditions reach their full potential.[1,2]

Protective factors include the following:

- Diagnosis before six years of age

- Loving, nurturing, and stable home environment during the school years

- Absence of violence

- Involvement in special education and social services

Get Help!

If you think your child might have an FASD, talk to your child's doctor and share your concerns. Don't wait!

If you or the doctor thinks there could be a problem, ask the doctor for a referral to a specialist (someone who knows about FASDs), such as a developmental pediatrician, child psychologist, or clinical geneticist. In some cities, there are clinics whose staffs have special training in diagnosing and treating children with FASDs.

At the same time, call your state's public early childhood system to ask for a free evaluation to find out if your child qualifies for treatment services. This is sometimes called a Child Find evaluation. You do not need to wait for a doctor's referral or a medical diagnosis to make this call.

Where to call for a free evaluation from the state depends on your child's age:

- If your child is younger than three years old, contact your local early intervention system.

- If your child is three years old or older, contact your local public school system.

Even if your child is not old enough for kindergarten or is not enrolled in a public school, call your local elementary school or board of education and ask to speak with someone who can help you have your child evaluated.

References

1. Streissguth, A.P., Bookstein, F.L., Barr, H.M., Sampson, P.D., O'Malley, K., and Young, J.K. (2004). Risk factors for adverse life outcomes in fetal alcohol syndrome and fetal alcohol effects. *Developmental and Behavioral Pediatrics*, 5(4), 228–38.

2. Streissguth, A.P., Barr, H.M., Kogan, J. and Bookstein, F. L., Understanding the occurrence of secondary disabilities in clients with fetal alcohol syndrome (FAS) and fetal alcohol effects (FAE). Final report to the Centers for Disease Control and Prevention (CDC). Seattle: University of Washington, Fetal Alcohol & Drug Unit; August 1996. Tech. Rep. No. 96-06.

Section 20.2

Fetal Alcohol Exposure and the Brain

Reprinted from the National Institute on Alcohol Abuse and Alcoholism, National Institutes of Health, December 2000. Reviewed by David A. Cooke, M.D., FACP, January 2012.

Nearly thirty years ago, scientists first coined the term "fetal alcohol syndrome" (FAS) to describe a pattern of birth defects found in children of mothers who consumed alcohol during pregnancy.[1,2] Today, FAS remains the leading known preventable cause of mental retardation.[3] Behavioral and neurological problems associated with prenatal alcohol exposure may lead to poor academic performance as well as legal and employment difficulties in adolescence and adulthood.[4] Despite attempts to increase public awareness of the risks involved, increasing numbers of women are drinking during pregnancy.[5] This section provides data on the prevalence and nature of the neurobehavioral problems associated with alcohol use during pregnancy, explores potential mechanisms underlying alcohol-induced damage to the developing brain, and discusses prevention research.

Definitions and Incidence

FAS is defined by four criteria: maternal drinking during pregnancy; a characteristic pattern of facial abnormalities; growth retardation; and brain damage, which often is manifested by intellectual difficulties or behavioral problems.[3] When signs of brain damage appear following fetal alcohol exposure in the absence of other indications of FAS, the condition is termed "alcohol-related neurodevelopmental disorder" (ARND).[3]

Investigators have used both passive and active methods to determine the overall incidence of FAS and ARND. The passive approach uses data collected from existing medical records, which are often based on information recorded at birth. However, the criteria required for these diagnoses may not be apparent at birth and often develop gradually from infancy through the first few years of grade school.[6] In the active approach, investigators use a defined set of diagnostic criteria to screen all members of a selected population for FAS and other alcohol-related problems. Although both strategies have limitations, active ascertainment provides more accurate prevalence data for the study population, especially if children are examined at elementary school age.[3] For example, a comprehensive survey of 992 first-grade students in twelve of the thirteen elementary schools in a South African community revealed an FAS incidence of more than 40 FAS cases per 1,000 births among children ages five to nine.[7] In the United States, a preliminary active ascertainment of FAS in a single county in Washington State yielded a minimum estimate of 3.1 per 1,000 first-grade students.[8] By comparison, passive estimates of FAS rates range from 0.33 to 3 infants per 1,000 births.[3,9]

Specific Cognitive and Behavioral Impairments

The broad range of cognitive and behavioral disabilities associated with prenatal alcohol exposure was attributed by many researchers to a generalized impairment of mental functioning. However, recent studies on FAS and ARND reveal that specific neurobehavioral functions are consistently impaired, whereas others are spared.[10-13] Thus, the outlook for persons diagnosed with FAS or ARND should not be considered hopeless.[14,15] Some specific neurobehavioral impairments associated with prenatal alcohol exposure are discussed below.

Verbal learning: Children prenatally exposed to alcohol exhibit a variety of problems with language and memory.[3,10] For example, Mattson and colleagues[11] found that children with FAS ages five to sixteen learned fewer words compared with a group of children of comparable mental age who did not have FAS. However, both groups demonstrated equal ability to recall information learned previously. These findings indicate that FAS-related learning problems occur during the initial stages of memory formation (i.e., encoding). Once encoded, verbal information can be retained and recalled, subject to normal rates of forgetting.[11,13] Clinically, this pattern helps distinguish FAS from Down syndrome, in which learning and recall are equally impaired.[16]

Visual-spatial learning: Children of mothers who drank heavily during pregnancy perform poorly on tasks that involve learning spatial relationships among objects. In one experiment, groups of children with and without FAS were equal in their ability to recall common, small household and schoolroom objects (e.g., a paper clip or spoon) that had been placed within sight on a table and then removed.[17] However, children with FAS had greater difficulty subsequently restoring the objects to their original positions on the table.[17]

Attention: Attention problems have been considered a hallmark of prenatal alcohol exposure.[13] Consequently, FAS is often incorrectly diagnosed as attention deficit hyperactivity disorder (ADHD) and treated inappropriately.[18] Coles and colleagues[18] found that children with ADHD exhibited difficulty focusing and sustaining attention over time. In contrast, children who were exposed to alcohol prenatally were able to focus and maintain attention, but displayed difficulty in shifting attention from one task to another (i.e., set shifting).[18]

Reaction time: Individual differences in intelligence are based in part on how quickly the brain processes information. Prenatal alcohol exposure has been associated with slower, less efficient information processing in school-age children.[19] Jacobson and colleagues[20] found similar problems in children as young as six and a half months. These researchers recorded the eye movements of infants reacting to the appearance, movement, and disappearance of a repeating sequence of geometric designs and colors on a video screen. Maternal drinking during pregnancy was related to longer reaction times among the children, suggesting slower, less efficient information processing.[20]

Executive functions: Important deficits in FAS involve executive functions (i.e., activities that require abstract thinking, such as planning and organizing). For example, problems with set shifting are common, as noted earlier. Children prenatally exposed to alcohol respond poorly when asked to switch from naming animals to naming types of furniture, and then back to naming animals.[21] They also have difficulty abandoning demonstrably ineffective strategies when approaching problem-solving tasks,[21,22] a type of behavioral inflexibility referred to as perseveration. Perseveration and impaired set shifting are consistent with distractibility and impulsivity, factors that at least theoretically might contribute to attention and learning problems.[11,22,23]

Effects on Brain Structure

The behavioral and cognitive impairments associated with FAS reflect underlying structural or functional changes in the brain.[24] Techniques for viewing the living brain, such as magnetic resonance imaging (MRI), reveal reduced overall brain size in persons with FAS and disproportionate reductions in the size of specific brain structures.[24]

One such area is the deep-brain structure called the basal ganglia.[25,26] Damage to the basal ganglia impairs spatial memory and set shifting in animals[26,27] and various cognitive processes in humans.[28] Another common finding is reduced size of the cerebellum,[25,29] a structure involved in balance, gait, coordination, and cognition.[30] Finally, prenatal alcohol exposure is the major cause of impaired development[30] or complete absence[30,31] of the corpus callosum, a band of nerve fibers that forms the major communication link between the right and left halves of the brain. Approximately 7 percent of children with FAS may lack a corpus callosum, an incidence rate twenty times higher than that in the general population.[30]

Potential Causal Mechanisms

The mechanisms that underlie alcohol-induced fetal brain damage have been studied in experimental animals and in nerve cells (i.e., neurons) grown in culture.[32] Within the fetus, embryonic cells destined to become brain neurons grow in number, move to their ultimate locations, and mature into a wide variety of functionally distinct neuronal cell types, eventually forming connections with other brain cells in a predetermined pattern. Alcohol metabolism is associated with increased susceptibility to cell damage caused by potentially harmful substances called free radicals. Free radical damage can kill sensitive populations of brain cells at critical times of development in the first trimester of pregnancy.[33,34] Other animal experiments suggest that the third trimester may also represent a particularly sensitive period for brain cell damage associated with FAS.[35]

Alcohol or its metabolic breakdown products can also interfere with brain development by altering the production or function of natural regulatory substances that help promote the orderly growth and differentiation of neurons.[32] Research using animals or cell cultures shows that many of alcohol's adverse effects on brain cells can be prevented by treatments aimed at restoring the balance of regulatory substances upset by alcohol.[36,37] Promising results have also been obtained in similar experiments by administering substances (i.e., antioxidants) that help protect cells against free radical–induced cell damage.[38] This is only one of several potential mechanisms that may contribute to alcohol-related fetal injury. Further research is needed to determine if such an approach might prove both effective and safe in humans during pregnancy.

Effect of Maternal Drinking Levels

The minimum quantity of alcohol required to produce adverse fetal consequences is unknown.[22] Clinically significant deficits are not common in children whose mothers drank less than approximately five drinks per occasion once per week.[39] However, vulnerability to a given alcohol level during pregnancy varies markedly from person to person, possibly reflecting genetic factors, nutritional status, environmental factors, co-occurring diseases, and maternal age.[40]

Prospects for Prevention

FAS and ARND could be completely eliminated if pregnant women did not consume alcohol. Therefore, recent FAS prevention research has focused on finding and treating women who drink during pregnancy. For example, TWEAK[41]—a brief questionnaire for assessing alcohol problems in women—shows promise as a screening instrument for identifying risk drinking by pregnant women.[42]

Pregnant women who are consuming alcohol but are not "problem" drinkers may decrease their drinking level following such an assessment without subsequent treatment.[43] An overall decline in alcohol consumption has also been noted among pregnant women following a brief intervention, which can be conducted by a primary care provider.[43] Such sessions may include a discussion of the risks of maternal drinking and suggested alternatives to alcohol use. Pregnant women with higher drinking levels may benefit from a one-hour motivational interview focusing on the health of the unborn child.[44] Women who are alcohol dependent require intensive alcoholism treatment.[44]

Fetal Exposure and the Brain: A Commentary by NIAAA Director Enoch Gordis, M.D.

Since our last *Alcohol Alert* on FAS, the pace of research on the effects of alcohol on the fetus has accelerated appreciably. Progress has been made most notably in research aimed at understanding the basic mechanisms involved in the neurobiological damage that occurs in alcohol-exposed fetuses and in developing potential new therapies to prevent that damage. We also have increased our understanding of the long-term cognitive and physical challenges of children who were exposed to alcohol in the womb. As a result, clinicians and behavioral scientists are finding ways to identify these children early and ways to help.

Despite the many gains in knowledge, we still do not know if there is a "safe" dose of alcohol that can be consumed by pregnant women without risking damage to their unborn children. Until such a safe dose, if it exists, can be determined, the only responsible advice to women who wish to become pregnant and to those who are pregnant is to avoid alcohol use entirely. Unfortunately, many women continue to drink during pregnancy. Furthermore, many of the women who continue to drink during pregnancy are at highest risk for having children with fetal alcohol syndrome and related problems. Thus, finding potent new ways to reach populations at risk and to influence changes in their behavior remains a challenge for alcohol research.

References

1. Lemoine, P., Harousseau, H., Borteyru, J.P., and Menuet, J.C. Les enfants de parents alcooliques: Anomalies observées à propos de 127 cas. *Ouest Med* 21:476–82, 1968.

2. Jones, K.L., and Smith, D.W. Recognition of the fetal alcohol syndrome in early infancy. Lancet 2:999–1001, 1973.

3. Stratton, K.; Howe, C.; and Battaglia, F., eds. Fetal Alcohol Syndrome: Diagnosis, Epidemiology, Prevention, and Treatment. Washington, D.C.: National Academy Press, 1996.

4. Thomas, S.E., Kelly, S.J., Mattson, S.N., and Riley, E.P. Comparison of social abilities of children with fetal alcohol syndrome to those of children with similar IQ scores and normal controls. Alcohol Clin Exp Res 22(2):528–33, 1998.

5. Ebrahim, S.H., Diekman, S.T., Floyd, R.L., and Decoufle, P. Comparison of binge drinking among pregnant and nonpregnant women, United States, 1991–1995. Am J Obstet Gynecol 180(1, Part 1):1–7, 1999.

6. Aase, J.M. Clinical recognition of FAS: Difficulties of detection and diagnosis. Alcohol Health Res World 18(1):5–9, 1994.

7. May, P.A., Brooke, L., Gossage, J.P., et al. Epidemiology of fetal alcohol syndrome in a South African community in the Western Cape Province. *Am J Pub Health* 90(12):1905–12, 2000.

8. Clarren, S.K., Randels, S.P., Sanderson, M., and Fineman, R.M. Screening for fetal alcohol syndrome in primary schools: A feasibility study. *Teratology* 63(1):3–10, 2001.

9. Abel, E.L., and Sokol, R.J. A revised conservative estimate of the incidence of FAS and its economic impact. *Alcoholism: Clin Exp Res* 15(3):514–24, 1991.

10. Janzen, L.A., Nanson, J.L., and Block, G.W. Neuropsychological evaluation of preschoolers with fetal alcohol syndrome. *Neurotoxicol Teratology* 17(3):273–79, 1995.

11. Mattson, S.N., Riley, E.P., Delis, D.C., Stern, C., and Jones, K.L. Verbal learning and memory in children with fetal alcohol syndrome. *Alcohol Clin Exp Res* 20(5):810–16, 1996a.

12. Olson, H.C., Feldman, J.J., Streissguth, A.P., Sampson, P.D., and Bookstein, F.L. Neuropsychological deficits in adolescents with fetal alcohol syndrome: Clinical findings. *Alcohol Clin Exp Res* 22(9):1998–2012, 1998.

13. Mattson, S.N., and Riley, E.P. A review of the neurobehavioral deficits in children with fetal alcohol syndrome or prenatal exposure to alcohol. *Alcohol Clin Exp Res* 22(2):279–94, 1998.

14. Mattson, S.N., Riley, E.P., Gramling, L., et al. Neuropsychological comparisons of alcohol-exposed children with or without physical features of fetal alcohol syndrome. *Neuropsychology* 12(1):146–53, 1998.

15. Ernhart, C.B., Greene, T., Sokol, R.J., et al. Neonatal diagnosis of fetal alcohol syndrome: Not necessarily a hopeless prognosis. *Alcohol Clin Exp Res* 19(6):1550–57, 1995.

16. Mattson, S.N., Goodman, A.M., Caine, C., Delis, D.C., and Riley, E.P. Executive functioning in children with heavy prenatal alcohol exposure. *Alcohol Clin Exp Res* 23(11):1808–15, 1999.

17. Uecker, A., and Nadel, L. Spatial locations gone awry: Object and spatial memory deficits in children with fetal alcohol syndrome. *Neuropsychologia* 34(3):209–23, 1996.

18. Coles, C.D., Platzman, K.A., Raskind-Hood, C.L., et al. A comparison of children affected by prenatal alcohol exposure and attention deficit, hyperactivity disorder. *Alcohol Clin Exp Res* 21(1):150–61, 1997.

19. Streissguth, A.P., Barr, H.M., Sampson, P.D., et al. Attention, distraction, and reaction time at age 7 years and prenatal

alcohol exposure. *Neurobehav Toxicol Teratology* 8(16):717–25, 1986.

20. Jacobson, S.W., Jacobson, J.L., and Sokol, R.J. Effects of fetal alcohol exposure on infant reaction time. *Alcohol Clin Exp Res* 18(5):1125–32, 1994.

21. Kodituwakku, P.W., Handmaker, N.S., Cutler, S.K., Weathersby, E.K., and Handmaker, S.D. Specific impairments in self-regulation in children exposed to alcohol prenatally. *Alcohol Clin Exp Res* 19(6):1558–64, 1995.

22. Roebuck, T.M., Mattson, S.N., and Riley, E.P. Behavioral and psychosocial profiles of alcohol-exposed children. *Alcohol Clin Exp Res* 23(6):1070–76, 1999.

23. Hunt, E., Streissguth, A.P., Kerr, B., and Olson, H.C. Mothers' alcohol consumption during pregnancy: Effects on spatial-visual reasoning in 14-year-old children. *Psychol Science* 6(6):339–42, 1995.

24. Roebuck, T.M., Mattson, S.N., and Riley, E.P. A review of the neuroanatomical findings in children with fetal alcohol syndrome or prenatal exposure to alcohol. *Alcohol Clin Exp Res* 22(2):339–44, 1998.

25. Mattson, S.N., Riley, E.P., Jernigan, T.L., et al. A decrease in the size of the basal ganglia following prenatal alcohol exposure: A preliminary report. *Neurotoxicol Teratology* 16(3):283–89, 1994.

26. Mattson, S.N., Riley, E.P., Sowell, E.R., et al. A decrease in the size of the basal ganglia in children with fetal alcohol syndrome. *Alcohol Clin Exp Res* 20(6):1088–93, 1996b.

27. Mattson, S.N., and Riley, E.P. Implicit and explicit memory functioning in children with heavy prenatal alcohol exposure. *J Int Neuropsychol Soc* 5(5):462–71, 1999.

28. Bannister, R. *Brain and Bannister's Clinical Neurology. 7th ed.* New York: Oxford University Press, 1992.

29. Sowell, E.R., Jernigan, T.L., Mattson, S.N., et al. Abnormal development of the cerebellar vermis in children prenatally exposed to alcohol: Size reduction in lobules I–V. *Alcohol Clin Exp Res* 20(1):31–34, 1996.

30. Riley, E.P., Mattson, S.N., Sowell, E.R., et al. Abnormalities of the corpus callosum in children prenatally exposed to alcohol. *Alcohol Clin Exp Res* 19(5):1198–1202, 1995.

31. Swayze, II, V.W., Johnson, V.P., Hanson, J.W., et al. Magnetic resonance imaging of brain anomalies in fetal alcohol syndrome. *Pediatrics* 99(2):232–40, 1997.

32. Michaelis, E.K., and Michaelis, M.L. Cellular and molecular bases of alcohol's teratogenic effects. *Alcohol Health Res World* 18(1):17–21, 1994.

33. Cartwright, M.M., and Smith, S.M. Increased cell death and reduced neural crest cell numbers in ethanol-exposed embryos: Partial basis for the fetal alcohol syndrome. *Alcohol Clin Exp Res* 19(2):378–86, 1995.

34. Chen, S., and Sulik, K.K. Free radicals and ethanol-induced cytotoxicity in neural crest cells. *Alcohol Clin Exp Res* 20(6):1071–76, 1996.

35. Maier, S.E., Chen, W.-J.A., and West, J.R. The effects of timing and duration of alcohol exposure on development of the fetal brain. In: Abel, E.L., ed. *Fetal Alcohol Syndrome: From Mechanism to Prevention.* Boca Raton, Florida: CRC Press, 1996, 27–50.

36. Luo, J., West, J.R., and Pantazis, N.J. Nerve growth factor and basic fibroblast growth factor protect rat cerebellar granule cells in culture against ethanol-induced cell death. *Alcohol Clin Exp Res* 21(6):1108–20, 1997.

37. Tajuddin, N.F., and Druse, M.J. In utero ethanol exposure decreased the density of serotonin neurons: Maternal ipsapirone treatment exerted a protective effect. *Del Brain Res* 117(1):91–97, 1999.

38. Heaton, M.B., Mitchell, J.J., and Paiva, M. Amelioration of ethanol-induced neurotoxicity in the neonatal rat central nervous system by antioxidant therapy. *Alcohol Clin Exp Res* 24(4):512–18, 2000.

39. Jacobson, J.L., and Jacobson, S.W. Drinking moderately and pregnancy: Effects on child development. *Alcohol Res Health* 23(1):25–30, 1999.

40. Abel, E.L., and Hannigan, J.H. Maternal risk factors in fetal alcohol syndrome: Provocative and permissive influences. *Neurotoxicol Teratology* 17(4):445–62, 1995.

41. Russell, M. New assessment tools for risk drinking during pregnancy: T-ACE, TWEAK, and others. *Alcohol Health Res World* 18(1):55–61, 1994.

42. Chang, G., Wilkins-Haug, L., Berman, S., and Goetz, M.A. The TWEAK: Application in a prenatal setting. *J Stud Alcohol* 60(3):306–9, 1999a.

43. Chang, G., Wilkins-Haug, L., Berman, S., and Goetz, M.A. Brief intervention for alcohol use in pregnancy: A randomized trial. *Addict* 94(10):1499–1508, 1999b.

44. Handmaker, N.S., Miller, W.R., and Manicke, M. Findings of a pilot study of motivational interviewing with pregnant drinkers. *J Stud Alcohol* 60(2):285–87, 1999.

Chapter 21

Gerstmann Syndrome

What is Gerstmann syndrome?

Gerstmann syndrome is a cognitive impairment that results from damage to a specific area of the brain—the left parietal lobe in the region of the angular gyrus. It may occur after a stroke or in association with damage to the parietal lobe. It is characterized by four primary symptoms: a writing disability (agraphia or dysgraphia), a lack of understanding of the rules for calculation or arithmetic (acalculia or dyscalculia), an inability to distinguish right from left, and an inability to identify fingers (finger agnosia). The disorder should not be confused with Gerstmann-Sträussler-Scheinker disease, a type of transmissible spongiform encephalopathy.

In addition to exhibiting the above symptoms, many adults also experience aphasia, (difficulty in expressing oneself when speaking, in understanding speech, or in reading and writing).

There are few reports of the syndrome, sometimes called developmental Gerstmann syndrome, in children. The cause is not known. Most cases are identified when children reach school age, a time when they are challenged with writing and math exercises. Generally, children with the disorder exhibit poor handwriting and spelling skills, and difficulty with math functions, including adding, subtracting, multiplying, and dividing. An inability to differentiate right from left and to discriminate among individual fingers may also be apparent.

"Gerstmann's Syndrome Information Page," National Institute of Neurological Disorders and Stroke, National Institutes of Health, July 2, 2008.

In addition to the four primary symptoms, many children also suffer from constructional apraxia, an inability to copy simple drawings. Frequently, there is also an impairment in reading. Children with a high level of intellectual functioning as well as those with brain damage may be affected with the disorder.

Is there any treatment?

There is no cure for Gerstmann syndrome. Treatment is symptomatic and supportive. Occupational and speech therapies may help diminish the dysgraphia and apraxia. In addition, calculators and word processors may help schoolchildren cope with the symptoms of the disorder.

What is the prognosis?

In adults, many of the symptoms diminish over time. Although it has been suggested that in children symptoms may diminish over time, it appears likely that most children probably do not overcome their deficits, but learn to adjust to them.

What research is being done?

The National Institute of Neurological Disorders and Stroke (NINDS) supports research on disorders that result from damage to the brain, such as dysgraphia. The NINDS and other components of the National Institutes of Health also support research on learning disabilities. Current research avenues focus on developing techniques to diagnose and treat learning disabilities and increase understanding of the biological basis of them.

Chapter 22

Hearing Disabilities

Frequently Asked Questions about Hearing Loss

What causes minimal hearing loss?

Ear infection or otitis media is the most frequent cause of minimal hearing loss in children. It is an inflammation in the middle ear that usually causes fluctuating hearing loss averaging 21–40dB. However, many children are born with minimal hearing loss caused by problems in the inner ear. Because these hearing losses are mild they may go undiagnosed in the early years but they can cause significant problems educationally if they are not addressed.

This diagnosis is often missed and many children with hearing loss due to otitis media will pass a school screening test. Children with learning disabilities frequently have histories of chronic middle ear infection (four to five episodes over a six- to twelve-month period), causing reduced hearing over a significant part of the school year.

What causes hearing loss?

About 50 percent of deafness is hereditary. Genetic hearing loss is not necessarily passed from parent to child, but may appear in other family members. More than 90 percent of the parents of deaf children

---

are hearing people. Most hereditary hearing loss is recessive so both parents need to be carriers. Each parent carries a single copy of a deafness-causing mutation. The carrier rate in the general population for a recessive deafness-causing GJB2 mutation is about one in thirty-three.

Other factors that can cause hearing loss include accidents and injuries, constant high noise levels that eventually cause severe damage to the nerves of the ear, illness or infection, and drugs which adversely effect the organ of hearing. Rubella or other viral infections contracted by the pregnant mother may cause deafness in an unborn child. A problem during the birth process such as a cutoff in the supply of oxygen may affect hearing. Hearing loss may also be part of the aging process in older people and is more likely to be mild. In many cases there may be no clear reason for hearing loss and the cause may never be determined.

Is hearing loss permanent? Can It be corrected?

In order to understand the different types of hearing loss it is important to know something about how normal hearing occurs. Sound waves traveling through air are funneled into the external ear canal, which makes the eardrum with its attached ear bones (malleus = hammer, incus = anvil, stapes = stirrup) vibrate within the air-filled middle ear. This is the ears' conduction system. The piston-like movement of the three bones and eardrum stimulates a fluid wave in the liquid-filled inner ear. The movement of the inner ear fluid bends microscopic nerve endings called hair cells that are the ears' sensory structures. There are thirty thousand hair cells and when they are bent by the movement of the fluid they work like a switch turning on an electrical current that travels through the nerve of hearing to the central auditory centers in the brain.

Conductive hearing loss: Caused by a problem affecting the conduction system. Examples are excessive wax blocking the external ear canal, fluid in the middle ear preventing the eardrum from vibrating, or a disruption or fixation of the bones in the middle ear. Many conductive hearing losses can be treated and eliminated with medication or surgery. If a problem in the middle ear cannot be corrected, hearing aids and other assistive devices may be helpful.

Sensorineural hearing loss: Caused by a problem in the inner ear hair cells (sensory loss) or auditory nerve (neural loss). Some or all of the hair cells in the cochlea may be damaged or absent. It is also possible that the auditory nerve from the cochlea to the brain may be damaged, incompletely formed, or there may be problems with transmission of sound across the auditory nerve. Infrequently, the auditory nerve may have a tumor growing in it which is generally benign (acoustic neuroma). This type of loss is not reversible. Most people with sensorineural hearing loss benefit from hearing aids. If the hearing loss is severe or profound, a cochlear implant may be recommended. A cochlear implant can be thought of as a very strong hearing aid which is surgically implanted. Sensorineural hearing loss can be stable, can fluctuate or be progressive, and can even worsen as children get older. It is important to monitor children's hearing to determine the stability of their hearing loss. Young children should be tested at least twice yearly. Older children should be tested annually. Your child should always be retested if you suspect a change in his/her hearing ability.

Mixed hearing loss: A combination of conductive and sensorineural losses.

Will my child ever talk?

Almost all children who are deaf can learn to speak. With the use of powerful hearing aids and/or cochlear implant and speech therapy, a deaf child can learn to hear which is the first step to learning to talk.

Testing for Hearing Loss

When should my child be tested for hearing loss?

Children should be tested for hearing loss as early as possible. Ideally all newborns should be screened for hearing loss before they leave the hospital. The Center for Disease Control's Early Hearing Detection and Intervention (EHDI) program funds newborn hearing screening programs in many states. The EDHI website covers topics such as screening guidelines, state programs, and resources for parents and professionals.

Many things can affect hearing as a child gets older. Even if an infant passes newborn hearing screening, children should be tested again if any concern develops about hearing or speech and language development.

There are numerous testing measures available to determine the hearing status of children of all ages. Detecting deafness early enables children with hearing loss to receive services that promote language, cognitive development, and social interaction early, during the years that are crucial to academic and social development. Hearing should be screened at birth and two to three times a year during the first few years of life and yearly throughout schools years. This can be done in the pediatrician's office or at school. If there is a question about hearing, a child should have a diagnostic evaluation by an audiologist.

How are infants tested for hearing loss?

A baby's hearing can be tested hours after birth through two techniques: automated auditory brainstem response screening (ABR) and/or otoacoustic emissions screening (OAE). The ABR monitors brain activity that occurs in response to sound. OAE's are a quick, noninvasive probe measure that determines if the cochlear, or inner ear, is working normally. Both techniques are painless, easy to administer, relatively inexpensive, and accurate. They can be done while an infant is sleeping. Early diagnosis is of major importance because the earlier the hearing loss is diagnosed the sooner intervention can begin, leading to better communication skills in the child. It is important to remember that these are screening tests. If a concern develops about hearing it is important to have a diagnostic evaluation with an audiologist.

Why is it important to have my baby's hearing screened early?

The most important time for a child to be exposed to and learn language is in the first three years of life. Children hear even before they are born and begin learning speech and language in the first six months of life. Hearing is critical for developing speech and language. Even before a child begins to talk they are hearing speech around them and starting to learn to understand what the people around them are saying. Research suggests that children who have hearing impairment and receive early intervention before six months of age have better language skills than those who don't. The earlier you know about deafness or hearing loss, the sooner you can begin treatment approaches that will help your child learn to communicate.

Where can my child's hearing be tested?

Many hospitals automatically screen all newborns for hearing loss. Many hospitals have speech and hearing clinics with audiologists who can test your child's hearing. Your pediatrician or family physician can also provide a referral to an ear, nose, and throat or otology practice that has a licensed audiologist on staff or to an audiologist in a hospital or to an audiology practice where your child can be tested. Audiologists can perform hearing tests, refer patients for medical treatment to an otolaryngologist (a physician specializing in ear, nose, and throat problems), and provide hearing rehabilitation services. Audiologists work in hospitals, clinics, private doctor's offices, public and private schools, universities, speech and hearing centers, and nursing homes. They are also listed in the yellow pages. It is best to find a pediatric audiologist who has extensive experience working with children.

What is an audiologist?

An audiologist is a professional with a masters or doctoral degree who diagnoses, treats, and manages individuals with hearing loss or balance problems. Audiologists have special training in the prevention, identification, assessment, and nonmedical treatment of hearing disorders. Audiologists receive professional certification and licensure and are the most qualified professionals to perform hearing tests, refer patients for medical treatment, and provide hearing rehabilitation services including hearing aids.

Audiologists determine appropriate treatment through a complete medical history and a variety of specialized hearing and balance tests. Based on the diagnosis, the audiologist presents treatment options to patients with hearing impairment or balance problems. Audiologists dispense and fit hearing aids as part of a comprehensive treatment program. They refer patients to physicians when the hearing or balance problem requires medical or surgical evaluation or treatment.

What is a speech-language pathologist and how do they help children with hearing loss?

Speech-language pathologists work with a team that can include parents, audiologists, psychologists, social workers, classroom teachers, special education teachers, guidance counselors, and physicians to provide comprehensive language and speech assessments for children. These services help children with communication skills, cognitive abilities, and social interaction. Services provided by speech-language pathologists include memory retraining, cognitive skills, language development, and efforts to improve abstract thinking. These services can help children overcome their disabilities, gain self-esteem, and lead productive and meaningful lives.

Hearing Loss and Learning

How does hearing loss affect learning?

Good hearing is essential to the social and intellectual development of infants and young children. Hearing loss can affect learning, speech, attention, and emotional development. It also affects reading, writing, and academic performance. These deficits can occur as early as kindergarten and first grade. Most children with hearing loss begin to show significant learning difficulties by the third grade due to the increasing complexity of language, social interaction, and verbal communications. Some of these problems can even affect children with minimal hearing loss. Children with minimal hearing loss experience problems hearing faint or distant speech and can miss classroom instruction and subtle conversational cues that could cause a child to react inappropriately. They have difficulty following fast-paced verbal exchanges and hearing the fine word-sound distinctions such as plurality, tense, possessives, etc. In addition, a child with a minimal hearing loss may appear immature and tire more easily than normal-hearing children because of the extra effort needed to hear.

What are signs that a communication disorder is affecting school performance?

Often hearing problems are mistaken for attention and behavior problems and are not properly identified as hearing loss. Problems in language development can lead to difficulty in learning to listen, speak, read, or write. Children with communication disorders who do not receive treatment may perform at a poor academic level, struggle with reading, have difficulty understanding and expressing language, misunderstand social cues, avoid attending school, show poor judgment, and have difficulty taking tests.

What is auditory processing disorder and how does it affect my child's learning?

Auditory processing disorder (APD) refers to the process of how the brain takes in auditory information. Even though children with APD can hear well, they may have difficulty using those sounds in speech and language because their brain does not pick up the electrical signals coming from their ears. Children with APD may have trouble listening, following verbal directions, developing language, remembering auditory information, remaining attentive, and understanding speech. All of these difficulties may worsen in noisy acoustic environments, such as classrooms.

It is important to understand that APD cannot be diagnosed from a checklist of symptoms. No matter how many symptoms of APD a child may have, only careful and accurate diagnostic tests can determine the underlying cause. To diagnose APD, an audiologist administers a series of tests in a sound-treated room. Most of the tests for APD require that a child be at least five years of age so that test interpretation is possible. There are many types of auditory processing deficits so once a diagnosis is made individualized management and treatment activities can be recommended that address each child's specific areas of difficulty.

Hearing Aids

Does a hearing aid "fix" hearing?

Hearing aids cannot restore perfect or normal hearing because a sensorineural hearing loss involves damage to some part of the inner ear (usually the cochlear). Some degree of sound distortion usually occurs. A hearing aid can amplify the loudness of the sound, but even with the most current hearing aids speech may not be completely clear. Because young children have very plastic brains, children with hearing loss can learn to listen and speak through auditory training and speech and language therapy.

Do all children with hearing loss need to wear hearing aids?

Children with permanent hearing loss should be properly amplified. However, some children with severe to profound hearing loss in both ears may find that they do not get enough benefit from hearing aids. These children may be candidates for a cochlear implant. Other children may have conductive hearing loss that can be corrected or improved by surgical or medical intervention. If the hearing loss cannot be medically corrected, they may benefit from hearing aids. These children need to be carefully evaluated by medical professionals.

Why is it so important for babies to have hearing aids?

Babies begin developing the skills necessary for language as soon as they are born. Research suggests that there is a critical learning period during which babies learn language, from birth to about three years of age. Research also shows that when infants are aided early on they have the greatest chance of developing language skills comparable to their same-aged peers. Exposure to sound actually stimulates the development of the auditory neural synapses within the brain. If a child is unaided, it is important to begin using a visual form of language early to be certain that the child has a method of communication.

What types of hearing aids are there?

There are essentially two kinds of hearing aid technology: analog and digital.

Analog hearing aids use an analog signal to amplify sound. It is considered basic technology and offers limited adjustment capability. It is the least expensive and the least flexible. They may be very good for patients with more mild hearing loss and for patients who do not rely on listening to understand speech. As technology improves, fewer analog hearing aids are being developed.

Digital hearing aids make use of digital technology to control the auditory signal. They are usually able to provide a cleaner signal and can eliminate background noise. They are also the most expensive.

What styles of hearing aids are there?

Behind the ear (BTE) hearing aids: These are the most commonly dispensed hearing aids. They are available for people with mild to severe hearing losses. BTE hearing aids fit over the ear and use an ear mold to send sound into the ear. They are usually easy to manipulate and can easily be connected to an FM system so they are ideal for children in school.

In-the-ear (ITE) hearing aids: These are very popular with adults who have mild to moderately severe hearing loss because they are smaller than BTE hearing aids. They fill in the ear and usually have one or two small switches which are used to turn the hearing aid on and off or to change programs. These hearing aids are not good for children because they need to be remade every time the child grows (which can be more than once a year). In addition they are not compatible with FM systems.

Completely-in-the-canal (CIC) hearing aids: These are very small hearing aids that fit into the ear canal and are less visible than ITE hearing aids. Because they are so small they may not be able to have all the options that a BTE hearing aid has.

Cochlear Implants

What is a cochlear implant and how does it work?

A cochlear implant is very small, complex electronic device that can provide sound to a person who has a severe or profound hearing loss. One part is surgically placed inside the inner ear while the other external part is worn behind the ear. The cochlear implant delivers electrical stimulation to the inner ear (the cochlea) and bypasses the damaged hair cells, directly stimulating the hearing nerve. These electric currents activate the nerve, which then sends a signal to the brain. The brain learns to recognize this signal and the person experiences this as "hearing."

Unlike a hearing aid, which amplifies sound, the cochlear implant bypasses the damaged, nonworking hair cell parts of the inner ear. In normal hearing, the inner ear converts sound waves into electrical impulses that are sent to the brain, and a hearing person recognizes them as sound. The cochlear implant works in a similar way. It electronically finds useful sounds and then sends them to the brain. However, the result is not the same as normal hearing. Although an implant does not create normal hearing, it provides the person with a digitalized computerized version of sounds. It gives a person with a severe or profound hearing loss access to sound, and can help them to understand speech. With the help of intensive speech, language, and listening therapy, many children with cochlear implants develop excellent speech and language skills and can even communicate over the phone.

What is the ideal age for a deaf child to receive a cochlear implant?

There is no single ideal age for implantation in children. It depends on each family, each child, and the individual factors affecting each child. The best age for implantation is still being debated, but research has clearly indicated that children who receive cochlear implants early have the best results. In 2002 the FDA lowered the age for inclusion in pediatric clinical trials to twelve months. Many centers will implant children as early as six months if there is certainty as to the audiologic indications.

In general, because it is felt that there is a window of opportunity for learning the skills necessary for spoken language, the earlier the implant the better. Speech and language development occurs, for the most part, by age six. Progress does not occur as quickly or as easily after that age. The decision about whether to implant an older child is made individually. Factors to consider include use of hearing aids and auditory skills. If an older child has not worn hearing aids, benefit received from a cochlear implant may be limited.

Children implanted after the age of three years may require more frequent and more intensive speech and language therapy to progress at rates comparable to children implanted before age three. Implantation should always be weighed carefully against the child's educational and therapy environments, level of family involvement, and use of residual hearing with amplification, among other factors.

Who is a candidate for a cochlear implant?

Children and adults who have severe or profound sensorineural hearing loss and derive minimal benefit from hearing aids may be candidates for a cochlear implant.

The benefit that an adult receives from an implant depends on several factors: their degree of hearing loss, their ability to understand speech before receiving the implant, experience using a hearing aid, and the length of time they have been severely deaf. Generally the more experience a person has with hearing and the shorter the duration of their deafness, the more benefit they can expect to receive.

Young children are excellent candidates for cochlear implants because their nervous systems are able to learn easily, which allows them to make use of the sound the implant provides. Children implanted early, who do not have other significant development disabilities and who receive intensive post-implantation speech, language, and listening therapy, may acquire age-appropriate speech, language, developmental, and social skills. They are usually schooled in mainstream educational settings.

What happens after implementation?

Individuals who receive a cochlear implant require continual followup. Children, in particular, require a long period of rehabilitation to teach them to listen to the new sounds and to optimally tune the device.

How long does it take to get maximum benefit from a cochlear implant?

Many factors determine progress. It depends on how long you have had a severe to profound hearing loss and your ability to use hearing with hearing aids. Improvement is slow in the beginning and improves rapidly over the first few months. For adults, generally there are good benefits by three months and it may take about a year to achieve full benefit.

How much do cochlear implants cost?

The total cost is between $40,000 and $60,000. That includes the cost of the device itself and the surgery to implant it. In addition, cochlear implants need to be programmed on a regular basis after surgery. The fees for programming vary depending on individual needs.

Do insurance companies pay for cochlear implants?

Because cochlear implants are recognized as standard treatment for severe to profound nerve deafness, most insurance companies cover them. Medicare, Medicaid, the Veteran's Administration, and other public healthcare plans cover cochlear implants. More than 90 percent of all private health plans cover cochlear implants. Cochlear implant centers usually take the responsibility of obtaining prior authorization from the appropriate insurance company before proceeding with surgery.

My Child's Education

What kinds of schools are available for a hearing impaired child?

There are various options available to educate children who are deaf. The law mandates that public schools are responsible for providing a free and appropriate public school education for all students regardless of disability. School districts are required to provide adequate services to educate hearing-impaired students. Children may be mainstreamed in regular classes or provided special classes for students who are deaf or hard of hearing located in specific schools. A child may also attend a school for the deaf. These schools offer a variety of communication options for parents to choose for their child.

What is an IEP?

Federal law requires that an Individualized Educational Program (IEP) be developed for each child who is identified as having special needs. A hearing loss qualifies children for special education services if they have an educational deficit as a result of the hearing loss and require specially designed instruction to meet their educational needs. An evaluation by a multidisciplinary team will determine eligibility for special education services.

Once special education eligibility has been determined, a meeting will be convened to develop the IEP to help teachers determine exactly what your child needs and to set education goals for your child. The parent has the right to request reasonable services and placements for the child. If a parent disagrees with the services and/or assisted listening devices offered they have the right to appeal the decision.

Communication Options

What communication options are available for my child?

Auditory-verbal: Emphasizes the development and reliance upon auditory cues to receive and comprehend spoken language. Underlying this approach is the understanding of interdependency between listening and speaking. As a result, spoken language is expected as the response to being talked to.

Auditory-oral: Like auditory-verbal therapy, this approach emphasizes the development and reliance on auditory cues to receive and comprehend spoken language. However, this approach acknowledges that in some instances emphasis on visual or vibrotactile cues may be utilized. Spoken language is the expected response.

Total communication: This multi-sensory training approach emphasizes the combined use of spoken language with a manual communication system (signs). Sign alone or sign with vocalization are acceptable responses. Typically maintaining English word order is emphasized by service providers implementing this approach.

Manual communication: This approach emphasizes conveying meaning and eliciting responses based on a formal visual communication system. There are two sign systems typically used: ASL (American Sign Language) is the most common manual communication system. It is a formal language with its own syntax and grammar. SEE (Signed Exact English) is a system which uses signs but follows standard English syntax and marks English grammar forms with a set of endings. Adding auditory cues is compatible with SEE, as the word order is English word order and there is a match between what the child sees and hears. In contrast, the simultaneous presentation of speech and ASL results in a mismatch because ASL has a different word order from spoken English.

Cued speech: This training approach provides supplemental visual gestures or "cues" to distinguish between speech sounds that look the same on the lips. It is designed to supplement spoken language until the child has the opportunity to establish more precise auditory skills for distinguishing between similar-sounding or visually similar-looking sounds.

Chapter 23

Pervasive Developmental Disorders

Chapter Contents

Section 23.1

Autism

Reprinted from the National Dissemination
Center for Children with Disabilities, June 2010.

Ryan's Story

Ryan is a healthy, active two-year-old, but his parents are concerned because he doesn't seem to be doing the same things that his older sister did at this age. He's not really talking, yet, although sometimes he repeats, over and over, words that he hears others say. He doesn't use words to communicate, though. It seems he just enjoys the sounds of them. Ryan spends a lot of time playing by himself. He has a few favorite toys, mostly cars, or anything with wheels on it! And sometimes he spins himself around as fast as he does the wheels on his cars. Ryan's parents are really concerned, as he's started throwing a tantrum whenever his routine has the smallest change. More and more, his parents feel stressed, not knowing what might trigger Ryan's next upset.

Often, it seems Ryan doesn't notice or care if his family or anyone else is around. His parents just don't know how to reach their little boy, who seems so rigid and far too set in his ways for his tender young age. After talking with their family doctor, Ryan's parents call the Early Intervention office in their community and make an appointment to have Ryan evaluated.

When the time comes, Ryan is seen by several professionals who play with him, watch him, and ask his parents a lot of questions. When they're all done, Ryan is diagnosed with autism, one of the five disorders listed under an umbrella category of "Pervasive Developmental Disorders"—a category that's often referred to as simply the "autism spectrum."

As painful as this is for his parents to learn, the early intervention staff encourage them to learn more about the autism spectrum. By getting an early diagnosis and beginning treatment, Ryan has the best chance to grow and develop. Of course, there's a long road ahead, but his parents take comfort in knowing that they aren't alone and they're getting Ryan the help he needs.

What Are the Characteristics of Autism Spectrum Disorders?

Each of the disorders on the autism spectrum is a neurological disorder that affects a child's ability to communicate, understand language, play, and relate to others. They share some or all of the following characteristics, which can vary from mild to severe:

- Communication problems (for example, with the use or comprehension of language)

- Difficulty relating to people, things, and events

- Playing with toys and objects in unusual ways

- Difficulty adjusting to changes in routine or to familiar surroundings

- Repetitive body movements or behaviors.[1]

These characteristics are typically evident before the age of three.

Children with autism or one of the other disorders on the autism spectrum can differ considerably with respect to their abilities, intelligence, and behavior. Some children don't talk at all. Others use language where phrases or conversations are repeated. Children with the most advanced language skills tend to talk about a limited range of topics and to have a hard time understanding abstract concepts. Repetitive play and limited social skills are also evident. Other common symptoms of a disorder on the autism spectrum can include unusual and sometimes uncontrolled reactions to sensory information—for instance, to loud noises, bright lights, and certain textures of food or fabrics.

What Are the Specific Disorders on the Autism Spectrum?

There are five disorders classified under the umbrella category officially known as pervasive developmental disorders, or PDD. These are:

- autism;

- Asperger syndrome;

- Rett syndrome;

- childhood disintegrative disorder; and

- pervasive developmental disorder not otherwise specified (often referred to as PDDNOS).[2]

Although there are subtle differences and degrees of severity between these five conditions, the treatment and educational needs of a child with any of these disorders will be very similar. For that reason, the term "autism spectrum disorders"—or ASDs, as they are sometimes called— is used quite often now and is actually expected to become the official term to be used in the future.[3]

The five conditions are defined in the *Diagnostic and Statistical Manual, Fourth Edition, Text Revision (DSM-IV-TR)* of the American Psychiatric Society (2000). This is also the manual used to diagnose autism and its associated disorders, as well as a wide variety of other disabilities.

At the moment, according to the 2000 edition of the DSM-IV, a diagnosis of autistic disorder (or "classic" autism) is made when a child displays six or more of twelve symptoms across three major areas:

- Social interaction (such as the inability to establish or maintain relationships with peers appropriate to the level of the child's development

- Communication (such as the absence of language or delays in its development)

- Behavior (such as repetitive preoccupation with one or more areas of interest in a way that is abnormal in its intensity or focus)

When children display similar behaviors but do not meet the specific criteria for autistic disorder, they may be diagnosed as having one of the other disorders on the spectrum—Asperger, Rett, childhood disintegrative disorder, or PDDNOS. PDDNOS (pervasive developmental disorder not otherwise specified) is the least specific diagnosis and typically means that a child has displayed the least specific of autistic-like symptoms or behaviors and has not met the criteria for any of the other disorders.

How Common Are ASDs?

According to the National Institute of Mental Health (NIMH) and the Centers for Disease Control and Prevention (CDC), some form of autism affects 2 to 6 of every 1,000 children, with the most recent statistic being 1 in 110.[4] ASDs are four times more common in boys than in girls, although Rett syndrome has only been diagnosed in girls.[5]

What Causes an ASD?

The causes of autism and the other disorders on the spectrum are not known. Researchers are currently studying such areas as neurological damage and chemical imbalances within the brain. These disorders are not due, however, to psychological factors or, as has been widely reported in the press, to childhood vaccines.[6]

A Look at ASD Diagnoses in the Future

In early 2010, the American Psychiatric Association released draft revisions to its *Diagnostic and Statistical Manual of Mental Disorders* (*DSM-5*) and invited comments from both professionals and the general public. The final and official fifth revision of the *DSM* is expected to be published in May 2013.[7]

When published, the *DSM-5* is expected to affect how autism and associated disorders are diagnosed. Among the proposed revisions are the following:

- Changing the name of the diagnostic category to Autism spectrum disorders

- Including Asperger syndrome, childhood disintegrative disorder, and PDDNOS under the diagnosis of autism spectrum disorders, rather than defining them separately and a bit differently, as is now the case

- Removing Rett syndrome from the *DSM* entirely (and, thus, from the autism spectrum).[8]

All this is to say . . . stay tuned. The criteria for diagnoses of ASDs are in the process of changing.

Is There Help Available?

Yes, there's a lot of help available, beginning with the free evaluation of the child. The nation's special education law, the Individuals with Disabilities Education Act (IDEA), requires that all children suspected of having a disability be evaluated without cost to their parents to determine if they do have a disability and, because of the disability, need special services under IDEA. Those special services are as follows:

- **Early intervention:** A system of services to support infants and toddlers with disabilities (before their third birthday) and their families.

- **Special education and related services:** Services available through the public school system for school-aged children, including preschoolers (ages three to twenty-one).

Under IDEA, children with a disorder on the autism spectrum are usually found eligible for services under the category of "autism." In the fall of 2005, more than 160,000 school-aged children (three to twenty-one) received special education and related services in the public schools under the "autism" category.[9]

IDEA specifically defines "autism" as follows:

. . . a developmental disability significantly affecting verbal and nonverbal communication and social interaction, generally evident before age three, that adversely affects a child's educational performance.

A child who shows the characteristics of autism after age three could be diagnosed as having autism if the criteria above are satisfied. [34 CFR §300.8(c)(1)]

Other characteristics often associated with autism are engaging in repetitive activities and stereotyped movements, resistance to environmental change or change in daily routines, and unusual responses to sensory experiences. The term *autism* does not apply if the child's educational performance is adversely affected primarily because the child has an emotional disturbance, as defined in IDEA.

What about School?

Early diagnosis and intervention are very important for children with an ASD. As we've mentioned, under IDEA children with an ASD may be eligible for early intervention services (birth to three) and an educational program appropriate to their individual needs.

In addition to academic instruction, special education programs for students with ASDs focus on improving communication, social, academic, behavioral, and daily living skills. Behavior and communication problems that interfere with learning often require the assistance of a professional who is particularly knowledgeable in the autism field to develop and help implement a plan which can be carried out at home and school.

The classroom environment should be structured so that the program is consistent and predictable. Students with an ASD learn better and are less confused when information is presented visually as well as verbally. Interaction with nondisabled peers is also important, for these students provide models of appropriate language, social, and behavioral skills. Consistency and continuity are very important for children with an ASD, and parents should always be involved in the development of their child's program, so that learning activities, experiences, and approaches will be most effective and can be carried over into the home and community.

With educational programs designed to meet a student's individual needs and specialized adult support services in employment and living arrangements, many children and adults with a disability on the autism spectrum grow to live, work, and participate fully in their communities.

Tips for Parents

- Learn about autism spectrum disorders—especially the specific disorder of your child. The more you know, the more you can help yourself and your child.

- Be mindful to interact with and teach your child in ways that are most likely to get a positive response. Learn what is likely to trigger a meltdown for your child, so you can try to minimize them. Remember, the earliest years are the toughest, but it does get better!

- Learn from professionals and other parents how to meet your child's special needs, but remember your son or daughter is first and foremost a child; life does not need to become a never-ending round of therapies.

- If you weren't born loving highly structured, consistent schedules and routines, ask for help from other parents and professionals on how to make it second nature for you. Behavior, communication, and social skills can all be areas of concern for a child with autism and experience tells us that maintaining a solid, loving, and structured approach in caring for your child can help greatly.

- Learn about assistive technology (AT) that can help your child. This may include a simple picture communication board to help your child express needs and desires, or may be as sophisticated as an augmentative communication device.

- Work with professionals in early intervention or in your child's school to develop an Individualized Family Service Plan (IFSP) or an Individualized Education Program (IEP) that reflects your child's needs and abilities. Be sure to include related services, supplementary aids and services, AT, and a positive behavioral support plan, if needed.

- Be patient and stay optimistic. Your child, like every child, has a whole lifetime to learn and grow.

Tips for Teachers

- Learn more about the autism spectrum.

- Make sure directions are given step-by- step, verbally, visually, and by providing physical supports or prompts, as needed by the student. Students with autism spectrum disorders often have trouble interpreting facial expressions, body language, and tone of voice. Be as concrete and explicit as possible in your instructions and feedback to the student.

- Find out what the student's strengths and interests are and emphasize them. Tap into those avenues and create opportunities for success. Give positive feedback and lots of opportunities for practice.

- Build opportunities for the student to have social and collaborative interactions throughout the regular school day. Provide support, structure, and lots of feedback.

- If behavior is a significant issue for the student, seek help from expert professionals (including parents) to understand the meanings of the behaviors and to develop a unified, positive approach to resolving them.

- Have consistent routines and schedules. When you know a change in routine will occur (e.g., a field trip or assembly) prepare the student by telling him or her what is going to be different and what to expect or do.

- Work together with the student's parents and other school personnel to create and implement an educational plan tailored to meet the student's needs. Regularly share information about how the student is doing at school and at home.

References

1. Autism Society of America. (2008). About autism. Available online at: www.autism-society.org.

2. American Psychiatric Association. (2000). *Diagnostic and statistical manual of mental disorders fourth edition, text revision (DSM-IV-TR)*. Arlington, VA: Author.

3. American Psychiatric Association. (2010). DSM-5 proposed revisions include new category of autism spectrum disorders (press release). Available online at: www.dsm5.org/Newsroom/Documents/Autism%20Release%20FINAL%202.05.pdf.

4. Centers for Disease Control and Prevention (CDC). (2009). Autism spectrum disorders: Data and statistics. Available online at: www.cdc.gov/ncbddd/autism/data.html.

5. Centers for Disease Control and Prevention (CDC). (2009). Autism spectrum disorders: Research. Available online at: www .cdc.gov/ncbddd/autism/research.html.

6. Centers for Disease Control and Prevention (CDC). (2009). Concerns about autism: CDC statement on autism and thimerosal. Available online at: www.cdc.gov/vaccinesafety/Concerns/Autism/Index.html.

7. American Psychiatric Association. (2009). DSM-5 publication date moved to May 2013 (press release). Available at: www.dsm5.org/Newsroom/Documents/09-65%20DSM%20Timeline.pdf.

8. American Psychiatric Association. (2010). Proposed revision: Autistic disorder. Available online at: www.dsm5.org/Proposed Revisions/Pages/proposedrevision.aspx?rid=94#.

9. U.S. Department of Education. (2007). 27th annual report to Congress on the implementation of the Individuals with Disabilities Education Act, 2005 (Vol. 2). Washington, DC: Author.

Section 23.2

Asperger Syndrome

"Asperger Syndrome Fact Sheet," National Institute of Neurological Disorders and Stroke, National Institutes of Health, June 15, 2011.

What is Asperger syndrome?

Asperger syndrome (AS) is a developmental disorder that is characterized by the following:[1]

- Limited interests or an unusual preoccupation with a particular subject to the exclusion of other activities

- Repetitive routines or rituals

- Peculiarities in speech and language, such as speaking in an overly formal manner or in a monotone, or taking figures of speech literally

- Socially and emotionally inappropriate behavior and the inability to interact successfully with peers

- Problems with nonverbal communication, including the restricted use of gestures, limited or inappropriate facial expressions, or a peculiar, stiff gaze

- Clumsy and uncoordinated motor movements

AS is an autism spectrum disorder (ASD), one of a distinct group of neurological conditions characterized by a greater or lesser degree of impairment in language and communication skills, as well as repetitive or restrictive patterns of thought and behavior. Other ASDs include: classic autism, Rett syndrome, childhood disintegrative disorder, and pervasive developmental disorder not otherwise specified (usually referred to as PDD-NOS).

Parents usually sense there is something unusual about a child with AS by the time of his or her third birthday, and some children may exhibit symptoms as early as infancy. Unlike children with autism, children with AS retain their early language skills. Motor development delays—crawling or walking late, clumsiness—are sometimes the first indicator of the disorder.

The incidence of AS is not well established, but experts in population studies conservatively estimate that two out of every ten thousand children have the disorder. Boys are three to four times more likely than girls to have AS.

Studies of children with AS suggest that their problems with socialization and communication continue into adulthood. Some of these children develop additional psychiatric symptoms and disorders in adolescence and adulthood.

Although diagnosed mainly in children, AS is being increasingly diagnosed in adults who seek medical help for mental health conditions such as depression, obsessive-compulsive disorder (OCD), and attention deficit hyperactivity disorder (ADHD). No studies have yet been conducted to determine the incidence of AS in adult populations.

Why is it called Asperger syndrome?

In 1944, an Austrian pediatrician named Hans Asperger observed four children in his practice who had difficulty integrating socially. Although their intelligence appeared normal, the children lacked nonverbal communication skills, failed to demonstrate empathy with their peers, and were physically clumsy. Their way of speaking was either disjointed or overly formal, and their all-absorbing interest in a single topic dominated their conversations. Dr. Asperger called the condition "autistic psychopathy" and described it as a personality disorder primarily marked by social isolation.

Asperger's observations, published in German, were not widely known until 1981, when an English doctor named Lorna Wing published a series of case studies of children showing similar symptoms, which she called "Asperger's" syndrome. Wing's writings were widely published and popularized. AS became a distinct disease and diagnosis in 1992, when it was included in the tenth published edition of the World Health Organization's diagnostic manual, *International Classification of Diseases* (*ICD-10*), and in 1994 it was added to the *Diagnostic and Statistical Manual of Mental Disorders* (*DSM-IV*), the American Psychiatric Association's diagnostic reference book.

What are some common signs or symptoms?

The most distinguishing symptom of AS is a child's obsessive interest in a single object or topic to the exclusion of any other. Some children with AS have become experts on vacuum cleaners, makes and models of cars, even objects as odd as deep fat fryers. Children with AS want to know everything about their topic of interest and their conversations with others will be about little else. Their expertise, high level of vocabulary, and formal speech patterns make them seem like little professors.

Children with AS will gather enormous amounts of factual information about their favorite subject and will talk incessantly about it, but the conversation may seem like a random collection of facts or statistics, with no point or conclusion.

Their speech may be marked by a lack of rhythm, an odd inflection, or a monotone pitch. Children with AS often lack the ability to modulate the volume of their voice to match their surroundings. For example, they will have to be reminded to talk softly every time they enter a library or a movie theatre.

Unlike the severe withdrawal from the rest of the world that is characteristic of autism, children with AS are isolated because of their poor social skills and narrow interests. In fact, they may approach other people, but make normal conversation impossible by inappropriate or eccentric behavior, or by wanting only to talk about their singular interest.

Children with AS usually have a history of developmental delays in motor skills such as pedaling a bike, catching a ball, or climbing outdoor play equipment. They are often awkward and poorly coordinated with a walk that can appear either stilted or bouncy.

Many children with AS are highly active in early childhood, and then develop anxiety or depression in young adulthood. Other conditions that often coexist with AS are ADHD, tic disorders (such as Tourette syndrome), depression, anxiety disorders, and OCD.

What causes AS? Is it genetic?

Current research points to brain abnormalities as the cause of AS. Using advanced brain imaging techniques, scientists have revealed structural and functional differences in specific regions of the brains of normal versus AS children. These defects are most likely caused by the abnormal migration of embryonic cells during fetal development that affects brain structure and "wiring" and then goes on to affect the neural circuits that control thought and behavior.

For example, one study found a reduction of brain activity in the frontal lobe of AS children when they were asked to respond to tasks that required them to use their judgment. Another study found differences in activity when children were asked to respond to facial expressions. A different study investigating brain function in adults with AS revealed abnormal levels of specific proteins that correlate with obsessive and repetitive behaviors.

Scientists have always known that there had to be a genetic component to AS and the other ASDs because of their tendency to run in families. Additional evidence for the link between inherited genetic mutations and AS was observed in the higher incidence of family members who have behavioral symptoms similar to AS but in a more limited form. For example, they had slight difficulties with social interaction, language, or reading.

A specific gene for AS, however, has never been identified. Instead, the most recent research indicates that there are most likely a common group of genes whose variations or deletions make an individual vulnerable to developing AS. This combination of genetic variations or deletions will determine the severity and symptoms for each individual with AS.

How is it diagnosed?

The diagnosis of AS is complicated by the lack of a standardized diagnostic screen or schedule. In fact, because there are several screening instruments in current use, each with different criteria, the same child could receive different diagnoses, depending on the screening tool the doctor uses.

To further complicate the issue, some doctors believe that AS is not a separate and distinct disorder. Instead, they call it high-functioning autism (HFA), and view it as being on the mild end of the ASD spectrum with symptoms that differ—only in degree—from classic autism. Some clinicians use the two diagnoses, AS or HFA, interchangeably. This makes gathering data about the incidence of AS difficult, since some children will be diagnosed with HFA instead of AS, and vice versa.

Most doctors rely on the presence of a core group of behaviors to alert them to the possibility of a diagnosis of AS. These are as follows:

- Abnormal eye contact

- Aloofness

- The failure to turn when called by name

- The failure to use gestures to point or show

- A lack of interactive play

- A lack of interest in peers

Some of these behaviors may be apparent in the first few months of a child's life, or they may appear later. Problems in at least one of the areas of communication and socialization or repetitive, restricted behavior must be present before the age of three.

The diagnosis of AS is a two-stage process. The first stage begins with developmental screening during a "well-child" check-up with a family doctor or pediatrician. The second stage is a comprehensive team evaluation to either rule in or rule out AS. This team generally includes a psychologist, neurologist, psychiatrist, speech therapist, and additional professionals who have expertise in diagnosing children with AS.

The comprehensive evaluation includes neurologic and genetic assessment, with in-depth cognitive and language testing to establish intelligence quotient (IQ) and evaluate psychomotor function, verbal and nonverbal strengths and weaknesses, style of learning, and independent living skills. An assessment of communication strengths and weaknesses includes evaluating nonverbal forms of communication (gaze and gestures); the use of nonliteral language (metaphor, irony, absurdities, and humor); patterns of inflection, stress, and volume modulation; pragmatics (turn-taking and sensitivity to verbal cues); and the content, clarity, and coherence of conversation. The physician will look at the testing results and combine them with the child's developmental history and current symptoms to make a diagnosis.

Are there treatments available?

The ideal treatment for AS coordinates therapies that address the three core symptoms of the disorder: poor communication skills, obsessive or repetitive routines, and physical clumsiness. There is no single best treatment package for all children with AS, but most professionals agree that the earlier the intervention, the better.

An effective treatment program builds on the child's interests, offers a predictable schedule, teaches tasks as a series of simple steps, actively engages the child's attention in highly structured activities, and provides regular reinforcement of behavior. This kind of program generally includes the following:

- Social skills training, a form of group therapy that teaches children with AS the skills they need to interact more successfully with other children

- Cognitive behavioral therapy, a type of "talk" therapy that can help the more explosive or anxious children to manage their emotions better and cut back on obsessive interests and repetitive routines

- Medication, for coexisting conditions such as depression and anxiety

- Occupational or physical therapy, for children with sensory integration problems or poor motor coordination

- Specialized speech/language therapy, to help children who have trouble with the pragmatics of speech—the give and take of normal conversation

- Parent training and support, to teach parents behavioral techniques to use at home

Do children with AS get better? What happens when they become adults?

With effective treatment, children with AS can learn to cope with their disabilities, but they may still find social situations and personal relationships challenging. Many adults with AS are able to work successfully in mainstream jobs, although they may continue to need encouragement and moral support to maintain an independent life.

What research is being done?

The National Institute of Neurological Disorders and Stroke (NINDS) is one of the federal government's leading supporters of biomedical research on brain and nervous system disorders. The NINDS conducts research in its laboratories at the National Institutes of Health (NIH) in Bethesda, Maryland, and awards grants to support research at universities and other facilities. Many of the Institutes at the NIH, including NINDS, are sponsoring research to understand what causes AS and how it can be effectively treated.

One study is using functional magnetic resonance imaging (fMRI) to show how abnormalities in particular areas of the brain cause changes in brain function that result in the symptoms of AS and other ASDs. Another large-scale study is comparing neuropsychological and psychiatric assessments of children with possible diagnoses of AS or HFA to those of their parents and siblings to see if there are patterns of symptoms that link AS and HFA to specific neuropsychological profiles.

NINDS is also supporting a long-range international study that brings together investigators to collect and analyze DNA samples from children with AS and HFA, as well as their families, to identify associated genes and how they interact. Called the Autism Genome Project, it's a consortium of scientists from universities, academic centers, and

277

institutions around the world that functions as a repository for genetic data so that researchers can look for the genetic "building blocks" of AS and the other ASDs.

Since there are so many different forms of ASD, understanding the genetic basis of each opens the door to opportunities for more precise diagnosis and treatment. Knowing the genetic profile of a particular disorder could mean early identification of those at risk, and early intervention when treatments and therapies are likely to be the most successful.

Notes

1. Adapted from the *Diagnostic and Statistical Manual of Mental Disorders IV and the International Classification of Diseases—10.*

Section 23.3

Understanding the Differences between Learning Disabilities and Asperger Syndrome

Understanding the Differences

Given that children with specific learning disabilities (SLD) and Asperger syndrome sometimes share characteristics, parents and professionals must collaborate to make the correct diagnoses and put appropriate interventions in place. In addition to the guidelines provided below, adults should watch for the following behavioral clues.

For children with LD, when learning problems are not addressed, they may engage in impulsive or risk-taking acts, inappropriate classroom behavior, or associate with low-achieving peers. Constant frustration with learning tasks can trigger a range of behaviors including boredom and seeming carelessness; school withdrawal or avoidance;

disorganization, inattention or sloppiness; slow response to questions; and physical symptoms of stress (e.g., headaches or stomach aches).

Children with Asperger syndrome often exhibit their unique cognitive and behavioral profiles before formal schooling begins. Even as preschoolers they may deviate from peers in social and interpersonal skills, speech, language, communication, daily behaviors and routines, and general maturation and development.

When children with Asperger syndrome begin formal schooling they are usually impatient with the concerns of others. Despite a high intelligence quotient (IQ), they can look impulsive or emotionally unregulated, often failing to comprehend basic directions or procedures. Asperger syndrome is often mistaken for attention deficit hyperactivity disorder (ADHD) or SLD because many affected have trouble focusing and abiding by rules they interpret as illogical. Because they seem too bright to be unaware of typical demands, they are sometimes viewed as arrogant or oppositional. If treated appropriately, however, their intelligence, exceptional focus, and specific talents can lessen school anxiety and support academic performance.

They can also develop school phobia or behaviors related to low self-esteem, difficulty with novelty or transition, extreme literal interpretation, and easily triggered anxiety.

Regardless of a child's diagnosis—whether SLD, Asperger syndrome, or both—fundamental educational principles provide the keys to success. Parents and educators should search for schools that offer consistent understanding, individualized accommodation, and compassion. Settings with those attributes will always be the right settings for students with atypical and unique cognitive needs.

Tell-Tale Signs

Suspect LD if your child:

- works hard but gets poor grades;
- needs constant, step by step guidance;
- cannot solve problems, remember steps, comprehend tasks, or understand logic;
- has poor memory;
- has difficulty with reading, writing, or math;
- is frustrated by school and homework;
- has low self-esteem.

Suspect Asperger if your child:

- has difficulty making or sustaining eye contact;
- is isolated from family members and peers;
- doesn't understand the perspectives of others
- has trouble discussing feelings (his own or others')
- is interested in people, but lacks social skills;
- has an obsessive arcane interest;
- has a highly developed vocabulary with formal or peculiar speech patterns;
- is clumsy, uncoordinated, or unaware of personal space.

Chapter 24

Specific Language Impairment

Children with specific language impairment (SLI) have difficulties with oral language that first become apparent in the preschool years, prior to formal schooling. Although the pace of oral language development varies widely among typical youngsters, children with SLI have language difficulties that are clearly outside the typical range and that can be diagnosed by a speech-language pathologist. A variety of components of oral language may be affected by SLI, including grammatical and syntactic development (e.g., correct verb tense, word order, and sentence structure), semantic development (e.g., vocabulary knowledge), and phonological development (e.g., phonological awareness, or awareness of sounds in spoken language). Children may manifest receptive difficulties, that is, problems understanding language, or expressive difficulties, involving use of language. These difficulties usually do not revolve around the motor aspects of producing or articulating words; for example, a child whose sole difficulty is stuttering does not have SLI. Specific language impairment is relatively common, affecting as many as 5 to 10 percent of preschoolers, and it appears to have a genetic base in many families.

Differentiating Specific Language Impairment from Other Disabilities

Oral language difficulties are associated with a wide range of disabilities, including hearing impairment, broad cognitive delays or disabilities, and autism spectrum disorders. Specific language impairment differs from the preceding conditions. Although it is always important to rule out hearing problems as a source of language difficulties—including fluctuating hearing loss such as that associated with repeated ear infections—most children with SLI have normal hearing. Furthermore, specific language impairment does not involve global developmental delays; children with SLI function within the typical range in nonlinguistic areas, such as nonverbal social interaction, play, and self-help skills (e.g., feeding and dressing themselves). Children with autism spectrum disorders have core impairments in social interaction and communication, including both nonverbal and verbal skills, as well as certain characteristic behaviors (e.g., repetitive movements, lack of pretend play, and inflexible adherence to routines) that are not found in youngsters with SLI.

Specific Language Impairment and Learning Disabilities

Specific language impairment puts children at clear risk for later academic difficulties, in particular, for reading disabilities. Studies have indicated that as many as 40 to 75 percent of children with SLI will have problems in learning to read, presumably because reading depends upon a wide variety of underlying language skills, including all of the component language abilities mentioned above (grammar and syntax, semantics, and phonological skills). Moreover, children with continuing language problems at school entrance are not the only ones at risk; kindergartners with previous SLI who appear to have "caught up" to their age peers in language abilities still are at increased risk of reading difficulties, relative to children with no history of SLI. However, the preschoolers at greatest risk of future reading problems are those whose language difficulties are persistent over time, affect multiple components of language, or are severe, even if only in a single component of language.

What Parents and Schools Can Do

Parents who have concerns about the language development of their toddler or preschooler should seek an evaluation from a qualified speech-language specialist. These kinds of evaluations can be obtained in several ways. Parents can contact their local school district to request a developmental screening—no referral is needed. Also, speech-language evaluations may be provided pro bono or relatively inexpensively at many universities with departments that train speech-language pathologists. Young children with significant language difficulties are eligible for "Birth to Three" or preschool services at no cost to parents. Activities to facilitate language development may be done by a speech-language specialist in the home, at a clinic, or in an early childhood education program; parents generally are encouraged to be involved in the intervention and are given suggestions for ways to help their child. Early identification and intervention are extremely important in order to foster language and social growth and to give children the best possible foundation for formal schooling. Although preschool language intervention may not eliminate the risk of future reading difficulties, it can prevent or reduce many problems. For example, children with language impairment may have temper tantrums that occur due to frustration over their inability to communicate effectively; intervention that enables children to communicate their wishes and needs can help to avoid these kinds of behavior problems.

It should be noted that, although children with SLI are at substantially increased risk of reading difficulties compared to other children, they are by no means destined for poor reading; some youngsters with a preschool history of SLI go on to achieve normally in school, and those with ongoing difficulties can certainly be helped. Toward this end, there are a number of things schools can do. A comprehensive reading curriculum that provides explicit, systematic instruction in the abilities known to be important in reading—phonemic awareness, phonics, fluency, vocabulary, and comprehension—benefits all children, including those with language problems. In addition, information about whether children have a history of SLI and about their language abilities upon entry to kindergarten should be shared as they make the transition from preschool to formal schooling. Schools should be aware that a history of SLI increases the risk of reading problems even if children no longer meet eligibility criteria for speech-language services. These children must be monitored closely for early signs of reading difficulties—including difficulties in component reading-related skills such as phonemic awareness and knowledge of letter sounds—and provided with prompt intervention if it is needed. Children with continuing language difficulties will require speech-language services that are integrated and coordinated with reading instruction. A high-quality reading curriculum, careful monitoring, and prompt, appropriate intervention as needed can help children with SLI achieve success.

Chapter 25

Tourette Syndrome

Tourette syndrome (TS) is a neurological disorder characterized by repetitive, stereotyped, involuntary movements and vocalizations called tics. The disorder is named for Dr. Georges Gilles de la Tourette, the pioneering French neurologist who in 1885 first described the condition in an eighty-six-year-old French noblewoman.

The early symptoms of TS are almost always noticed first in childhood, with the average onset between the ages of seven and ten years. TS occurs in people from all ethnic groups; males are affected about three to four times more often than females. It is estimated that two hundred thousand Americans have the most severe form of TS, and as many as one in one hundred exhibit milder and less complex symptoms such as chronic motor or vocal tics or transient tics of childhood. Although TS can be a chronic condition with symptoms lasting a lifetime, most people with the condition experience their worst symptoms in their early teens, with improvement occurring in the late teens and continuing into adulthood.

What are the symptoms?

Tics are classified as either simple or complex. Simple motor tics are sudden, brief, repetitive movements that involve a limited number of muscle groups. Some of the more common simple tics include eye blinking and other vision irregularities, facial grimacing, shoulder

"Tourette Syndrome Fact Sheet," National Institute of Neurological Disorders and Stroke, National Institutes of Health, June 15, 2011.

shrugging, and head or shoulder jerking. Simple vocalizations might include repetitive throat clearing, sniffing, or grunting sounds. Complex tics are distinct, coordinated patterns of movements involving several muscle groups. Complex motor tics might include facial grimacing combined with a head twist and a shoulder shrug. Other complex motor tics may actually appear purposeful, including sniffing or touching objects, hopping, jumping, bending, or twisting. Simple vocal tics may include throat clearing, sniffing/snorting, grunting, or barking. More complex vocal tics include words or phrases. Perhaps the most dramatic and disabling tics include motor movements that result in self-harm such as punching oneself in the face or vocal tics including coprolalia (uttering swear words) or echolalia (repeating the words or phrases of others). Some tics are preceded by an urge or sensation in the affected muscle group, commonly called a premonitory urge. Some with TS will describe a need to complete a tic in a certain way or a certain number of times in order to relieve the urge or decrease the sensation.

Tics are often worse with excitement or anxiety and better during calm, focused activities. Certain physical experiences can trigger or worsen tics, for example tight collars may trigger neck tics, or hearing another person sniff or throat-clear may trigger similar sounds. Tics do not go away during sleep but are often significantly diminished.

What is the course of TS?

Tics come and go over time, varying in type, frequency, location, and severity. The first symptoms usually occur in the head and neck area and may progress to include muscles of the trunk and extremities. Motor tics generally precede the development of vocal tics and simple tics often precede complex tics. Most patients experience peak tic severity before the mid-teen years with improvement for the majority of patients in the late teen years and early adulthood. Approximately 10 percent of those affected have a progressive or disabling course that lasts into adulthood.

Can people with TS control their tics?

Although the symptoms of TS are involuntary, some people can sometimes suppress, camouflage, or otherwise manage their tics in an effort to minimize their impact on functioning. However, people with TS often report a substantial buildup in tension when suppressing their tics to the point where they feel that the tic must be expressed. Tics in response to an environmental trigger can appear to be voluntary or purposeful but are not.

What causes TS?

Although the cause of TS is unknown, current research points to abnormalities in certain brain regions (including the basal ganglia, frontal lobes, and cortex), the circuits that interconnect these regions, and the neurotransmitters (dopamine, serotonin, and norepinephrine) responsible for communication among nerve cells. Given the often complex presentation of TS, the cause of the disorder is likely to be equally complex.

What disorders are associated with TS?

Many with TS experience additional neurobehavioral problems including inattention; hyperactivity and impulsivity (attention deficit hyperactivity disorder—ADHD) and related problems with reading, writing, and arithmetic; and obsessive-compulsive symptoms such as intrusive thoughts/worries and repetitive behaviors. For example, worries about dirt and germs may be associated with repetitive hand washing, and concerns about bad things happening may be associated with ritualistic behaviors such as counting, repeating, or ordering and arranging. People with TS have also reported problems with depression or anxiety disorders, as well as other difficulties with living, that may or may not be directly related to TS. Given the range of potential complications, people with TS are best served by receiving medical care that provides a comprehensive treatment plan.

How is TS diagnosed?

TS is a diagnosis that doctors make after verifying that the patient has had both motor and vocal tics for at least one year. The existence of other neurological or psychiatric conditions[1] can also help doctors arrive at a diagnosis. Common tics are not often misdiagnosed by knowledgeable clinicians. But atypical symptoms or atypical presentation (for example, onset of symptoms in adulthood) may require specific specialty expertise for diagnosis. There are no blood or laboratory tests needed for diagnosis, but neuroimaging studies, such as magnetic resonance imaging (MRI), computerized tomography (CT), and electroencephalogram (EEG) scans, or certain blood tests may be used to rule out other conditions that might be confused with TS.

It is not uncommon for patients to obtain a formal diagnosis of TS only after symptoms have been present for some time. The reasons for this are many. For families and physicians unfamiliar with TS, mild and even moderate tic symptoms may be considered inconsequential, part of a developmental phase, or the result of another condition. For example, parents may think that eye blinking is related to vision problems or that sniffing is related to seasonal allergies. Many patients are self-diagnosed after they, their parents, other relatives, or friends read or hear about TS from others.

How is TS treated?

Because tic symptoms do not often cause impairment, the majority of people with TS require no medication for tic suppression. However, effective medications are available for those whose symptoms interfere with functioning. Neuroleptics are the most consistently useful medications for tic suppression; a number are available but some are more effective than others (for example, haloperidol and pimozide). Unfortunately, there is no one medication that is helpful to all people with TS, nor does any medication completely eliminate symptoms. In addition, all medications have side effects. Most neuroleptic side effects can be managed by initiating treatment slowly and reducing the dose when side effects occur. The most common side effects of neuroleptics include sedation, weight gain, and cognitive dulling. Neurological side effects such as tremor, dystonic reactions (twisting movements or postures), parkinsonian-like symptoms, and other dyskinetic (involuntary) movements are less common and are readily managed with dose reduction. Discontinuing neuroleptics after long-term use must be done slowly to avoid rebound increases in tics and withdrawal dyskinesias. One form of withdrawal dyskinesia called tardive dyskinesia is a movement disorder distinct from TS that may result from the chronic use of neuroleptics. The risk of this side effect can be reduced by using lower doses of neuroleptics for shorter periods of time.

Other medications may also be useful for reducing tic severity, but most have not been as extensively studied or shown to be as consistently useful as neuroleptics. Additional medications with demonstrated efficacy include alpha-adrenergic agonists such as clonidine and guanfacine. These medications are used primarily for hypertension but are also used in the treatment of tics. The most common side effect from these medications that precludes their use is sedation.

Effective medications are also available to treat some of the associated neurobehavioral disorders that can occur in patients with TS. Recent research shows that stimulant medications such as methylphenidate and dextroamphetamine can lessen ADHD symptoms in people with TS without causing tics to become more severe. However, the product labeling for stimulants currently contraindicates the use of these drugs in children with tics/TS and those with a family history of tics. Scientists hope that future studies will include a thorough discussion of the risks and benefits of stimulants in those with TS or a family history of TS and will clarify this issue. For obsessive-compulsive symptoms that significantly disrupt daily functioning, the serotonin reuptake inhibitors (clomipramine, fluoxetine, fluvoxamine, paroxetine, and sertraline) have been proven effective in some patients.

Psychotherapy may also be helpful. Although psychological problems do not cause TS, such problems may result from TS. Psychotherapy can help the person with TS better cope with the disorder and deal with the secondary social and emotional problems that sometimes occur. More recently, specific behavioral treatments that include awareness training and competing response training, such as voluntarily moving in response to a premonitory urge, have shown effectiveness in small controlled trials. Larger and more definitive National Institutes of Health (NIH)–funded studies are underway.

Is TS inherited?

Evidence from twin and family studies suggests that TS is an inherited disorder. Although early family studies suggested an autosomal dominant mode of inheritance (an autosomal dominant disorder is one in which only one copy of the defective gene, inherited from one parent, is necessary to produce the disorder), more recent studies suggest that the pattern of inheritance is much more complex. Although there may be a few genes with substantial effects, it is also possible that many genes with smaller effects and environmental factors may play a role in the development of TS. Genetic studies also suggest that some forms of ADHD and OCD are genetically related to TS, but there is less evidence for a genetic relationship between TS and other neurobehavioral problems that commonly co-occur with TS. It is important for families to understand that genetic predisposition may not necessarily result in full-blown TS; instead, it may express itself as a milder tic disorder or as obsessive-compulsive behaviors. It is also possible that the gene-carrying offspring will not develop any TS symptoms.

The sex of the person also plays an important role in TS gene expression. At-risk males are more likely to have tics and at-risk females are more likely to have obsessive-compulsive symptoms.

People with TS may have genetic risks for other neurobehavioral disorders such as depression or substance abuse. Genetic counseling of individuals with TS should include a full review of all potentially hereditary conditions in the family.

What is the prognosis?

Although there is no cure for TS, the condition in many individuals improves in the late teens and early twenties. As a result, some may actually become symptom-free or no longer need medication for tic suppression. Although the disorder is generally lifelong and chronic, it is not a degenerative condition. Individuals with TS have a normal life expectancy. TS does not impair intelligence. Although tic symptoms tend to decrease with age, it is possible that neurobehavioral disorders such as depression, panic attacks, mood swings, and antisocial behaviors can persist and cause impairment in adult life.

What is the best educational setting for children with TS?

Although students with TS often function well in the regular classroom, ADHD, learning disabilities, obsessive-compulsive symptoms, and frequent tics can greatly interfere with academic performance or social adjustment. After a comprehensive assessment, students should be placed in an educational setting that meets their individual needs. Students may require tutoring, smaller or special classes, and in some cases special schools.

All students with TS need a tolerant and compassionate setting that both encourages them to work to their full potential and is flexible enough to accommodate their special needs. This setting may include a private study area, exams outside the regular classroom, or even oral exams when the child's symptoms interfere with his or her ability to write. Untimed testing reduces stress for students with TS.

What research is being done?

Within the federal government, the leading supporter of research on TS and other neurological disorders is the National Institute of Neurological Disorders and Stroke (NINDS). The NINDS, a part of the National Institutes of Health (NIH), is responsible for supporting and conducting research on the brain and central nervous system.

NINDS sponsors research on TS both in its laboratories at the NIH and through grants to major medical institutions across the country. The National Institute of Mental Health, the National Center for Research Resources, the National Institute of Child Health and Human Development, the National Institute on Drug Abuse, and the National Institute on Deafness and Other Communication Disorders also support research of relevance to TS. And another component of the Department of Health and Human Services, the Centers for Disease

Control and Prevention, funds professional education programs as well as TS research.

Knowledge about TS comes from studies across a number of medical and scientific disciplines, including genetics, neuroimaging, neuropathology, clinical trials (medication and nonmedication), epidemiology, neurophysiology, neuroimmunology, and descriptive/diagnostic clinical science.

Genetic studies: Currently, NIH-funded investigators are conducting a variety of large-scale genetic studies. Rapid advances in the technology of gene finding will allow for genome-wide screening approaches in TS, and finding a gene or genes for TS would be a major step toward understanding genetic risk factors. In addition, understanding the genetics of TS genes will strengthen clinical diagnosis, improve genetic counseling, lead to the clarification of pathophysiology, and provide clues for more effective therapies.

Neuroimaging studies: Within the past five years, advances in imaging technology and an increase in trained investigators have led to an increasing use of novel and powerful techniques to identify brain regions, circuitry, and neurochemical factors important in TS and related conditions.

Neuropathology: Within the past five years, there has been an increase in the number and quality of donated postmortem brains from TS patients available for research purposes. This increase, coupled with advances in neuropathological techniques, has led to initial findings with implications for neuroimaging studies and animal models of TS.

Clinical trials: A number of clinical trials in TS have recently been completed or are currently underway. These include studies of stimulant treatment of ADHD in TS and behavioral treatments for reducing tic severity in children and adults. Smaller trials of novel approaches to treatment such as dopamine agonist and GABAergic medications also show promise.

Epidemiology and clinical science: Careful epidemiological studies now estimate the prevalence of TS to be substantially higher than previously thought with a wider range of clinical severity. Furthermore, clinical studies are providing new findings regarding TS and coexisting conditions. These include subtyping studies of TS and OCD, an examination of the link between ADHD and learning problems in children with TS, a new appreciation of sensory tics, and the role of coexisting disorders in rage attacks. One of the most important and controversial areas of TS science involves the relationship between TS and autoimmune brain injury associated with group A beta-hemolytic streptococcal infections or other infectious processes. There are a number of epidemiological and clinical investigations currently underway in this intriguing area.

Notes

1. These include childhood-onset involuntary movement disorders such as dystonia, or psychiatric disorders characterized by repetitive behaviors/movements (for example, stereotypic behaviors in autism and compulsive behaviors in obsessive-compulsive disorder—OCD).

Chapter 26

Traumatic Brain Injury

What Is Traumatic Brain Injury?

A traumatic brain injury (TBI) is an injury to the brain caused by the head being hit by something or shaken violently. (The exact definition of TBI, according to special education law, is given below.) This injury can change how the person acts, moves, and thinks. A traumatic brain injury can also change how a student learns and acts in school. The term TBI is used for head injuries that can cause changes in one or more areas, such as the following:

- Thinking and reasoning

- Understanding words

- Remembering things

- Paying attention

- Solving problems

- Thinking abstractly

- Talking

- Behaving

- Walking and other physical activities

Excerpted from "Traumatic Brain Injury," National Dissemination Center for Children with Disabilities, March 2011.

- Seeing and/or hearing

- Learning

The term TBI is not used for a person who is born with a brain injury. It also is not used for brain injuries that happen during birth.

How Is TBI Defined?

The definition of TBI below comes from the Individuals with Disabilities Education Act (IDEA). The IDEA is the federal law that guides how schools provide special education and related services to children and youth with disabilities.

IDEA's Definition of "Traumatic Brain Injury"

Our nation's special education law, the Individuals with Disabilities Education Act (IDEA) defines traumatic brain injury as:

. . . an acquired injury to the brain caused by an external physical force, resulting in total or partial functional disability or psychosocial impairment, or both, that adversely affects a child's educational performance. The term applies to open or closed head injuries resulting in impairments in one or more areas, such as cognition; language; memory; attention; reasoning; abstract thinking; judgment; problem-solving; sensory, perceptual, and motor abilities; psycho-social behavior; physical functions; information processing; and speech. The term does not apply to brain injuries that are congenital or degenerative, or to brain injuries induced by birth trauma. [34 Code of Federal Regulations §300.8(c)(12)]

What Are the Signs of Traumatic Brain Injury?

The signs of brain injury can be very different depending on where the brain is injured and how severely. Children with TBI may have one or more difficulties, including the following:

- **Physical disabilities:** Individuals with TBI may have problems speaking, seeing, hearing, and using their other senses. They may have headaches and feel tired a lot. They may also have trouble with skills such as writing or drawing. Their muscles may suddenly contract or tighten (this is called spasticity). They may also have seizures. Their balance and walking may also be affected. They may be partly or completely paralyzed on one side of the body, or both sides.

- **Difficulties with thinking:** Because the brain has been injured, it is common that the person's ability to use the brain changes. For example, children with TBI may have trouble with short-term memory (being able to remember something from one minute to the next, like what the teacher just said). They may also have trouble with their long-term memory (being able to remember information from a while ago, like facts learned last month). People with TBI may have trouble concentrating and only be able to focus their attention for a short time. They may think slowly. They may have trouble talking and listening to others. They may also have difficulty with reading and writing, planning, understanding the order in which events happen (called sequencing), and judgment.

- **Social, behavioral, or emotional problems:** These difficulties may include sudden changes in mood, anxiety, and depression. Children with TBI may have trouble relating to others. They may be restless and may laugh or cry a lot. They may not have much motivation or much control over their emotions.

A child with TBI may not have all of the above difficulties. Brain injuries can range from mild to severe, and so can the changes that result from the injury. This means that it's hard to predict how an individual will recover from the injury. Early and ongoing help can make a big difference in how the child recovers.

It's also important to know that, as the child grows and develops, parents and teachers may notice new problems. This is because, as students grow, they are expected to use their brain in new and different ways. The damage to the brain from the earlier injury can make it hard for the student to learn new skills that come with getting older. Sometimes parents and educators may not even realize that the student's difficulty comes from the earlier injury.

Is There Help Available?

Yes, there's a lot of help available, beginning with the free evaluation of the child. The nation's special education law, IDEA, requires that all children suspected of having a disability be evaluated without cost to their parents to determine if they do have a disability and, because of the disability, need special services under IDEA. Those special services are as follows:

- **Early intervention:** A system of services to support infants and toddlers with disabilities (before their third birthday) and their families.

- **Special education and related services:** Services available through the public school system for school-aged children, including preschoolers (ages three to twenty-one).

To access special education and related services, we recommend that you get in touch with your local public school system. Calling the elementary school in your neighborhood is an excellent place to start. The school should be able to tell you the next steps to having your child evaluated free of charge. If found eligible, he or she can begin receiving services specially designed to address your child's needs.

In the fall of 2007, nearly twenty-five thousand school-aged children (ages three to twenty-one) received special education and related services in our public schools under the category of "traumatic brain injury."[3]

What about School?

Although TBI is very common, many medical and education professionals may not realize that some difficulties can be caused by a childhood brain injury. Often, students with TBI are thought to have a learning disability, emotional disturbance, or mental retardation. As a result, they don't receive the type of educational help and support they really need.

When children with TBI return to school, their educational and emotional needs are often very different than before the injury. Their disability has happened suddenly and traumatically. They can often remember how they were before the brain injury. This can bring on many emotional and social changes. The child's family, friends, and teachers also recall what the child was like before the injury. These other people in the child's life may have trouble changing or adjusting their expectations of the child.

Therefore, it is extremely important to plan carefully for the child's return to school. Parents will want to find out ahead of time about special education services at the school. This information is usually available from the school's principal or special education teacher. The school will need to evaluate the child thoroughly. This evaluation will let the school and parents know what the student's educational needs are. The school and parents will then develop an Individualized Education Program (IEP) that addresses those educational needs.

It's important to remember that the IEP is a flexible plan. It can be changed as the parents, the school, and the student learn more about what the student needs at school.

Tips for Parents

- Learn about TBI. The more you know, the more you can help yourself and your child.

- Work with the medical team to understand your child's injury and treatment plan. Don't be shy about asking questions. Tell them what you know or think. Make suggestions.

- Keep track of your child's treatment. A three-ring binder or a box can help you store this history. As your child recovers, you may meet with many doctors, nurses, and others. Write down what they say. Put any paperwork they give you in the notebook or throw it in the box. You can't remember all this! Also, if you need to share any of this paperwork with someone else, make a copy. Don't give away your original.

- Talk to other parents whose children have TBI. There are parent groups all over the United States. Parents can share practical advice and emotional support.

- If your child was in school before the injury, plan for his or her return to school. Get in touch with the school. Ask the principal about special education services. Have the medical team share information with the school.

- When your child returns to school, ask the school to test your child as soon as possible to identify his or her special education needs. Meet with the school and help develop a plan for your child called an Individualized Education Program (IEP).

- Keep in touch with your child's teacher. Tell the teacher about how your child is doing at home. Ask how your child is doing in school.

Tips for Teachers

- Find out as much as you can about the child's injury and his or her present needs.

- Give the student more time to finish schoolwork and tests.

- Give directions one step at a time. For tasks with many steps, it helps to give the student written directions.

- Show the student how to perform new tasks. Give examples to go with new ideas and concepts.

- Have consistent routines. This helps the student know what to expect. If the routine is going to change, let the student know ahead of time.

- Check to make sure that the student has actually learned the new skill. Give the student lots of opportunities to practice the new skill.

- Show the student how to use an assignment book and a daily schedule. This helps the student get organized.

- Realize that the student may get tired quickly. Let the student rest as needed.

- Reduce distractions.

- Keep in touch with the student's parents. Share information about how the student is doing at home and at school.

- Be flexible about expectations. Be patient. Maximize the student's chances for success.

References

1.   National Center for Injury Prevention and Control. (2009). What is traumatic brain injury? Available online at the Centers for Disease Prevention and Control (CDC) website: http://www.cdc.gov/ncipc/tbi/TBI.htm.

2.   Ibid.

3.   Data Accountability Center. (2009). Data tables for OSEP state reported data. Available online at:

      - http://www.ideadata.org/TABLES31ST/AR_1-2.htm

      - http://www.ideadata.org/TABLES31ST/AR_1-3.htm

Chapter 27

Visual Impairment

Throughout grade school, the demands placed on children in the classroom are great. However, no task is more challenging in those early years of school than learning to read.

Reading requires children to accurately use all of their language, decoding, phonetic, and visual skills to successfully recognize words and gather meaning from the written text. Unfortunately, about 20 percent of school-aged children struggle to read. Some of these children suffer from learning disabilities or dyslexia, the inability of the brain's verbal language or auditory processing centers to accurately decode print or phonetically make the connection between the word's written symbols and their appropriate sounds. However, a large portion of children struggling to read are not dyslexic at all; their phonetic awareness and language processing skills are fine. It's their vision that is interfering with their ability to read.

Vision plays a vital role in the reading process. First of all, children must have crisp, sharp eyesight in order to see the print clearly. School vision screenings routinely check children's sharpness of vision at distance—measured by the 20/20 line on the eye chart—and refer children for glasses if they have blurry far-away vision and can't see the board from the back of the room. Unfortunately, this is all school vision screenings are designed to check, and children's vision involves so much more.

Excerpted from "Vision and Reading," © 2012 Children's Vision Information Network. All rights reserved. Reprinted with permission. For additional information, visit www.childrensvision.com.

For success in school, children must have other equally important visual skills besides their sharpness of sight, or visual acuity. They must also be able to coordinate their eye movements as a team. They must be able to follow a line of print without losing their place. They must be able to maintain clear focus as they read or make quick focusing changes when looking up to the board and back to their desks. And they must be able to interpret and accurately process what they are seeing. If children have inadequate visual skills in any of these areas, they can experience great difficulty in school, especially in reading.

Children who lack good basic visual skills often struggle in school unnecessarily. Their "hidden" vision problem is keeping them from performing at grade level, yet teachers and parents often fail to make the connection between poor reading and the child's vision.

The following information summarizes each of the major areas which can interfere with a child's school performance.

Eye Teaming Problems

Our eyes are designed to work as a team, but each eye functions independently. When we look at something, the right eye records the image and the left eye records the image. Then the two separate images are transmitted up the optic nerves to the brain, which combines them into a single picture. For the visual system to work correctly, each eye must aim at the exact same point in space so that the images being recorded are identical. This allows the brain to combine, or "fuse," the two incoming images for clear, comfortable single vision. However, if the eyes aren't aiming together, then the images being recorded are slightly different. If the disparity is great enough, the brain can't combine the two pictures. The result is double vision.

Unfortunately, about 10 percent of school-aged children have eye teaming problems—technically, called convergence insufficiency or convergence excess. At the close up distances required for reading, children with eye teaming problems are only able to aim their eyes together correctly for short periods of time. As their ability to accurately aim their eyes breaks down, their eyes end up pointing at slightly different places on the page. The result is a great deal of visual strain and eventually blurred, scrambled, or double print.

Of course, reading and comprehension become increasingly difficult as the child strains to aim both eyes at the same place to keep the print from blurring, jumping, or splitting apart.

In addition, children with eye teaming problems can be highly distractible, finding it difficult to concentrate and remain on task when the strain on their eyes is so great. (In fact, many of these children are often misdiagnosed with attention deficit disorder.) Other symptoms of eye teaming problems include loss of place as the print "swims" and moves, eyestrain, fatigue, headaches, and frustration.

To keep from seeing double, many children with eye teaming problems end up suppressing an eye. In other words, their brain "turns off" one eye by neurologically blocking its visual input. This allows them to maintain single vision because they're just using one eye. While suppression helps the child cope, it's extremely tiring and robs the child of concentration.

Because these children have always seen this way, their vision seems normal to them. They don't recognize that they're fighting their eyes harder than anyone else just to maintain a clear, single picture. Very rarely do children realize something is wrong and report transient double vision or the eye strain and fatigue which usually accompanies suppression.

Left undiagnosed and untreated, eye teaming problems can appear to be a learning disability or dyslexia. They are not. Eye teaming disorders are visual problems, not language-based reading dysfunctions. The symptoms, however, are similar and only a complete eye exam by an developmental optometrist trained to diagnose and treat eye teaming problems can determine for certain if vision is the basis of the child's struggle to read.

The good news, however, is that eye teaming problems can be treated very successfully. One type of teaming problem called convergence excess is often corrected with reading glasses. Another teaming problem called convergence insufficiency is usually corrected through vision therapy. Vision therapy is a series of special eye exercises and treatment procedures prescribed by doctors of optometry that correct problems that glasses alone can't help. During therapy, the child learns to gain control of his or her eye muscle coordination and builds the eye teaming skills necessary for success in school.

Tracking

Tracking skills, or the ability to control the fine eye movements required to follow a line of print, are especially important in reading. Children with tracking problems will often lose their place, skip or transpose words, and have difficulty comprehending because of their difficulty moving their eyes accurately. Many are forced to use their fingers to follow the line because their eyes can't.

When we read, our eyes don't move smoothly across the line. Instead, our eyes make a series of jumps and pauses as we read. The small jumps between words or groups of words are called saccades. The brief pause we make while looking at the words is called a fixation. After a fixation, we move our eyes to the next word or group of words—another saccade.

This very precise coordination of jumps and pauses is controlled by our central and peripheral visual systems. Our central vision processes what we're seeing in clear detail and defines what we're looking at. Our peripheral, or side vision, simultaneously locates surrounding objects and lets us know where to look. (These two systems are sometimes referred to as the "Where is it?" and "What is it?" systems.) In reading, our central vision processes the word, while our side vision locates the following word and tells us where to aim our eyes next. The integration of these two systems is what allows us to efficiently move our eyes along a line of print without overshooting or undershooting, or mistakenly aiming our eyes at lines above or below. If there is not continuous, fluid, simultaneous integration between these two systems, reading will be jerky, loss of place will be common, and comprehension will be poor.

Focusing

Our focusing system, technically called accommodation, allows us to see clearly, especially up close. Our eyes are designed for distance vision, so when we look at something up close, the natural lens in our eye has to change shape to redirect light rays on the retina for near objects. At the close ranges required for reading, this is the visual skill needed to maintain clear sharp images for extended periods of time. It also includes the ability to quickly shift focus when looking from near to far, such as when looking from our desk to the board. For children with accommodation problems, print will become progressively blurry as they read for longer periods of time, and their eyes will fatigue from the strain of trying to keep the print clear. Sometimes children with focusing problems will hold their books very closely or lay their heads down. Headaches are very common. Reading glasses are often prescribed to help shore up inadequate focusing systems, but sometimes therapy is need to improve a child's focusing stamina.

Visual Perception

Visual perception is the ability to interpret, analyze, and give meaning to what is seen. Visual perception skills can be broken down into the following areas:

- **Visual discrimination:** The ability to determine exact characteristics and distinctive features among similar objects or forms. In reading, this skill helps children distinguish between similarly spelled words, such as was/saw, then/when, on/one, or run/ran.

- **Visual memory:** The ability to remember for immediate recall the characteristics of a given object or form. This skill helps children remember what they read and see by adequately processing information through their short-term memory, from where it is filtered out into the long-term memory. Children with poor visual memory may struggle with comprehension. They often subvocalize, or softly whisper to themselves, as they read in order to help compensate auditorily. They may have difficulty remembering what a word looks like or fail to recognize the same word on another page. They may also take longer copying assignments because they must frequently review the text.

- **Visual sequential memory:** The ability to remember forms or characters in correct order. This skill is particularly important in spelling. Letter omissions, additions, or transpositions within words are common for children who struggle with this skill. They often subvocalize (whisper or talk aloud) as they write. Recognizing and remembering patterns may also be a problem.

- **Visual spatial relations:** The ability to distinguish differences among similar objects or forms. This skill helps children in understanding relationships and recognizing underlying concepts. This area is closely related to the problem solving and conceptual skills required for higher level science and math.

- **Visual spatial orientation:** This helps us with letter reversals. Many parents and educators consider letter reversals after age seven to be a symptom of dyslexia. While this can be true, the most common cause of reversals in older children is a lack of visual spatial development—consistently knowing left from right, either in relationship to their own bodies or in the world around them. Children with poor visual processing have not developed adequate skills in visual perception and spatial orientation, such as laterality and directionality. Also, children who experience frequent double vision deal with such visual confusion that their brains often misinterpret their visual input.

- **Visual form constancy:** The ability to mentally manipulate forms and visualize the resulting outcomes. This skill helps children distinguish differences in size, shape, and orientation.

Children with poor form-constancy may frequently reverse letters and numbers.

- **Visual closure:** The ability to visualize a complete whole when given incomplete information or a partial picture. This skill helps children read and comprehend quickly; their eyes don't have to individually process every letter in every word for them to quickly recognize the word by sight. This skill can also help children recognize inferences and predict outcomes. Children with poor visual closure may have difficulty completing a thought. They may also confuse similar objects or words, especially words with close beginning or endings.

- **Visual figure ground:** The ability to perceive and locate a form or object within a busy field without getting confused by the background or surrounding images. This skill keeps children from getting lost in details. Children with poor figure-ground become easily confused with too much print on the page, affecting their concentration and attention. They may also have difficulty scanning text to locate specific information.

Visual Motor Integration

Twenty percent of the raw visual data coming off the retina does not go back to the visual cortex for imaging but breaks away and travels up to the brain's motor centers to help with balance, coordination, and movement. Visual motor integration, commonly called eye-body or eye-hand coordination, is a critical component of vision. Think of it as a visual "follow the leader": the eyes go first and tell the muscles where to follow:

- **Gross motor eye-body coordination:** The efficient visual input to the body's relationship with its surrounding space, commonly referred to as eye-body coordination. Good visual motor and bilateral integration skills allow children to use their visual systems to monitor and adjust placement of their body weight against the gravitational forces on both sides of their body's midline, allowing for good balance and coordination. Children with poor eye-body skills may have difficulty in such areas as sports, learning to ride a bicycle, or general "clumsiness."

- **Fine motor eye-hand coordination:** The efficient visual input into the body's fine motor system. Children with poor eye-hand coordination may have poor handwriting and take longer to complete written assignments. They usually become frustrated over time and lose concentration, resulting in less time on task.

Help for Children who Struggle

There is help for children who struggle to read and learn because of poor vision skills. A developmental optometrist who specializes in children's vision can run a complete diagnostic workup to determine to what extent a child's visual skills are hindering school performance and prescribe vision therapy to correct the problems. Vision therapy is the science of remediating inadequate visual systems by improving function and performance. Vision therapy is highly successful, supported by decades of research and the testimony of countless parents and children whose lives have been changed when dysfunctional vision systems are restored to normal. Remove a child's stumbling block to learning, and you allow him the opportunity to succeed.

Part Four

Learning Disabilities
and the Educational Process

Chapter 28

Early Intervention Strategies

Chapter Contents

Section 28.1

Early Intervention: An Overview

"Overview of Early Intervention," National Dissemination
Center for Children with Disabilities, September 2010.

Early intervention services are concerned with all the basic and brand new skills that babies typically develop during the first three years of life, such as the following:

- Physical (reaching, rolling, crawling, and walking)
- Cognitive (thinking, learning, solving problems)
- Communication (talking, listening, understanding)
- Social/emotional (playing, feeling secure and happy)
- Self-help (eating, dressing)

Early intervention services are designed to meet the needs of infants and toddlers who have a developmental delay or disability. Sometimes it is known from the moment a child is born that early intervention services will be essential in helping the child grow and develop. Often this is so for children who are diagnosed at birth with a specific condition or who experience significant prematurity, very low birth weight, illness, or surgery soon after being born. Even before heading home from the hospital, this child's parents may be given a referral to their local early intervention office.

Some children have a relatively routine entry into the world, but may develop more slowly than others, experience setbacks, or develop in ways that seem very different from other children. For these children, a visit with a developmental pediatrician and a thorough evaluation may lead to an early intervention referral. However a child comes to be referred, assessed, and determined eligible—early intervention services provide vital support so that children with developmental needs can thrive and grow. Eligible children can receive early intervention services from birth through the third birthday.

Let's take a closer look at the early intervention process. This overview will discuss actions you can take to find help for your child, including contacting the early intervention program in your community.

Part 1: So You're Concerned about Your Child's Development

It's not uncommon for parents and family members to become concerned when their beautiful baby or growing toddler doesn't seem to be developing according to the normal schedule of "baby" milestones—"He hasn't rolled over yet," or "the little girl next door is already sitting up on her own!" or "she should be saying a few words by now." And while it's true that children develop differently, at their own pace, and that the range of what's "normal" development is quite broad, it's hard not to worry and wonder.

If you think that your child is not developing at the same pace or in the same way as most children his or her age, it is often a good idea to talk first to your child's pediatrician. Explain your concerns. Tell the doctor what you have observed with your child. Your child may have a disability or a developmental delay, or he or she may be at risk of having a disability or delay. You can also get in touch with your community's early intervention program, and ask to have your little one evaluated to see if he or she has a developmental delay or disability. This evaluation is free of charge, won't hurt your child, and looks at his or her basic skills. Based on that evaluation, your child may be eligible for early intervention services, which will be designed to address your child's special needs or delays.

Where do I go for help?

How might you find out about early intervention services in your community? Here are two ways:

- Ask your child's pediatrician to put you in touch with the early intervention system in your community or region.

- Contact the Pediatrics branch in a local hospital and ask where you should call to find out about early intervention services in your area.

It is very important to write down the names and phone numbers of everyone you talk to. Having this information available will be helpful to you later on.

Make sure you get copies of all written information about your child (records, reports, etc.). This will help you become an important coordinator of services and a better advocate for your child. Remember, as time goes on, you'll probably have more information to keep track of, so it's a good idea to keep it together in one place.

What do I say to the early intervention contact person?

Explain that you are concerned about your child's development. Say that you think your child may need early intervention services. Explain that you would like to have your child evaluated under IDEA (the nation's special education law). Write down any information the contact person gives you.

The person may refer you to what is known as Child Find. One of Child Find's purposes is to identify children who need early intervention services. Child Find operates in every state and conducts screenings to identify children who may need early intervention services. These screenings are provided free of charge.

Each state has one agency that is in charge of the early intervention system for infants and toddlers with special needs. This agency is known as the lead agency. It may be the state education agency or another agency, such as the health department. Each state decides which agency will serve as the lead agency.

What happens next?

Once you are in contact with the early intervention system, the system will assign someone to work with you and your child through the evaluation and assessment process. This person will be your temporary service coordinator. He or she should have a background in early childhood development and ways to help young children who may have developmental delays. The service coordinator should also know the policies for early intervention programs and services in your state.

The early intervention system will need to determine if your child is eligible for early intervention services. To do this, the staff will set up and carry out a multidisciplinary evaluation and assessment of your child. Read on for more information about this process.

Part 2: Your Child's Evaluation

What is a multidisciplinary evaluation and assessment?

The law IDEA requires that your child receive a timely, comprehensive, multidisciplinary evaluation and assessment. The purposes of the evaluation and assessment are to find out the following:

- The nature of your child's strengths, delays, or difficulties

- Whether or not your child is eligible for early intervention services

Multidisciplinary means that the evaluation group is made up of qualified people who have different areas of training and experience. Together, they know about children's speech and language skills, physical abilities, hearing and vision, and other important areas of development. They know how to work with children, even very young ones, to discover if a child has a problem or is developing within normal ranges. Group members may evaluate your child together or individually.

Evaluation refers to the procedures used by these professionals to find out if your child is eligible for early intervention services. As part of the evaluation, the team will observe your child, ask your child to do things, talk to you and your child, and use other methods to gather information. These procedures will help the team find out how your child functions in five areas of development: cognitive development, physical development, communication, social-emotional development, and adaptive development.

Following your child's evaluation, you and a team of professionals will meet and review all of the data, results, and reports. The people on the team will talk with you about whether your child meets the criteria under IDEA and state policy for having a developmental delay, a diagnosed physical or mental condition, or being at risk for having a substantial delay. If so, your child is generally found to be eligible for services.

If found eligible, he or she will then be assessed. Assessment refers to the procedures used throughout the time your child is in early intervention. The purposes of these ongoing procedures are to do the following:

- Identify your child's unique strengths and needs

- Determine what services are necessary to meet those needs

With your consent, your family's needs will also be identified. This process, which is family-directed, is intended to identify the resources, priorities, and concerns of your family. It also identifies the supports and services you may need to enhance your family's capacity to meet your child's developmental needs. The family assessment is usually conducted through an interview with you, the parents.

When conducting the evaluation and assessment, team members may get information from some or all of the following:

- Doctor's reports

- Results from developmental tests and performance assessments given to your child

- Your child's medical and developmental history
- Direct observations and feedback from all members of the multi-disciplinary team, including you, the parents
- Interviews with you and other family members or caretakers
- Any other important observations, records, and/or reports about your child

Who pays for the evaluation and assessment?

Under IDEA, evaluations and assessments are provided at no cost to parents. They are funded by state and federal monies.

Who is eligible for services?

Under the IDEA, "infants and toddlers with disabilities" are defined as children from birth to the third birthday who need early intervention services because they are experiencing developmental delays, as measured by appropriate diagnostic instruments and procedures, in one or more of the following areas:

- Cognitive development
- Physical development, including vision and hearing
- Communication development
- Social or emotional development
- Adaptive development

or who have a diagnosed physical or mental condition that has a high probability of resulting in developmental delay.

The term may also include, if a state chooses, children from birth through age two who are at risk of having substantial developmental delays if early intervention services are not provided. (34 Code of Federal Regulations §303.16)

My child has been found eligible for services. What's next?

If your child and family are found eligible, you and a team will meet to develop a written plan for providing early intervention services to your child and, as necessary, to your family. This plan is called the Individualized Family Service Plan, or IFSP. It is a very important document, and you, as parents, are important members of the team that develops it.

Part 3: Your Child's Early Intervention Services

What is an Individualized Family Service Plan, or IFSP?

The IFSP is a written document that, among other things, outlines the early intervention services that your child and family will receive. One guiding principal of the IFSP is that the family is a child's greatest resource, that a young child's needs are closely tied to the needs of his or her family. The best way to support children and meet their needs is to support and build upon the individual strengths of their family. So, the IFSP is a whole family plan with the parents as major contributors in its development. Involvement of other team members will depend on what the child needs. These other team members could come from several agencies and may include medical people, therapists, child development specialists, social workers, and others.

Your child's IFSP must include the following:

- Your child's present physical, cognitive, communication, social/emotional, and adaptive development levels and needs

- Family information (with your agreement), including the resources, priorities, and concerns of you, as parents, and other family members closely involved with the child

- The major results or outcomes expected to be achieved for your child and family; the specific services your child will be receiving

- Where in the natural environment (e.g., home, community) the services will be provided (if the services will not be provided in the natural environment, the IFSP must include a statement justifying why not)

- When and where your son or daughter will receive services

- The number of days or sessions he or she will receive each service and how long each session will last

- Whether the service will be provided on a one-on-one or group basis

- Who will pay for the services

- The name of the service coordinator overseeing the implementation of the IFSP

- The steps to be taken to support your child's transition out of early intervention and into another program when the time comes

The IFSP may also identify services your family may be interested in, such as financial information or information about raising a child with a disability. The IFSP is reviewed every six months and is updated at least once a year. The IFSP must be fully explained to you, the parents, and your suggestions must be considered. You must give written consent before services can start. If you do not give your consent in writing, your child will not receive services. Each state has specific guidelines for the IFSP. Your service coordinator can explain what the IFSP guidelines are in your state.

What's included in early intervention services?

Under IDEA, early intervention services must include a multidisciplinary evaluation and assessment, a written Individualized Family Service Plan, service coordination, and specific services designed to meet the unique developmental needs of the child and family. Early intervention services may be simple or complex depending on the child's needs. They can range from prescribing glasses for a two-year-old to developing a comprehensive approach with a variety of services and special instruction for a child, including home visits, counseling, and training for his or her family. Depending on your child's needs, his or her early intervention services may include the following:

- Family training, counseling, and home visits
- Special instruction
- Speech-language pathology services (sometimes referred to as speech therapy)
- Audiology services (hearing impairment services)
- Occupational therapy
- Physical therapy
- Psychological services; medical services (only for diagnostic or evaluation purposes)
- Health services needed to enable your child to benefit from the other services
- Social work services
- Assistive technology devices and services
- Transportation
- Nutrition services
- Service coordination services

How are early intervention services delivered?

Early intervention services may be delivered in a variety of ways and in different places. Sometimes services are provided in the child's home with the family receiving additional training. Services may also be provided in other settings, such as a clinic, a neighborhood daycare center, hospital, or the local health department. To the maximum extent appropriate, the services are to be provided in natural environments or settings. Natural environments, broadly speaking, are where the child lives, learns, and plays. Services are provided by qualified personnel and may be offered through a public or private agency.

Will I have to pay for services?

Whether or not you, as parents, will have to pay for any services for your child depends on the policies of your state. Under IDEA, the following services must be provided at no cost to families:

- Child Find services

- Evaluations and assessments

- The development and review of the Individualized Family Service Plan

- Service coordination

Depending on your state's policies, you may have to pay for certain other services. You may be charged a "sliding-scale" fee, meaning the fees are based on what you earn. Check with the contact person in your area or state. Some services may be covered by your health insurance, by Medicaid, or by Indian Health Services. Every effort is made to provide services to all infants and toddlers who need help, regardless of family income. Services cannot be denied to a child just because his or her family is not able to pay for them.

Section 28.2

Recognition and Response: Response to Intervention in the Preschool Years

Background and Origins

Recognition and Response (R&R) is a model of RTI (Response to Intervention) for pre-k developed by researchers at the FPG Child Development Institute. It is designed to enhance teaching practices of language, literacy, and math with three- to five-year-olds enrolled in center-based early childhood programs. The instructional principles that serve as the foundation for R&R are consistent with those widely acknowledged in early childhood, namely, the emphasis on high-quality curriculum and instruction and the importance of intervening early using research-based practices. There is now a body of evidence for the effectiveness of using RTI to improve reading and math skills with school-age children and emerging evidence for its effectiveness in language and literacy with pre-k children.

A Framework for Linking Assessment and Instruction

R&R is a tiered model of instruction comprised of three components congruent with RTI:

- Universal screening and progress monitoring (Recognition)

- Effective core curriculum, intentional teaching, and targeted interventions (Response)

- Collaborative problem-solving to support data-based decision-making

Recognition: Universal screening and progress monitoring.
The recognition component consists of the systematic use of assessment data gathered through universal screening and progress monitoring. Universal screening involves teachers periodically gathering assessment information on all children in their pre-k classroom to determine which children might benefit from targeted interventions to master certain skills. Progress monitoring is a systematic process used to further assess the progress of those children receiving targeted interventions. Teachers monitor children's progress by assessing their skills during the intervention period to see how well they are responding to interventions over time. Teachers use the assessment results from both universal screening and progress monitoring to help them determine whether individual children require additional instructional supports at various points.

Response: Curriculum, intentional teaching, and targeted interventions. The response component refers to the core instruction offered to all children as well as the targeted interventions that are provided for some children who require additional help to learn. In R&R, classroom instruction and interventions are implemented through a tiered approach. They are organized hierarchically from least to most intensive to show how directive and involved teachers should be in their instruction for children who need various levels of support. Tier 1 involves providing a high-quality, effective core curriculum along with intentional teaching of key school readiness skills for all children in the classroom. Intentional teaching occurs through the purposeful organization of the classroom environment and the provision of planned, developmentally appropriate activities to help children learn key skills. At Tier 2, teachers make adjustments to their instruction for children who require additional supports on the basis of universal screening results. To enhance learning, teachers implement targeted interventions with small groups of children (generally three to six children) who have similar learning goals. The Tier 2 interventions involve small-group lessons that take place for approximately fifteen minutes a day over a two-month period, complemented by embedded learning opportunities designed to complement and extend learning outside of small-group time. Tier 3 consists of more intensive scaffolding strategies such as response prompting, modeling, and peer supports to further promote children's learning within the Tier 2 interventions.

Collaborative problem-solving to support data-based decision-making. Collaborative problem-solving offers a process by which teachers, parents, specialists, and others can work together to plan various levels of instructional supports and assess how well children respond to them. A core problem-solving team is established to interpret assessment results, develop an intervention plan, and to evaluate the effectiveness of the instructional supports that teachers implement for children. The problem-solving team also determines the methods for documenting and sharing information with others, including parents, administrators, and other professionals.

Considerations for Implementation

Because R&R (and RTI approaches more broadly) represents a set of related practices (assessment, instructional, and problem-solving) in early childhood, a number of decisions must be made to support its implementation in pre-k classrooms. Key decisions such as selecting a universal screening and progress monitoring tool and identifying standardized tiered interventions are best made at the program level. Furthermore, to use R&R effectively, teachers generally will need administrative oversight to establish core problem-solving teams. In the meantime, programs can get started by determining which assessment approaches, instructional strategies, and methods for collaborating with families and professionals are already being used in pre-k classrooms and how these could be reorganized in accordance with the R&R framework.

Chapter 29

Understanding Your Child's Right to Special Education Services

Chapter Contents

Section 29.1

Section 504

If your child has diagnosed learning disabilities, you're probably aware that she is eligible for services under the Individuals with Disabilities Education Act (IDEA 2004). What you may not realize is that she may also qualify for protection and services under Section 504 of the Rehabilitation Act of 1973.

What is Section 504?

Section 504 is a federal civil rights law that prohibits discrimination against persons with disabilities. It ensures that a student with a disability has equal access to an education and to benefits and services comparable to those given to peers without disabilities.

Who does Section 504 protect?

Section 504 applies to students, employees, and the parents of students who attend public schools or any program operated by an organization that receives federal funds.

All students eligible under IDEA are automatically protected under Section 504. However the reverse is not necessarily the case: a child that does not qualify for services under IDEA may still be protected under 504 if she has a physical or mental impairment that substantially limits a major life activity.

For example, a student with attention deficit hyperactivity disorder (ADHD) who does not require special education services would not be eligible for IDEA, but may still be entitled to reasonable accommodations under 504 if it's shown that her disability limits a major life activity.

What are "life activities?"

Major life activities include caring for oneself, performing manual tasks, walking, seeing, hearing, speaking, breathing, working, and learning (reading, writing, performing math calculations).

It is important for parents of students with Individualized Education Programs (IEPs) to know that 504 extends beyond IDEA to housing, employment, and post-secondary education.

What does 504 require?

Like IDEA, Section 504 has specific procedural requirements for the identification, evaluation, placement, and safeguards for preschool, elementary, and secondary students, and encompasses Child Find, which mandates school systems to identify and locate students with disabilities throughout a community's school system.

Do 504 students have an IEP?

Students under 504 are not entitled to an Individualized Education Program (IEP). However, a group of people knowledgeable about a 504-eligible student must identify the services or accommodations necessary for her to access an education and, subsequently, develop and implement a written 504 Plan. Like an IEP, a 504 Plan is driven by the needs of the child as identified by formal and informal assessments and evaluations.

Section 29.2

Additional 2009 Provisions to Section 504

Did you know that, effective January 2009, eligibility for protection under Section 504 of the Rehabilitation Act became broader? Some students who did not qualify for Section 504 in the past, or who were not eligible for services and supports under the Individuals with Disabilities Education Act (IDEA) may now qualify for Section 504 plans. Students with Section 504 plans may now qualify for additional supports, services, auxiliary aids, and/or accommodations in public schools. For many students with learning disabilities (LD) and/or ADHD (Attention Deficit Hyperactivity Disorder), this is good news! These positive changes are the result of recent amendments to the Americans with Disabilities Act (ADA), a broad civil rights law that also impacts Section 504.

You'll be especially interested in these developments if:

- your child was evaluated under IDEA but was found ineligible;

- your child was previously evaluated for Section 504 but was found ineligible;

- your child is currently receiving informal accommodations in school;

- your child has a Section 504 plan in place (if your child has an IEP, he is automatically considered to have a 504 plan);

- your child needs accommodations on the Scholastic Aptitude Test (SAT) or American College Test (ACT);

- your teenager is getting ready to go college.

What's the Connection between Section 504 and the ADA?

What does the ADA Amendments Act of 2008 (ADAAA) have to do with Section 504? Both are civil rights laws that protect individuals with disabilities from discrimination. Section 504 was enacted in 1973 and applies to all programs and activities that receive federal financial assistance. This includes public schools, colleges, and universities as well as certain employers, state and local government programs, and places of public accommodation (such as a public library). So the "common denominator" between Section 504 and ADAAA related to school-age students is protecting students with disabilities from being discriminated against in our public schools.

The ADAAA includes a "conforming amendment" to Section 504 of the Rehabilitation Act; meaning that the newly expanded coverage under ADAAA also applies to Section 504. Matt Cohen, an attorney who works on behalf of children with disabilities in disputes with public schools, explains, "Because ADA and 504 are interpreted in parallel, the ADAAA will be applied to the public schools in their interpretation of both the ADAAA and Section 504."

How Things Have Changed with ADAAA

Because of the ADAAA, more students may now qualify as persons with disabilities entitled to protection from discrimination based on their disabilities. They also may now be eligible to receive special education or general education with related services and reasonable accommodations, including auxiliary aids and services in school, under Section 504.

The ADA Amendments Act of 2008 includes several significant changes, which also apply to Section 504:

- The definition of "major life activities" was expanded to include learning, reading, concentrating, and thinking. Also, the definition of "major bodily functions" has been expanded to include neurological and brain functions. This change makes it much easier for individuals with LD and/or ADHD to qualify for protections under ADAAA.

- ADAAA requires that the limitation on a "major" life activity be broadly, rather than narrowly, interpreted.

- Conditions that are episodic or in remission are covered when they are active. For example, a student with ADHD may be affected by his symptoms differently and at different times and under different conditions. ADAAA does not disqualify him from protection on that basis alone.

- Under ADAAA a person cannot be denied protection simply because he uses a mitigating measure, such as taking medication for ADHD, or being allowed extra time when taking tests to accommodate for an LD. (The only exception to this is corrective lenses that fully correct a vision problem.)

- Limitation in one major life activity need not impact other major life activities in order to trigger ADAAA protection. Some students with disabilities struggle in just one academic area, such as reading or writing, but excel in other skills or subjects, and shine in extra-curricular activities. Such students might now qualify for ADAAA protection, whereas before 2009 they would have been found ineligible because they struggled in only one major life activity.

What Does This Mean for Your Child?

Now that you have a sense of how the ADAAA affects the interpretation of Section 504, you're probably eager to know how these changes might help your child. While every situation—and every child—is unique, we'll provide answers and action steps for some of the most common questions here.

My child receives informal accommodations that his teacher or other school personnel (e.g., counselor, nurse) provides. Should I request these accommodations be formalized through a 504 plan?

Yes. By documenting that your child has a disability which substantially limits a major life activity (e.g., learning or concentrating), you are ensuring the legal protections provided by federal law. You're also providing documentation that will be important in the case of transition to a new school/setting, a new teacher, or some other life event.

My child was previously found ineligible for services under IDEA, but a 504 plan was not discussed at that time. Since ADAAA has broadened eligibility requirements, should we reapply?

Yes, you should request a 504 evaluation if you believe your child could benefit from a 504 plan. Because of the similarities between the IDEA and Section 504 "child find" requirement to provide a free, appropriate public education, schools should begin to pay particular attention to students found ineligible for services under IDEA and be willing to discuss whether accommodations under a 504 plan are appropriate for the child.

My child was previously found ineligible for a 504 plan. Should we reapply?

Yes, especially if you believe the denial was directly related to the old interpretation of the law, such as finding that there was no substantial limitation of a major life activity, or denial due to use of a mitigating measure such as medication.

My child already has a Section 504 plan. Should I ask if he is allowed additional (or different) accommodations under ADAAA?

Yes, if you believe that your child will benefit from additional or different reasonable accommodations, auxiliary aids, supports, or services. Once your child has a 504 plan, the school should be willing to have regular discussions about the effectiveness of the plan and whether adjustments need to be made to support your child's success.

My child has been eligible for services under IDEA and now the school proposes to end that eligibility. Should there be a discussion about a 504 plan?

Yes. Every year, about sixty-six thousand students in special education (3 percent) are declassified, which means their eligibility for services and supports under IDEA is terminated. It's very likely that many of these children need accommodations for both classroom instruction and testing in order to succeed in general education. In those cases, a Section 504 plan might provide such accommodations.

My teenager has a 504 plan and will soon be taking Advanced Placement tests and/or college entrance exams. What accommodations might he be allowed to use during those exams?

This is where the ADAAA and Section 504 intersect. National testing services are required under the ADAAA to provide reasonable accommodations, and most have information on their websites about how to document a disability and request accommodations. However, all documentation must be prepared well in advance. You and your teen will want to talk to his high school counselor about the required paperwork and the timeline for submission to the College Board, the ACT, or Education Testing Service.

My teenager has a 504 plan and is applying to college. What are the most important steps in assuring she gets what she needs in the college setting?

The most important thing to teach your teenager is to advocate for herself—to communicate what her disability is and what accommodations she needs to succeed. Because each college establishes its own procedures based on its interpretation of the ADAAA and Section 504, it's important to check with the college about its policies.

Federal Funding and Regulations

While public schools receive federal financial assistance under IDEA, they don't receive any such financial assistance to provide Section 504 plans. Schools may therefore view providing a Section 504 plan as a financial burden. Because there's no requirement to collect data on how many students actually have 504 plans (Zirkel and Holler report in 2008 that 1.2 percent of students on average nationally have 504 plans), some schools and districts don't track how many students benefit from Section 504 or the cost associated with serving those students.

The new law intends to expand eligibility and coverage; however, while new regulations are forthcoming from the Equal Employment Opportunity Commission on the ADAAA, Congress has urged the U.S. Department of Education, Office for Civil Rights (OCR) to maintain the current regulations and guidance related to Section 504. This means that parents will need to advocate for their children's rights and schools are obligated to ensure their current policies and practices are in full compliance with the new law.

Remain Vigilant in the Face of Victory

While the ADAAA represents a victory for students with disabilities, you'll want to be vigilant to ensure your child is treated fairly and appropriately. Through the ADAAA, Congress has intentionally expanded the ADA, which, in turn, broadens the interpretation of who should have access to 504 plans. Students with LD and ADHD should directly benefit from the new law because the use of mitigating measures can no longer be the basis for denying 504 plans to students. If your child already has a 504 plan, you should work with your school's 504 team, guidance counselor, and other school personnel to make any appropriate changes.

Section 29.3

Individuals with Disabilities Education Act (IDEA)

Reprinted from the following documents from the National Dissemination Center for Children with Disabilities: "Q and A on IDEA 2004: Purposes and Key Definitions," April 2009, and "Parental Rights under IDEA," December 2010.

Q and A on IDEA 2004: Purposes and Key Definitions

More than 6.8 million children with disabilities in our public schools receive special education and related services as part of their publicly funded education.[1] But:

- What is special education?
- What are related services?
- Who's considered a "child with a disability?"

This section is designed to answer these questions—looking in detail at the mandates and requirements of our nation's special education law, the Individuals with Disabilities Education Act (IDEA), as amended in 2004.

IDEA's Purposes

We'd like to start by taking a brief look at IDEA's purposes, for they underpin and guide its many detailed requirements. Those purposes have their roots in the past, when children with disabilities were often excluded from schools. This history can be clearly seen in the Findings that Congress states at the very beginning of the law, as most recently amended in 2004.

Public Law 108-446 states:

Findings.—Congress finds the following:

1. Disability is a natural part of the human experience and in no way diminishes the right of individuals to participate

in or contribute to society. Improving educational results for children with disabilities is an essential element of our national policy of ensuring equality of opportunity, full participation, independent living, and economic self-sufficiency for individuals with disabilities.

2. Before the date of enactment of the Education for All Handicapped Children Act of 1975 (Public Law 94–142), the educational needs of millions of children with disabilities were not being fully met because: (A) the children did not receive appropriate educational services; (B) the children were excluded entirely from the public school system and from being educated with their peers; (C) undiagnosed disabilities prevented the children from having a successful educational experience; or (D) a lack of adequate resources within the public school system forced families to find services outside the public school system.[2]

These words reveal why IDEA was originally passed in 1975 as Public Law 94-142. Then, it was called the Education for All Handicapped Children Act and gave grants to States for the education of children with disabilities. Since then, it has been amended many times, while always maintaining its original purpose—to ensure that children with disabilities have access to a free appropriate public education.

In August 2006, the U.S. Department of Education released final regulations for the amended IDEA passed by Congress in 2004. The regulations officially state that the major purposes of IDEA are as follows:

- To ensure that all children with disabilities have available to them a "free appropriate public education" that emphasizes special education and related services designed to meet their unique needs and prepare them for further education, employment, and independent living

- To ensure that the rights of children with disabilities and their parents are protected

- To help states, localities, educational service agencies, and federal agencies provide for the education of all children with disabilities

- To assess and ensure the effectiveness of efforts to educate children with disabilities.[3]

Within these purposes, you can see several key terms—children with disabilities, free appropriate public education, special education, related services—all of which are defined within the regulations. The next section will share those definitions with you. They're important to know, because they drive how states design their own special education policies and procedures, including their governing legislation.

Key Definitions

As we've said, IDEA requires that a free appropriate public education—which includes special education and related services—be made available to each eligible child with a disability. This is a sweeping mandate that contains four key terms frequently used in IDEA:

- A free appropriate public education, or FAPE
- Child with a disability
- Special education
- Related services

Understanding what each of these terms means is a crucial part of implementing IDEA. For parents, these terms will be central in determining their child's eligibility for special education and related services and what those services may include. Accordingly, we will now focus on how IDEA defines these four terms.

Special Symbols in This Issue

As you read the explanations about IDEA, you will find footnotes referencing specific sections of the federal regulations, such as §300.1. You can use these references to locate the precise sections in the federal regulations that address the issue being discussed. For example, in the discussion of IDEA's purposes, you are given the reference 34 CFR §300.1. (The § symbol means "section.") This reference tells you that, to read the exact words the regulations use to define IDEA's purposes, you would look under section 300.1 of the Code of Federal Regulations (CFR) for Title 34 (sometimes referred to as 34 CFR).

What Is a Free Appropriate Public Education?

In IDEA, a free appropriate public education (FAPE) means special education and related services that:

- are provided to children and youth with disabilities at public expense, under public supervision and direction, and without charge;

- meet the standards of the state educational agency (SEA), including the requirements of IDEA;

- include preschool, elementary school, or secondary school education in the state involved; and

- are provided in keeping with an individualized education program (IEP) that meets the requirements of IDEA.[4]

Those are practically IDEA's exact words. Note that they make direct reference to what FAPE itself stands for, word by word:

- **Free:** "without charge" to parents or children

- **Appropriate:** "in keeping with an individualized education program"

- **Public:** "at public expense, under public supervision and direction"

- **Education:** "preschool, elementary . . . or secondary school"

We'd like to elaborate for a moment on "appropriate," because it is a highly influential term in IDEA. You'll see it a lot, used in different contexts but generally meaning the same thing. It means whatever's suitable, fitting, or right for a specific child, given that child's specific needs, specific strengths, established goals, and the supports and services that will be provided to help the child reach those goals.

Thus, an "appropriate" education differs for each child with a disability because it is based on his or her individual needs. IDEA specifies in some detail how school systems and parents are to plan the education that each child receives so that it is appropriate—meaning, responsive to the child's needs.[5] The plan that parents and school staff develop is documented in writing through the individualized education program (IEP), which the school is then responsible for carrying out.[6]

How Does IDEA Define "Child with a Disability"?

"Child with a disability" is definitely one of the most important terms in IDEA, because it shapes whether or not a specific child is eligible for special education and related services (which we'll define in a moment). Every time IDEA uses the term "child with a disability," it means the same thing—the definition we're about to provide. That definition is long, so we'll break it down, factor by factor.

Factor A: Evaluation

IDEA's definition of a "child with a disability" begins like this:

(a) General. (1) Child with a disability means a child evaluated in accordance with §§300.304 through 300.311 . . .[7]

Thus, in order for your child to be considered a "child with a disability" in IDEA, he or she must first receive a full and individual evaluation as described within IDEA.

Factor B: The Disabilities

IDEA's definition goes on to say that, through the evaluation we just mentioned, the child is found to have one or more of the following disabilities:

- Mental retardation

- A hearing impairment, including deafness

- A speech or language impairment

- A visual impairment, including blindness

- A serious emotional disturbance (hereafter referred to as emotional disturbance)

- An orthopedic impairment

- Autism

- Traumatic brain injury

- Other health impairment

- A specific learning disability

- Deaf-blindness

- Multiple disabilities[8]

Each of these disabilities is also individually defined in the regulations for IDEA. These are important to know, because they add substantive detail to the meaning of "child with a disability."

Factor C: State Definitions

It's also important to understand that state definitions of individual disabilities can play a critical role in whether or not a child meets the definition of a "child with a disability." As long as state definitions are consistent with IDEA's, states may establish additional criteria in the disability areas and frequently do, setting policies that explain each of the thirteen disabilities in their own terms.[9]

Specific learning disability is an excellent example. States differ in how they define this term; in one state a child may be considered to have a specific learning disability, while in another state the child will not.[10]

Thus, while the term "child with a disability" is defined within IDEA 2004, the term also has an operational definition at the state level. So what the term really means, and whether or not a group of people decide that a child has a particular disability, is a matter of how IDEA's definition intersects with state definitions and policies.

Factor D: "By Reason Thereof"

Another influential part of IDEA's definition of a "child with a disability" is found in how the general definition ends, which is:

> . . . and who, by reason thereof, needs special education and related services.[11]

It's the "by reason thereof" that sometimes causes confusion and even gets forgotten in IDEA's definition of "child with a disability." This short phrase adds another level to what it means for a child with a disability to be eligible for special education and related services under IDEA 2004. It's not enough for a child to be evaluated in keeping with IDEA's requirements and found to have one of the disabilities listed in IDEA. "By reason thereof" is also a condition to be met—in other words, because of the disability, the child needs special education and related services. Many disabilities don't result in the need for special education. If a child is found to need only a related service and not special education, then he or she does not meet the definition of a "child with a disability."[12]

Factor E: Use of "Developmental Delays"

IDEA allows states, at their discretion, to adopt a definition of "child with a disability" that includes children aged three through nine (or any subset of that age range) who are experiencing "developmental delays" and "who, by reason thereof," need special education and related services.[13]

This provision allows states to find three- through nine-year-olds (or any subset of that age range) with developmental delays to be eligible children with a disability and to provide them with special education and related services without having to classify them under a specific disability category. This provision of law is intended to address the often-difficult process of determining the precise nature of a child's disability in the early years of his or her development.[14]

According to IDEA, as measured by appropriate diagnostic instruments and procedures, "developmental delays" must be in one or more of the following areas:

- Physical development
- Cognitive development
- Communication development
- Social or emotional development
- Adaptive development[15]

States do not have to adopt use of the term "developmental delay" in their definitions of "child with a disability." It's an option for states. Even if the state adopts the term (which includes defining the age range of children to which it applies), it can't force any of its local education agencies (LEAs) to do so. If the state does not adopt the term, its LEAs may not independently decide they will use the term. It's only an option for LEAs if the state adopts the term—and then, the LEA must use the state's definition, including the age range specified by the state.[16]

As you can see, the definition of "child with a disability" is intricate. Several factors must be met before a child can be considered to meet IDEA's definition—and you must also consider the specifics of your state's policies and definitions.

What Is Special Education?

Special education is defined as instruction that is specially designed, at no cost to you as parents, to meet your child's unique needs.[17] Specially designed instruction means adapting the content, methodology, or delivery of instruction:

- to address the unique needs of your child that result from his or her disability, and
- to ensure your child's access to the general education curriculum so that he or she can meet the educational standards that apply to all children within the jurisdiction of the school system.[18]

Special education can include instruction conducted in the classroom, in the home, in hospitals and institutions, and in other settings. It can include instruction in physical education as well. Speech-language pathology services or any other related service can be considered special education rather than a related service under state standards if the instruction is specially designed, at no cost to the parents, to meet the unique needs of a child with a disability. Travel training and vocational education also can be considered special education if these standards are met.[19]

Where Is Special Education Instruction Provided?

As listed above, special education instruction can be provided in a number of settings, such as: in the classroom, in the home, in hospitals and institutions, and in other settings.[20] School systems must ensure that a continuum of alternative placements is available to meet the needs of children with disabilities.[21] This continuum must include the placements just mentioned (instruction in regular classes, special classes, special schools, home instruction, and instruction in hospitals and institutions) and make provision for supplementary services (such as resource room or itinerant instruction) to be provided in conjunction with regular class placement.[22] Unless a child's IEP requires some other arrangement, the child must be educated in the school he or she would attend if he or she did not have a disability.[23]

Special education instruction must be provided to students with disabilities in what is known as the least restrictive environment, or LRE.[24] IDEA's LRE provisions ensure that children with disabilities are educated with children who do not have disabilities, to the maximum extent appropriate. IDEA's LRE requirements apply to students in public or private institutions or other care facilities.[25] Each state must further ensure that special classes, separate schooling, or other removal of children with disabilities from the regular educational environment occurs only if the nature or severity of the disability is such that education in regular classes with the use of supplementary aids and services cannot be achieved satisfactorily.[26]

What Are Related Services?

Related services are defined in IDEA's regulations as transportation and such developmental, corrective, and other supportive services as are required to assist a child with a disability to benefit from special education.[27] Related services may include the following:

- Audiology services
- Counseling services, including rehabilitation counseling

- Early identification and assessment of disabilities in children
- Interpreting services
- Medical services for diagnostic or evaluation purposes only
- Orientation and mobility services
- Parent counseling and training
- Physical therapy and occupational therapy
- Psychological services
- Recreation, including therapeutic recreation
- School health services and school nurse services
- Social work services in schools
- Speech-language pathology services[28]

The list of related services in IDEA is not intended to be exhaustive, which means that other developmental, corrective, or support services can be provided as "related services" if they are required to help a child benefit from special education.

However, related services may not include a medical device (such as a cochlear implant) that is surgically implanted, optimizing how the device functions, maintaining the device, or replacing it.[29] The public agency does remain responsible for appropriately monitoring and maintaining medical devices that are needed to maintain your child's health and safety, including breathing, nutrition, or operation of other bodily functions, while your child is at school or being transported to and from school.[30] The public agency is also responsible for routinely checking children's hearing aids and the external component of a surgically implanted device to make sure they are functioning properly.[31]

Endnotes

1. U.S. Department of Education. (2009). *28th annual report to Congress on the implementation of the Individuals with Disabilities Education Act, 2006* [Vol. 2]. Washington, DC: Author. (Available online at http://www.ed.gov/about/reports/annual/osep/2006/parts-b-c/index.html).

2. Public Law 108-446, Section 601(c)(1) and (2).

3. 34 CFR §300.1—Purposes.

4. 34 CFR §300.17—Free appropriate public education.

5. Drawn from page 1-51 of Küpper, L. (2007, July). The top 10 basics of special education (Module 1). *Building the legacy: IDEA 2004 training curriculum.* Washington, DC: National Dissemination Center for Children with Disabilities. Available online at: http://www.nichcy.org/wp-content/uploads/docs/legacy/1B-Slides13-end.pdf.

6. NICHCY. (2009, April). 10 basic steps in special education. Available online at: http://www.nichcy.org/schoolage/steps/.

7. 34 CFR §300.8(a)(1)—Child with a disability: General.

8. 34 CFR §300.8(a)(1)—Child with a disability: General.

9. Adapted from pages 1-26 through 1-28 of Küpper, L. (2007, July). The top 10 basics of special education (Module 1). *Building the legacy: IDEA 2004 training curriculum.* Washington, DC: National Dissemination Center for Children with Disabilities. Available online at: http://www.nichcy.org/wp-content/uploads/docs/legacy/1A-Slides1-12.pdf.

10. Ibid.

11. 34 CFR §300.8(a)(1)—Child with a disability: General.

12. 34 CFR §300.8(a)(2)—Child with a disability: General. Additional Note: If the related service the child needs is defined by the state as special education (and not as a related service, as within IDEA), then the child would be considered as a "child with a disability" after all.

13. 34 CFR §300.8(b)—Child with a disability: Children aged three through nine experiencing developmental delays.

14. Same as footnote 9. Adapted from page 1-28.

15. 34 CFR §300.8(b)—Child with a disability: Children aged three through nine experiencing developmental delays.

16. 34 CFR §300.111(b)—Child find: Use of the term developmental delay.

17. 34 CFR §300.39(a)—Special education: General.

18. 34 CFR §300.39(b)(3)—Special education: Individual special education terms defined: Specially designed instruction.

19. 34 CFR §300.39—Special education.

20. Ibid.

21. 34 CFR §300.115—Continuum of alternative placements.

22. 34 CFR §300.115(b)(2)—Continuum of alternative placements.

23. 34 CFR §300.116(c)—Placements.

24. 34 CFR §§300.114-300.120—Least Restrictive Environment (LRE).

25. 34 CFR §300.114(a)(2)(i)—LRE requirements.

26. 34 CFR §300.114(a)(2)(ii)—LRE requirements.

27. 34 CFR §300.34—Related services.

28. Ibid.

29. 34 CFR §300.34(b)—Related services: Exception.

30. 34 CFR §300.34(b)(2)(ii)—Related services: Exception.

31. 34 CFR §300.113—Routine checking of hearing aids and external components of surgically implanted medical devices.

Parental Rights under IDEA

The federal regulations for IDEA 2004 include a section (Subpart E) called Procedural Safeguards. These safeguards are designed to protect the rights of parents and their child with a disability and, at the same time, give families and school systems several mechanisms by which to resolve their disputes.

The most notable procedural safeguards include the following:

- The right of parents to receive a complete explanation of all the procedural safeguards available under IDEA and the procedures in the state for presenting complaints

- Confidentiality and the right of parents to inspect and review the educational records of their child

- The right of parents to participate in meetings related to the identification, evaluation, and placement of their child, and the provision of FAPE (a free appropriate public education) to their child

- The right of parents to obtain an independent educational evaluation (IEE) of their child

- The right of parents to receive "prior written notice" on matters relating to the identification, evaluation, or placement of their child, and the provision of FAPE to their child

- The right of parents to give or deny their consent before the school may take certain action with respect to their child

- The right of parents to disagree with decisions made by the school system on those issues

- The right of parents and schools to use IDEA's mechanisms for resolving disputes, including the right to appeal determinations

These are not the only procedural safeguards under IDEA, but they are the most relevant to the majority of parents.

Section 29.4

No Child Left Behind (NCLB)

"No Child Left Behind Act (NCLB): An Overview," copyright 2012 by National Center for Learning Disabilities, Inc. All rights reserved. Reprinted with permission. For more information, visit LD.org.

What is the No Child Left Behind Act?

The No Child Left Behind Act of 2001 (NCLB) is the current version of the Elementary and Secondary Education Act (ESEA)—the principal federal law affecting public education from kindergarten through high school in the United States. The ESEA was originally passed in 1965. NCLB is important legislation for students with learning disabilities (LD), because it ensures that they reach high levels of academic standards, just like other children in America's public schools today.

NCLB is based on four principles of educational reform:

- stronger accountability for results;

- increased flexibility and local control;

- expanded options for parents; and

- an emphasis on teaching qualifications and methods.

Of these four, accountability for results is the principle that has the potential to greatly improve the educational results for children with LD.

How does NCLB hold schools accountable for results?

Several critical elements in NCLB ensure that schools are held accountable for educational results so that the best education possible is provided to each and every student. The three most critical elements to understand are:

- academic content standards (what students should learn);

- academic achievement standards (how well they should learn);

- state assessments (whether a school is teaching all students successfully).

Academic content standards and academic achievement standards in reading/language arts, mathematics, and science have been defined by each state. These standards define what all children should know and be able to do to be considered "proficient." Information about each state's standards should be available on the state's education department website and in print materials.

State assessments are the way schools must prove that they have successfully taught their students. Beginning in 2005–2006, all states must provide annual assessments that are appropriate for all students in grades three through eight and once in high school in both reading/language arts and math (science assessments must be added beginning in 2007–2008). These assessments must include students with disabilities. Schools must also provide the accommodations and alternate assessments that may be needed by students with disabilities. Accommodations are changes to the assessment materials or procedures that allow for students to demonstrate their knowledge and skills rather than the effects of their disabilities. Students with learning disabilities should be participating in the regular state assessments with or without accommodations. Alternate assessments are assessments designed to measure the performance of students with disabilities who are unable to participate in state and district assessments even with appropriate accommodations. These alternate assessments are typically designed for students with complex disabilities and probably would not be appropriate for most students with learning disabilities.

How does NCLB work with the Individuals with Disabilities Education Act (IDEA)?

IDEA specifically provides services to students with disabilities. Each student served under IDEA has an Individualized Education

Program (IEP) that defines the special education and related services needed by the student. NCLB holds schools accountable for the educational outcomes of those children, as well as all others. In the past, students with disabilities were frequently left out of state and district level assessment and accountability systems, and in many cases did not have access to the general curriculum on which these assessments are based. Because this type of access and assessment did not happen, there was no external measure to indicate whether special education students were learning enough to move on to a post-secondary education or to get a job.

The IEP that is designed for each individual IDEA-eligible student must address how that student will participate in state assessments. Students with disabilities may participate in state assessments in the same way as other students, or with accommodations or by participating in alternate assessments. The IEP team should not be deciding whether a student will participate in state assessments, but how, so as to hold the educational system responsible for the student's learning. If the IEP team determines that an accommodation or modification needed by a child will invalidate a test's results for state accountability (such as, perhaps, having questions read aloud to the student), the team should decide how that student can appropriately be assessed through alternate methods.

Why is it so important that children with learning disabilities be included in state assessments?

No Child Left Behind is intended to improve the education of all children. As part of the law, all states are required to release easy-to-read, detailed report cards every year that provide parents and the general public with a measure of how schools are doing. These report cards must include information on how students in each district, as well as each school, performed on state assessments. The report cards must state student performance on three levels: basic, proficient, and advanced. The data must also be broken down by various student subgroups, including students with disabilities. Just like all other subgroups, NCLB requires that students with disabilities reach proficient levels of achievement. This is not extra pressure on the children. This is a mandate for schools to provide a better education for students with disabilities, including learning disabilities.

In addition, each state is required to set Adequate Yearly Progress (AYP) standards that schools must meet. In defining AYP, each state must set the minimum levels of improvement, measurable in terms of student performance, that school districts and schools must achieve within the time frame specified by the law. Basically, states have to continue to raise the bar on academic achievement, and by 2013–2014 all subgroups in all schools in all states must be achieving proficient levels in reading and math on state assessments. This includes students with learning disabilities. Unlike in the past, NCLB is setting a way (the state assessments) for schools to be held accountable for what their students with learning disabilities are learning and achieving.

How else does NCLB set out to improve public education?

Here is a brief summary of other ways NCLB will ensure a better education for students with LD.

Increased flexibility and local control: NCLB gives both states and local school districts greater flexibility in the use of federal funds than they previously had. This flexibility allows for the reallocation of certain funds to programs dedicated to teacher quality improvement, technology, safe and drug-free schools, and many others. This flexibility is dependent on improved results on state assessments and does not include IDEA funds, or the possibility of transferring money out of Title 1 programs.

Expanded options for parents: Under NCLB, all parents must receive local and district report cards before the beginning of every school year. If a Title 1 school fails to meet its AYP goal for two consecutive years, parents may choose to place their children in nonfailing schools in their district. Under NCLB, school districts must pay the cost of transporting students to the other public school. After three years of failure to meet AYP goals, schools must also offer supplemental services to the children remaining there, including tutoring, after-school programs, and summer school paid for by the district.

Improved teaching qualifications: NCLB requires that all teachers be highly qualified. That means they hold at least a bachelor's degree and have passed a state test of subject knowledge. Elementary school teachers must demonstrate knowledge of teaching math and reading, while teachers in higher grades must demonstrate knowledge of the subject they teach, or must have majored in the subject. Special education teachers must be knowledgeable about the content area(s) they teach as well as special education, unless they provide consultative services to highly qualified general education teachers.

Chapter 30

Understanding the Special Education Process: An Overview

When a child is having trouble in school, it's important to find out why. The child may have a disability. By law, schools must provide special help to eligible children with disabilities. This help is called special education and related services.

There's a lot to know about the process by which children are identified as having a disability and in need of special education and related services.

Here, we've distilled the process into ten basic steps. Once you have the big picture of the process, it's easier to understand the many details under each step.

Step 1. Child is identified as possibly needing special education and related services.

There are two primary ways in which children are identified as possibly needing special education and related services: the system known as Child Find (which operates in each state), and by referral of a parent or school personnel.

Child Find: Each state is required by the Individuals with Disabilities Education Act (IDEA) to identify, locate, and evaluate all children with disabilities in the state who need special education and related services. To do so, states conduct what are known as Child Find activities.

Excerpted from "Ten Basic Steps in Special Education," National Dissemination Center for Children with Disabilities, September 2010.

When a child is identified by Child Find as possibly having a disability and as needing special education, parents may be asked for permission to evaluate their child. Parents can also call the Child Find office and ask that their child be evaluated.

Referral or request for evaluation: A school professional may ask that a child be evaluated to see if he or she has a disability. Parents may also contact the child's teacher or other school professional to ask that their child be evaluated. This request may be verbal, but it's best to put it in writing.

Parental consent is needed before a child may be evaluated. Under the federal IDEA regulations, evaluation needs to be completed within sixty days after the parent gives consent. However, if a state's IDEA regulations give a different timeline for completion of the evaluation, the state's timeline is applied.

Step 2. Child is evaluated.

Evaluation is an essential early step in the special education process for a child. It's intended to answer these questions:

- Does the child have a disability that requires the provision of special education and related services?

- What are the child's specific educational needs?

- What special education services and related services, then, are appropriate for addressing those needs?

By law, the initial evaluation of the child must be "full and individual"—which is to say, focused on that child and that child alone. The evaluation must assess the child in all areas related to the child's suspected disability.

The evaluation results will be used to decide the child's eligibility for special education and related services and to make decisions about an appropriate educational program for the child.

If the parents disagree with the evaluation, they have the right to take their child for an Independent Educational Evaluation (IEE). They can ask that the school system pay for this IEE.

Step 3. Eligibility is decided.

A group of qualified professionals and the parents look at the child's evaluation results. Together, they decide if the child is a "child with a disability," as defined by IDEA. If the parents do not agree with the eligibility decision, they may ask for a hearing to challenge the decision.

Step 4. Child is found eligible for services.

If the child is found to be a child with a disability, as defined by IDEA, he or she eligible for special education and related services. Within thirty calendar days after a child is determined eligible, a team of school professionals and the parents must meet to write an individualized education program (IEP) for the child.

Step 5. IEP meeting is scheduled.

The school system schedules and conducts the IEP meeting. School staff must do the following things:

- Contact the participants, including the parents
- Notify parents early enough to make sure they have an opportunity to attend
- Schedule the meeting at a time and place agreeable to parents and the school
- Tell the parents the purpose, time, and location of the meeting
- Tell the parents who will be attending
- Tell the parents that they may invite people to the meeting who have knowledge or special expertise about the child

Step 6. IEP meeting is held and the IEP is written.

The IEP team gathers to talk about the child's needs and write the student's IEP. Parents and the student (when appropriate) are full participating members of the team. If the child's placement (meaning, where the child will receive his or her special education and related services) is decided by a different group, the parents must be part of that group as well.

Before the school system may provide special education and related services to the child for the first time, the parents must give consent. The child begins to receive services as soon as possible after the IEP is written and this consent is given.

If the parents do not agree with the IEP and placement, they may discuss their concerns with other members of the IEP team and try to work out an agreement. If they still disagree, parents can ask for mediation, or the school may offer mediation. Parents may file a state complaint with the state education agency or a due process complaint, which is the first step in requesting a due process hearing, at which time mediation must be available.

Step 7. After the IEP is written, services are provided.

The school makes sure that the child's IEP is carried out as it was written. Parents are given a copy of the IEP. Each of the child's teachers and service providers has access to the IEP and knows his or her specific responsibilities for carrying out the IEP. This includes the accommodations, modifications, and supports that must be provided to the child, in keeping with the IEP.

Step 8. Progress is measured and reported to parents.

The child's progress toward the annual goals is measured, as stated in the IEP. His or her parents are regularly informed of their child's progress and whether that progress is enough for the child to achieve the goals by the end of the year. These progress reports must be given to parents at least as often as parents are informed of their nondisabled children's progress.

Step 9. IEP is reviewed.

The child's IEP is reviewed by the IEP team at least once a year, or more often if the parents or school ask for a review. If necessary, the IEP is revised. Parents, as team members, must be invited to participate in these meetings. Parents can make suggestions for changes, can agree or disagree with the IEP, and can agree or disagree with the placement.

If parents do not agree with the IEP and placement, they may discuss their concerns with other members of the IEP team and try to work out an agreement. There are several options, including additional testing, an independent evaluation, or asking for mediation, or a due process hearing. They may also file a complaint with the state education agency.

Step 10. Child is reevaluated.

At least every three years the child must be reevaluated. This evaluation is sometimes called a "triennial." Its purpose is to find out if the child continues to be a child with a disability, as defined by IDEA, and what the child's educational needs are. However, the child must be reevaluated more often if conditions warrant or if the child's parent or teacher asks for a new evaluation.

Chapter 31

Individualized Education Programs

What's an Individualized Education Plan (IEP)?

Kids with delayed skills or other disabilities might be eligible for special services that provide individualized education programs in public schools, free of charge to families. Understanding how to access these services can help parents be effective advocates for their kids.

The passage of the updated version of the Individuals with Disabilities Education Act (IDEA 2004) made parents of kids with special needs even more crucial members of their child's education team.

Parents can now work with educators to develop a plan—the individualized education program (IEP)—to help kids succeed in school. The IEP describes the goals the team sets for a child during the school year, as well as any special support needed to help achieve them.

Who Needs an IEP?

A child who has difficulty learning and functioning and has been identified as a special needs student is the perfect candidate for an IEP.

Kids struggling in school may qualify for support services, allowing them to be taught in a special way, for reasons such as:

- learning disabilities;

- attention deficit hyperactivity disorder (ADHD);

- emotional disorders;

- cognitive challenges;

- autism;

- hearing impairment;

- visual impairment;

- speech or language impairment;

- developmental delay.

How Are Services Delivered?

In most cases, the services and goals outlined in an IEP can be provided in a standard school environment. This can be done in the regular classroom (for example, a reading teacher helping a small group of children who need extra assistance while the other kids in the class work on reading with the regular teacher) or in a special resource room in the regular school. The resource room can serve a group of kids with similar needs who are brought together for help.

However, kids who need intense intervention may be taught in a special school environment. These classes have fewer students per teacher, allowing for more individualized attention.

In addition, the teacher usually has specific training in helping kids with special educational needs. The children spend most of their day in a special classroom and join the regular classes for nonacademic activities (like music and gym) or in academic activities in which they don't need extra help.

Because the goal of IDEA is to ensure that each child is educated in the least restrictive environment possible, effort is made to help kids stay in a regular classroom. However, when needs are best met in a special class, then kids might be placed in one.

The Referral and Evaluation Process

The referral process generally begins when a teacher, parent, or doctor is concerned that a child may be having trouble in the classroom, and the teacher notifies the school counselor or psychologist.

The first step is to gather specific data regarding the student's progress or academic problems. This may be done through:

- a conference with parents;

- a conference with the student;

- observation of the student;

- analysis of the student's performance (attention, behavior, work completion, tests, class work, homework, etc.).

This information helps school personnel determine the next step. At this point, strategies specific to the student could be used to help the child become more successful in school. If this doesn't work, the child would be tested for a specific learning disability or other impairment to help determine qualification for special services.

It's important to note, though, that the presence of a disability doesn't automatically guarantee a child will receive services. To be eligible, the disability must affect functioning at school.

To determine eligibility, a multidisciplinary team of professionals will evaluate the child based on their observations; the child's performance on standardized tests; and daily work such as tests, quizzes, class work, and homework.

Who's on the Team?

The professionals on the evaluation team can include:

- a psychologist;

- a physical therapist;

- an occupational therapist;

- a speech therapist;

- a special educator;

- a vision or hearing specialist;

- others, depending on the child's specific needs.

As a parent, you can decide whether to have your child assessed. If you choose to do so, you'll be asked to sign a permission form that will detail who is involved in the process and the types of tests they use. These tests might include measures of specific school skills, such as reading or math, as well as more general developmental skills, such as speech and language. Testing does not necessarily mean that a child will receive services.

Once the team members complete their individual assessments, they develop a comprehensive evaluation report (CER) that compiles their findings, offers an educational classification, and outlines the skills and support the child will need.

The parents then have a chance to review the report before the IEP is developed. Some parents will disagree with the report, and they will have the opportunity to work together with the school to come up with a plan that best meets the child's needs.

Developing an IEP

The next step is an IEP meeting at which the team and parents decide what will go into the plan. In addition to the evaluation team, a regular teacher should be present to offer suggestions about how the plan can help the child's progress in the standard education curriculum.

At the meeting, the team will discuss your child's educational needs—as described in the CER—and come up with specific, measurable short-term and annual goals for each of those needs. If you attend this meeting, you can take an active role in developing the goals and determining which skills or areas will receive the most attention.

The cover page of the IEP outlines the support services your child will receive and how often they will be provided (for example, occupational therapy twice a week). Support services might include special education, speech therapy, occupational or physical therapy, counseling, audiology, medical services, nursing, vision or hearing therapy, and many others.

If the team recommends several services, the amount of time they take in the child's school schedule can seem overwhelming. To ease that load, some services may be provided on a consultative basis. In these cases, the professional consults with the teacher to come up with strategies to help the child but doesn't offer any hands-on instruction. For instance, an occupational therapist may suggest accommodations for a child with fine-motor problems that affect handwriting, and the classroom teacher would incorporate these suggestions into the handwriting lessons taught to the entire class.

Other services can be delivered right in the classroom, so the child's day isn't interrupted by therapy. The child who has difficulty with handwriting might work one on one with an occupational therapist while everyone else practices their handwriting skills. When deciding how and where services are offered, the child's comfort and dignity should be a top priority.

The IEP should be reviewed annually to update the goals and make sure the levels of service meet your child's needs. However, IEPs can be changed at any time on an as-needed basis. If you think your child needs more, fewer, or different services, you can request a meeting and bring the team together to discuss your concerns.

Your Legal Rights

Specific time lines ensure that the development of an IEP moves from referral to providing services as quickly as possible. Be sure to ask about this time frame and get a copy of your parents' rights when your child is referred. These guidelines (sometimes called procedural safeguards) outline your rights as a parent to control what happens to your child during each step of the process.

The parents' rights also describe how you can proceed if you disagree with any part of the CER or the IEP—mediation and hearings both are options. You can get information about low-cost or free legal representation from the school district or, if your child is in early intervention (for kids ages three to five), through that program.

Attorneys and paid advocates familiar with the IEP process will provide representation if you need it. You also may invite anyone who knows or works with your child whose input you feel would be helpful to join the IEP team.

A Final Word

Parents have the right to choose where their kids will be educated. This choice includes public or private elementary schools and secondary schools, including religious schools. It also includes charter schools and home schools.

However, it is important to understand that the rights of children with disabilities who are placed by their parents in private elementary schools and secondary schools are not the same as those of kids with disabilities who are enrolled in public schools or placed by public agencies in private schools when the public school is unable to provide a free appropriate public education (FAPE).

Two major differences that parents, teachers, other school staff, private school representatives, and the kids need to know about are:

1. Children with disabilities who are placed by their parents in private schools may not get the same services they would receive in a public school.

2. Not all kids with disabilities placed by their parents in private schools will receive services.

The IEP process is complex, but it's also an effective way to address how your child learns and functions. If you have concerns, don't hesitate to ask questions about the evaluation findings or the goals recommended by the team. You know your child best and should play a central role in creating a learning plan tailored to his or her specific needs.

Chapter 32

Supports, Modifications, and Accommodations for Students with Disabilities

For many students with disabilities—and for many without—the key to success in the classroom lies in having appropriate adaptations, accommodations, and modifications made to the instruction and other classroom activities.

Some adaptations are as simple as moving a distractible student to the front of the class or away from the pencil sharpener or the window. Other modifications may involve changing the way that material is presented or the way that students respond to show their learning.

Adaptations, accommodations, and modifications need to be individualized for students, based upon their needs and their personal learning styles and interests. It is not always obvious what adaptations, accommodations, or modifications would be beneficial for a particular student, or how changes to the curriculum, its presentation, the classroom setting, or student evaluation might be made. This chapter is intended to help teachers and others find information that can guide them in making appropriate changes in the classroom based on what their students need.

Part 1: A Quick Look at Terminology

You might wonder if the terms *supports*, *modifications*, and *adaptations* all mean the same thing. The simple answer is: No, not completely, but yes, for the most part. (Don't you love a clear answer?)

"Supports, Modifications, and Accommodations for Students," National Dissemination Center for Children with Disabilities, September 2010.

People tend to use the terms interchangeably, to be sure, and we will do so here, for ease of reading, but distinctions can be made between the terms.

Sometimes people get confused about what it means to have a modification and what it means to have an accommodation. Usually a modification means a change in what is being taught to or expected from the student. Making an assignment easier so the student is not doing the same level of work as other students is an example of a modification.

An accommodation is a change that helps a student overcome or work around the disability. Allowing a student who has trouble writing to give his answers orally is an example of an accommodation. This student is still expected to know the same material and answer the same questions as fully as the other students, but he doesn't have to write his answers to show that he knows the information.

What is most important to know about modifications and accommodations is that both are meant to help a child to learn.

Part 2: Different Types of Supports

Special Education

By definition, special education is "specially designed instruction" (§300.39). And the Individuals with Disabilities Education Act (IDEA) defines that term as follows:

> (3) Specially designed instruction means adapting, as appropriate to the needs of an eligible child under this part, the content, methodology, or delivery of instruction—
>
> (i) To address the unique needs of the child that result from the child's disability; and
>
> (ii) To ensure access of the child to the general curriculum, so that the child can meet the educational standards within the jurisdiction of the public agency that apply to all children. [§300.39(b)(3)]

Thus, special education involves adapting the "content, methodology, or delivery of instruction." In fact, the special education field can take pride in the knowledge base and expertise it's developed in the past thirty-plus years of individualizing instruction to meet the needs of students with disabilities. It's a pleasure to share some of that knowledge with you now.

Adapting Instruction

Sometimes a student may need to have changes made in class work or routines because of his or her disability. Modifications can be made to:

- what a child is taught; and/or
- how a child works at school.

For example: Jack is an eighth-grade student who has learning disabilities in reading and writing. He is in a regular eighth-grade class that is team-taught by a general education teacher and a special education teacher. Modifications and accommodations provided for Jack's daily school routine (and when he takes state or district-wide tests) include the following:

- Jack will have shorter reading and writing assignments.
- Jack's textbooks will be based upon the eighth-grade curriculum but at his independent reading level (fourth grade).
- Jack will have test questions read/explained to him, when he asks.
- Jack will give his answers to essay-type questions by speaking, rather than writing them down.

Modifications or accommodations are most often made in the following areas:

- Scheduling. For example:
  - giving the student extra time to complete assignments or tests;
  - breaking up testing over several days.
- Setting. For example:
  - working in a small group;
  - working one-on-one with the teacher.
- Materials. For example:
  - providing audiotaped lectures or books;
  - giving copies of teacher's lecture notes;
  - using large-print books, Braille, or books on CD (digital text).
- Instruction. For example:
  - reducing the difficulty of assignments;

- reducing the reading level;

- using a student/peer tutor.

- Student response. For example:

- allowing answers to be given orally or dictated;

- using a word processor for written work;

- using sign language, a communication device, Braille, or native language if it is not English.

Because adapting the content, methodology, and/or delivery of instruction is an essential element in special education and an extremely valuable support for students, it's equally essential to know as much as possible about how instruction can be adapted to address the needs of an individual student with a disability. The special education teacher who serves on the Individualized Education Program (IEP) team can contribute his or her expertise in this area, which is the essence of special education.

Related Services

One look at IDEA's definition of related services at §300.34 and it's clear that these services are supportive in nature, although not in the same way that adapting the curriculum is. Related services support children's special education and are provided when necessary to help students benefit from special education. Thus, related services must be included in the treasure chest of accommodations and supports we're exploring. That definition begins:

§300.34 Related services.

(a) General. Related services means transportation and such developmental, corrective, and other supportive services as are required to assist a child with a disability to benefit from special education, and includes . . .

Here's the list of related services in the law:

- Speech-language pathology and audiology services

- Interpreting services

- Psychological services

- Physical and occupational therapy

- Recreation, including therapeutic recreation

- Early identification and assessment of disabilities in children
- Counseling services, including rehabilitation counseling
- Orientation and mobility services
- Medical services for diagnostic or evaluation purposes
- School health services and school nurse services
- Social work services in schools

This is not an exhaustive list of possible related services. There are others (not named here or in the law) that states and schools routinely make available under the umbrella of related services. The IEP team decides which related services a child needs and specifies them in the child's IEP.

Supplementary Aids and Services

One of the most powerful types of supports available to children with disabilities are the other kinds of supports or services (other than special education and related services) that a child needs to be educated with nondisabled children to the maximum extent appropriate. Some examples of these additional services and supports, called supplementary aids and services in IDEA, are as follows:

- Adapted equipment, such as a special seat or a cutout cup for drinking
- Assistive technology, such as a word processor, special software, or a communication system
- Training for staff, student, and/or parents
- Peer tutors
- A one-on-one aide
- Adapted materials, such as books on tape, large print, or high-lighted notes
- Collaboration/consultation among staff, parents, and/or other professionals

The IEP team, which includes the parents, is the group that decides which supplementary aids and services a child needs to support his or her access to and participation in the school environment. The IEP team must really work together to make sure that a child gets the supplementary aids and services that he or she needs to be successful. Team members talk about the child's needs, the curriculum, and school routine, and openly explore all options to make sure the right supports for the specific child are included.

Program Modifications or Supports for School Staff

If the IEP team decides that a child needs a particular modification or accommodation, this information must be included in the IEP. Supports are also available for those who work with the child, to help them help that child be successful. Supports for school staff must also be written into the IEP. Some of these supports might include the following:

- Attending a conference or training related to the child's needs

- Getting help from another staff member or administrative person

- Having an aide in the classroom

- Getting special equipment or teaching materials

Accommodations in Large Assessments

IDEA requires that students with disabilities take part in state or district-wide assessments. These are tests that are periodically given to all students to measure achievement. It is one way that schools determine how well and how much students are learning. IDEA now states that students with disabilities should have as much involvement in the general curriculum as possible. This means that, if a child is receiving instruction in the general curriculum, he or she could take the same standardized test that the school district or state gives to nondisabled children. Accordingly, a child's IEP must include all modifications or accommodations that the child needs so that he or she can participate in state or district-wide assessments.

The IEP team can decide that a particular test is not appropriate for a child. In this case, the IEP must include the following:

- An explanation of why that test is not suitable for the child

- How the child will be assessed instead (often called alternate assessment)

Ask your state and/or local school district for a copy of their guidelines on the types of accommodations, modifications, and alternate assessments available to students.

Conclusion

Even a child with many needs is to be involved with nondisabled peers to the maximum extent appropriate. Just because a child has severe disabilities or needs modifications to the general curriculum does not mean that he or she may be removed from the general education class. If a child is removed from the general education class for any part of the school day, the IEP team must include in the IEP an explanation for the child's nonparticipation.

Because accommodations can be so vital to helping children with disabilities access the general curriculum, participate in school (including extracurricular and nonacademic activities), and be educated alongside their peers without disabilities, IDEA reinforces their use again and again, in its requirements, in its definitions, and in its principles. The wealth of experience that the special education field has gained over the years since IDEA was first passed by Congress is the very resource you'll want to tap for more information on what accommodations are appropriate for students, given their disability, and how to make those adaptations to support their learning.

Chapter 33

Specialized Teaching Techniques

Chapter Contents

Section 33.1

Differentiated Instruction

Differentiation is responsive teaching rather than one-size-fits-all teaching (Tomlinson 2005). To put it yet another way, it means that teachers proactively plan varied approaches to what students need to learn, how they will learn it, and/or how they will show what they have learned in order to increase the likelihood that each student will learn as much as he or she can, as efficiently as possible (Tomlinson 2003).

The Differentiated Instruction Model

Students come to our classrooms with unique differences as people and therefore as learners. Our students have varied degrees of background knowledge and readiness to learn, different life experiences, cultural orientations, languages, interests, and preferences for how they learn best, and different feelings about themselves as learners and about school. Just as medical doctors don't prescribe the same medications for every one of their patients, teachers who differentiate instruction are mindful of the varied learning needs of their students and plan instruction accordingly.

Differentiated instruction (DI) is both a philosophy and a way of teaching that respects the different learning needs of students and expects all students to experience success as learners. Learning activities may be differentiated on the basis of students' readiness for learning the specific content or skill, their interests, or their preferred ways of learning. In a differentiated classroom, students experience learning in many configurations—working in small groups (with peers having similar or different readiness, interests, or learning preferences), with a partner, individually, and as a whole group.

The differentiated instruction model is based on effective educational practice (research base for DI) and is framed around several key elements:

- High-quality curriculum
- Respectful tasks
- Flexible grouping
- Continual assessment
- Building community
- Teaching up

High-Quality Curriculum

High-quality curriculum means planning with the end in mind. It begins with clearly defining where we want students to go before thinking about how we want them to get there. What do we want them to know, understand, and be able to do (KUD) as a result of the learning experience?

Designing good curriculum starts with identifying the essential Understandings—the concepts, principles, or big ideas of the unit topic. Understandings that are meaningful, intriguing, and thought provoking allow students to see the relevance of what they are studying to other subjects and to the world around them.

Knowledge includes the key facts (names, dates, places, etc.), vocabulary, and examples that you want students to know. In isolation, this knowledge is easily forgotten. But when linked with the understandings, the knowledge items help students to uncover and make sense of the understandings.

What you want students to be able to do might include basic skills such as literacy and numeracy, thinking skills such as reasoning and synthesizing, discipline-based skills such as graphing, planning skills such as goal-setting and project planning, and social skills such as collaboration and leadership.

High-quality curriculum engages students in exploring important ideas and challenges students to develop the skills and attitudes needed to do rigorous, quality work.

Continual Assessment

Assessment is the element that steers instruction in the differentiated classroom. Using ungraded tests or surveys to pre-assess students' readiness and interests before or at the start of a unit will help you determine where each student is in relation to the unit KUDs and guide you in identifying initial student groupings and task assignments in the beginning of the unit.

During the unit, continually assessing each students' progress toward the learning goals (KUDs) guides the teacher in planning the next instructional steps in the classroom. Formative assessments such as exit cards, questions for the day, journal prompts, observation, and one-on-one conversations with students all help in identifying when there is a need to re-teach something to certain students or to raise the challenge higher for some students. Formative assessments can be differentiated as long as they are aligned with the unit KUDs.

Summative assessments can also be differentiated based on readiness, interest, and learning profile. It is critical, however, that all variations of the summative assessment allow students to demonstrate what they have learned in reference to the unit KUDs.

Respectful Tasks

Students come into our classrooms seeking affirmation, contribution, challenge, power, and purpose. Respectful tasks are responsive to those needs.

In any classroom, it is critically important that the task we ask students to do is respectful—that it is challenging, interesting, and worth doing. In a differentiated classroom, students often work on different tasks simultaneously. The tasks may be adjusted for different readiness levels, interests, or learning preferences, but regardless of which task a student is assigned to (or selects) it should be respectful. If some students look like they are doing a task that is challenging, engaging, and thought-provoking to them while other students work on filling in a simplistic worksheet, the activities are not effectively differentiated and will affect how students perceive their status in the classroom.

Building Community

In an effectively differentiated classroom, the teacher focuses on building a learning community where students feel safe, accepted, and supported. One where students treat one another with respect, help one another to be productive, and share in one another's successes.

In a differentiated classroom, students understand what differentiation is all about and everyone feels they play an important role in the community. Students have a voice in how the community works and take responsibility for identifying and solving problems in the classroom.

Flexible Grouping

An effectively differentiated classroom is characterized by the practice of flexible grouping. This means that students work in a variety of arrangements—students may work:

- in small groups with students of similar readiness, interest, or learning profile;

- in small groups with students of different readiness, interest, or learning profile;

- with a partner of similar readiness, interest, or learning profile;

- with a partner of different readiness, interest, or learning profile;

- individually;

- as a whole class.

Grouping assignments may be selected by the teacher, by the student, or randomly. In this way, students have the opportunity to work with a variety of students on a frequent basis.

Teaching Up

Teaching up means raising the "ceiling" for all students. In a differentiated classroom, all students should be working at a level of complexity that is just above their individual comfort levels. By providing each student with reasonable levels of challenge and instructional scaffolding as needed, students learn that hard work results in successful growth.

One tip for achieving this is to plan the most complex learning activity first—one that would challenge the most advanced learner in your class. Then modify that activity for students who are currently at lower readiness levels.

Section 33.2

Effective Reading Interventions for Kids with Learning Disabilities

A worried mother says, "There's so much publicity about the best programs for teaching kids to read. But my daughter has a learning disability and really struggles with reading. Will those programs help her? I can't bear to watch her to fall further behind."

Fortunately, in recent years, several excellent, well-publicized re-search studies (including the Report of the National Reading Panel) have helped parents and educators understand the most effective guidelines for teaching all children to read. But, to date, the general public has heard little about research on effective reading interventions for children who have learning disabilities (LD). Until now, that is!

This section will describe the findings of a research study that will help you become a wise consumer of reading programs for kids with reading disabilities.

Research Reveals the Best Approach to Teaching Kids with LD to Read

You'll be glad to know that, over the past thirty years, a great deal of research has been done to identify the most effective reading inter-ventions for students with learning disabilities who struggle with word recognition and/or reading comprehension skills. Between 1996 and 1998, a group of researchers led by H. Lee Swanson, Ph.D., professor of educational psychology at the University of California at Riverside, set out to synthesize (via meta-analysis) the results of ninety-two such re-search studies (all of them scientifically based). Through that analysis, Dr. Swanson identified the specific teaching methods and instruction components that proved most effective for increasing word recognition and reading comprehension skills in children and teens with LD.

Some of the findings that emerged from the meta-analysis were surprising. For example, Dr. Swanson points out, "Traditionally, one-on-one reading instruction has been considered optimal for students with LD. Yet we found that students with LD who received reading instruction in small groups (e.g., in a resource room) experienced a greater increase in skills than did students who had individual instruction."

In this section, we'll summarize and explain Dr. Swanson's research findings. Then, for those of you whose kids have LD related to reading, we'll offer practical tips for using the research findings to "size up" a particular reading program. Let's start by looking at what the research uncovered.

A Strong Instructional Core

Dr. Swanson points out that, according to previous research reviews, sound instructional practices include: daily reviews, statements of an instructional objective, teacher presentations of new material, guided practice, independent practice, and formative evaluations (i.e., testing to ensure the child has mastered the material). These practices are at the heart of any good reading intervention program and are reflected in several of the instructional components mentioned in this section.

Improving Word Recognition Skills: What Works?

"The most important outcome of teaching word recognition," Dr. Swanson emphasizes, "is that students learn to recognize real words, not simply sound out 'nonsense' words using phonics skills."

What other terms might teachers or other professionals use to describe a child's problem with "word recognition":

- Decoding
- Phonics
- Phonemic awareness
- Word attack skills

Direct instruction appears the most effective approach for improving word recognition skills in students with learning disabilities. Direct instruction refers to teaching skills in an explicit, direct fashion. It involves drill/repetition/practice and can be delivered to one child or to a small group of students at the same time.

The three instruction components that proved most effective in increasing word recognition skills in students with learning disabilities are described in Table 33.1. Ideally, a reading program for word recognition will include all three components.

Table 33.1. Increasing Word Recognition Skills in Students with LD

Instruction component	Program activities and techniques*
Sequencing	The teacher:
	Breaks down the task (e.g., starts by having the child break an unknown word into separate sounds or parts they can sound out).
	Gradually reduces prompts or cues.
	Matches the difficulty level to the task and to the student.
	Sequences short activities (e.g., first spends ten minutes reviewing new words from a previous lesson, then five minutes underlining new words in the passage, and finally five minutes practicing blends).
	Uses step-by-step prompts.
Segmentation	The teacher:
	Breaks down the targeted skill (e.g., identifying a speech or letter sound) into smaller units or component parts (e.g., sounding out each speech or letter sound in that word).
	Segments or synthesizes component parts (e.g., sounds out each phoneme in a word, then blends the sounds together).
Advanced organizers	The teacher:
	Directs children to look over material prior to instruction.
	Directs children to focus on particular information.
	Provides students with prior information about tasks.
	Tells students the objectives of instruction up front.

Note: * May be called "treatment description" in research studies.

Table 33.2. Improving Reading Comprehension in Students with LD

Instruction component	Program activities and techniques*
Directed response/ questioning	The teacher:
	Asks questions.
	Encourages students to ask questions.
	The teacher and student(s):
	Engage in dialogue.
Control difficulty of processing demands of task	The teacher:
	Provides assistance (as needed).
	Gives a simplified demonstration.
	Sequences tasks from easy to difficult.
	Presents easy steps or concepts first and moves on to progressively more difficult steps or concepts (a technique called task analysis).
	Allows student to control level of difficulty.
	The activities:
	Are short.
Elaboration	The activities:
	Provide student with additional information or explanation about concepts, steps, or procedures.
	Use redundant text or repetition within text.
Modeling of steps by the teacher	Teacher demonstrates the processes and/or steps the students are to follow.
Group instruction	Instruction and/or verbal interaction takes place in a small group composed of students and teacher.
Strategy cues	The teacher:
	Reminds the student to use strategies or multiple steps.
	Explains steps or procedures for solving problems.
	The activities:
	Use "think aloud" models.
	List the benefits of strategy use or procedures.

Note: *May be called "treatment description" in research studies.

371

Improving Reading Comprehension Skills: What Works?

The most effective approach to improving reading comprehension in students with learning disabilities appears to be a combination of direct instruction and strategy instruction. Strategy instruction means teaching students a plan (or strategy) to search for patterns in words and to identify key passages (paragraph or page) and the main idea in each. Once a student learns certain strategies, he can generalize them to other reading comprehension tasks. The instruction components found most effective for improving reading comprehension skills in students with LD are shown in Table 33.2. Ideally, a program to improve reading comprehension should include all the components shown.

Evaluating Your Child's Reading Program

Now you are well equipped with research-based guidelines on the best teaching methods for kids with reading disabilities. These guidelines will serve you well even as new reading programs become available. To evaluate the reading program used in your child's classroom, follow these steps:

1. Ask for detailed literature on your child's reading program. Some schools voluntarily provide information about the reading programs they use. If they don't do this—or if you need more detail than what they provide—don't hesitate to request it from your child's teacher, special education teacher, resource specialist, or a school district administrator. In any school—whether public or private—it is your right to have access to such information.

2. Once you have literature on a specific reading program, locate the section(s) that describe its instruction components. Take note of where your child's reading program "matches" and where it "misses" the instruction components recommended in this section.

3. Find out if the instruction model your child's teacher uses is direct instruction, strategy instruction, or a combination approach. Some program literature states which approach a teacher should use; in other cases, it's up to the teacher to decide. Compare the approach used to what this section describes as being most effective for addressing your child's area of need.

4. Once you've evaluated your child's reading program, you may feel satisfied that her needs are being met. If not, schedule a conference with her teacher (or her IEP team, if she has one) to present your concerns and discuss alternative solutions.

Hope and Hard Work—Not Miracles

Finally, Dr. Swanson cautions, "There is no 'miracle cure' for reading disabilities. Even a reading program that has all the right elements requires both student and teacher to be persistent and work steadily toward reading proficiency."

But knowledge is power, and the findings of Dr. Swanson's study offer parents and teachers a tremendous opportunity to evaluate and select reading interventions most likely to move kids with LD toward reading success.

Section 33.3

Strategies for Tackling Writing Problems

"Tackling Writing Problems," by Miriam Cherkes-Julkowski, Ph.D.
© 2011 Smart Kids with LD. All rights reserved. Reprinted with permission.
For additional information, visit www.smartkidswithld.org.

Writing can be particularly challenging for children with learning disabilities. Those who have difficulties with reading and language, spelling, memory, attention, organization, sequencing, and fine motor coordination often struggle with both handwriting and written expression. As kids move up in school, the situation is further complicated by the need to acquire, prioritize, and organize information in a meaningful way. Helping children master these important skills requires understanding their specific problems and addressing them with strategies that have proved to be successful.

Early Skills

Children in elementary school are encouraged to write the way they speak. The focus is on writing legibly and invented spelling is acceptable, as long as the word is recognizable. But these tasks can be challenging for children with LD, who often need explicit instruction in letter formation, which is rarely taught in today's classroom.

For students struggling to form letters and words correctly on the page, first make sure they are using pens or pencils that are comfortable for them. Consult with an occupational or physical therapist who can teach your child how to grip the pencil properly and sit with good posture, both of which can make the act of writing easier.

Letter and word-spacing problems can be caused by fine motor or space-perception difficulties. Many young children benefit from writing and pasting individual words onto a page.

Children with reading disabilities (dyslexia) also tend to have problems with spelling. The child who has difficulties in phonological processing (discriminating among the sound components of language) is likely to have problems with both reading and spelling.

Multisensory structured language (MSL) programs help children learn the sounds of letters and how they are blended into syllables and words through instruction in listening, speaking, and writing. An MSL program addressing reading and writing together needs to be taught by a trained professional. Children who struggle with reading and writing also benefit from explicit instruction in spelling, since not knowing how to spell is a major roadblock to writing.

Finally, children who have persistent difficulties with telling stories (oral narrative) should be prompted with questions to extend their thinking ("Why?" "What happened next?"). Persistent difficulty with an oral narrative suggests the need for a speech-language evaluation.

Process Writing

By the time kids get to middle school they may have good ideas, but getting them down on paper can be challenging. It requires not only remembering and putting their ideas in order, but also managing handwriting, spelling, punctuation, vocabulary, and grammar. To make writing easier, the tasks can be handled one at a time.

The first challenge is coming up with ideas or thoughts and getting them down on paper, with no regard for spelling, punctuation, or organization. Children who have difficulty forming letters find the task easier if they use a computer or dictate their thoughts to someone acting as a scribe. Those who have trouble thinking and writing at the same time can brainstorm ideas on a tape recorder before beginning to write on paper.

The next step is to organize the ideas, grouping the ones that belong together, and omitting any that don't fit. Going back over the material to fill in any missing points should follow.

Finally, the material must be edited for clarity, adding introductory and transitional phrases where needed. The last step is to check spelling and punctuation, which computer software can do. Computers, however, aren't perfect, so a final read is still required to ensure that the paper reflects the writer's intent. The process may be easier if done over the course of several days.

Putting It All Together

As children go through school the writing demands become greater. By the time they're in high school they're expected to read and comprehend varied and difficult texts and to integrate a great deal of information into long, complex papers.

Students write best when they're engaged in the topic. Topic selection may have to be negotiated with the classroom teacher.

Virtually all aspects of writing including the development of ideas and organization as well as spelling have been facilitated greatly by assistive technology. But it's still wise to work closely with the teacher throughout these phases to get feedback as the paper is being developed.

While students should be encouraged to develop their writing skills, some with learning difficulties find that oral or graphic presentations are a viable alternative to a lengthy written report.

As Dr. Mel Levine observes in *Keeping a Head in School*, despite the difficulty involved, writing can be a great way for students with learning problems to explore their personal ideas. "If you have good ideas," he notes, "writing is worth the struggle."

Individualized Education Program (IEP) Modifications

Depending on your child's needs, the following modifications may be helpful:

1. Shorter writing assignments

2. Acceptance of imperfect spelling or punctuation that can be corrected later

3. Use of word processing

4. Extra time for class writing or homework assignments

5. No classmate review of papers to avoid embarrassment

6. Access to a computer for tests

7. Alternative presentation formats (oral or graphic)

Section 33.4

Multisensory Teaching Techniques

"The Benefits of Multisensory Teaching and Sensory Words," Performance Learning PLUS, December 2007. © Performance Learning Systems, Inc. (www.plsweb.com). Reprinted with permission. Reviewed by David A. Cooke, M.D., FACP, February 2012.

Research shows that effective teachers make a conscious effort to design instruction that incorporates a broad variety of learning preferences beyond their own (Doolan & Honigsfeld, 2000; Sadler-Smith & Smith, 2004).

Research shows that varying teaching strategies to address all sensory preferences increases learning, regardless of the individual student's primary preference (Thomas, Cox, & Kojima, 2000).

Research shows that by using multisensory strategies, teachers can engage and sustain the attention of all students. By employing a variety of strategies, the teacher may address the mixed efficiencies of those students as well as the dominant and secondary preferences of others. Thus, they reinforce strong preferences and strengthen weaker ones (Silver et al., 2000; Haggart, 2003).

> "I had a great feeling of relief when I began to understand that a youngster needs more than just subject matter. Oh, I know mathematics well, and I teach it well. I used to think that that was all I needed to do. Now I teach children, not math."
> —ChicEverett Shostrom in *Man, the Manipulator*

As a teacher, you know that students learn differently. Some prefer to learn by doing. Others like to watch a demonstration of what they need to do. Some want to listen to what is expected. Most students appreciate a combination of methods: a little bit of doing it, a little bit of seeing it, and a little bit of hearing it. When you teach using a combination of methods that appeal to different learning styles (kinesthetic, tactual, auditory, and visual), you are using multisensory teaching.

Below is an overview of the four major learning styles and their representation in the general population. As you read, you will probably think of past or present students who demonstrate characteristics of each style.

Kinesthetic style: Learning through doing. The kinesthetic learner must "do" something to learn it. This person is actively involved in learning and loves to flex those large motor muscles. There is a lot of body movement going on when these learners are in the throes of learning. Research in the learning styles area shows that 25 to 35 percent of the general population are kinesthetic learners.

Tactual style: Learning through sensations and feelings. The tactual learner learns through the sense of touch and small motor experiences. Tactual learners are also often very aware of the emotional signals, subtle and blatant, that others send. They may be sensitive to odors in their environment. They often are adept at using their hands, and they benefit from touching things to get to know them better. These are the true "hands-on" learners. Research indicates that 15 to 25 percent of the general population prefers the tactual modality.

Auditory style: Learning through hearing and speaking. The auditory learner is very focused on speaking and listening. This person enjoys discussions and often needs to "say it to learn it." This individual is tuned in to all the sounds in her environment and often benefits when trying to concentrate from soft music or white noise in the background. This person frequently needs to "say it to herself" or move her lips as though talking to herself to process the material in the most efficient way. Auditory learners compose about 10 to 15 percent of the general population.

Visual style: Learning through seeing. Visual learners process information best when they see it. They enjoy videos, movies, CD-ROMs, and watching demonstrations. Colors attract the attention of this person. This person must see it to believe it and see it to learn it. Visualization often comes easily to this individual, and he might also have a good visual-spatial sense. Maps, graphic organizers, and pictures of all kinds are this learner's best friends. In the general population, about 35 to 40 percent of people share this learning preference.

Chances are high that you have students representing each of these four learning styles in varying degrees in your classroom. Ideally, teachers create multisensory activities that appeal to kinesthetic, tactual, auditory, and visual learners.

Activities can also become multisensory—appealing to more than one learning style—by adding sensory words to them.

Read on for tips to use sensory words in your classroom.

Using Sensory Words to Reach All Students

Sensory Words are words that appeal to the senses associated with the four main learning styles—kinesthetic, tactual, auditory, and visual:

- **Kinesthetic:** jump, kick, run
- **Tactual:** pat, write, hold
- **Auditory:** whisper, cheer, growl
- **Visual:** glance, peek, notice

There are four occasions when you can use sensory words to enhance your teaching:

- When lack of time limits an opportunity for sensory experiences. When there is no time to create a multisensory experience, and you want students to understand something through their senses, using sensory words can provide a comparable experience for students.

- When a real sensory experience is not possible. For example, you want to study the ocean but you are living four hundred miles away.

- For example, when you are teaching an interpersonal skill such as "participate," tell what it looks like, sounds like, and feels like when you are "participating."

- To build rapport, mirror verbs. Use action-oriented words to describe nonphysical things—if a person is kinesthetic, say, "Let's slam our ideas together!" when suggesting action for a cerebral activity.

Vary sensory words when you communicate with students.

For example, the rule "Walk in the halls" is kinesthetic. If students continue to run or horse around in the halls, you might change how you present the rule by varying sensory words. For instance:

- When I see you running in the hall, it looks like a herd of elephants. Please slow down. (Visual)

- It sounds like thunder when you run in the hall! Please tread quietly! (Auditory)

- It feels like the building is shaking when you run in the hall. Please walk gently! (Tactual)

- Running in the hall distracts people from learning. Please walk. (Neutral/Kinesthetic)

Encourage students to vary sensory words when they communicate with one another and work on projects.

Learning to communicate with others, including those whose learning styles are different from their own, is a life skill that will benefit students during their education as well as when they enter the workforce. As a teacher, varying sensory words is an essential part of our jobs. You can take this skill a step further by encouraging your students to practice it as well.

Put students in groups of three or four and ask them to help create or modify classroom rules. If your students are not versed in learning styles, simply hand out a list of sensory words from which they can choose. Groups must choose at least one word from each KTAV (kinesthetic, tactual, auditory, and visual) category.

When students respond to one another or to questions you ask in class, ask them to stretch their responses to include a variety of KTAV responses. For example, rather than "I hear what you are saying" (auditory), a student could respond, "That feels right to me" (tactual).

For Younger Students

Use a kinesthetic activity where students toss a ball to one another. Each time the ball is caught, the student has to make a kinesthetic, tactual, auditory, or visual statement such as: "I saw that ball coming!" then toss it to someone else, who might make a tactual comment such as: "That catch felt great!" Students can choose from a list of words you write on the board, or can even use vocabulary words when appropriate.

For Older Students

1. Put students in groups to practice rotating sensory words:

    *   Person 1 makes a statement beginning with "fortunately, . . ." using a K word.

    *   Person 2 makes a statement beginning with "unfortunately, . . ." using a T word.

    *   Person 3 makes a statement beginning with "fortunately, . . ." using an A word.

    *   Back to Person 1, this time for a statement beginning with "unfortunately, . . ." and using a V word.

    *   Person 2 makes a statement beginning with "fortunately, . . ." using a neutral word.

2. Each person uses the previous statement as a springboard, so that each statement connects with the previous one and the group's statements make a continuing conversation.

3. Have students do four rounds of this activity. An added challenge is to make the responses content-specific.

Here is an example for health class:

- Fortunately, I am up and moving around after my bout with chicken pox. (K)

- Unfortunately, I sense that my older brother is getting it, as he has a fever and a rash. (T)

- Fortunately, I heard him say that he thinks it won't be so bad for him. (A)

- Unfortunately, I picture him being in pretty bad shape, like a human polka dot. (V)

- Fortunately, I will be back at school by then. (Neutral)

References

Doolan, L.S., and Honigsfeld, A. (2000). Illuminating the new standards with learning style: Striking a perfect match. *Clearing House*, 73(5), 274–78.

Haggart, W. (2003). *Discipline and learning styles: An educator's guide.* Nevada City, CA: Performance Learning Systems.

Sadler-Smith, E., and Smith, J. P. (2004). Strategies for accommodating individuals' styles and preferences in flexible learning programmes. *British Journal of Educational Technology*, 35(4), 395–412.

Silver, H.F., Strong, R.W., and Perini, M.J. (2000). *So each may learn: Integrating learning styles and multiple intelligences.* Alexandria, VA: Association for Supervision and Curriculum Development.

Thomas, H., Cox, R., and Kojima, T. (2000). Relating preferred learning style to student achievement. Paper presented at the Annual Meeting of the Teachers of English to Speakers of Other Languages, Vancouver, BC [Canada]. (ERIC Document Reproduction Service No. 445 513).

Section 33.5

Speech-Language Therapy

In a recent parent-teacher conference, the teacher expressed concern that your child may have a problem with certain speech or language skills. Or perhaps while talking to your child, you noticed an occasional stutter.

Could your child have a problem? And if so, what should you do?

It's wise to intervene quickly. An evaluation by a certified speech-language pathologist can help determine if your child is having difficulties. Speech-language therapy is the treatment for most kids with speech and/or language disorders.

Speech Disorders and Language Disorders

A speech disorder refers to a problem with the actual production of sounds, whereas a language disorder refers to a difficulty understanding or putting words together to communicate ideas.

Speech disorders include:

- **Articulation disorders:** Difficulties producing sounds in syllables or saying words incorrectly to the point that listeners can't understand what's being said.

- **Fluency disorders:** problems such as stuttering, in which the flow of speech is interrupted by abnormal stoppages, repetitions (st-st-stuttering), or prolonging sounds and syllables (sssstuttering).

- **Resonance or voice disorders:** problems with the pitch, volume, or quality of the voice that distract listeners from what's being said. These types of disorders may also cause pain or discomfort for a child when speaking.

- **Dysphagia/oral feeding disorders:** these include difficulties with drooling, eating, and swallowing.

Language disorders can be either receptive or expressive:

- **Receptive disorders:** difficulties understanding or processing language.

- **Expressive disorders:** difficulty putting words together, limited vocabulary, or inability to use language in a socially appropriate way.

Specialists in Speech-Language Therapy

Speech-language pathologists (SLPs), often informally known as speech therapists, are professionals educated in the study of human communication, its development, and its disorders. They hold at least a master's degree and state certification/licensure in the field, and a certificate of clinical competency from the American Speech-Language-Hearing Association (ASHA).

SLPs assess speech, language, cognitive-communication, and oral/feeding/swallowing skills to identify types of communication problems (articulation; fluency; voice; receptive and expressive language disorders, etc.) and the best way to treat them.

Remediation

In speech-language therapy, an SLP will work with a child one-on-one, in a small group, or directly in a classroom to overcome difficulties involved with a specific disorder.

Therapists use a variety of strategies, including:

- **Language intervention activities:** The SLP will interact with a child by playing and talking, using pictures, books, objects, or ongoing events to stimulate language development. The therapist may also model correct pronunciation and use repetition exercises to build speech and language skills.

- **Articulation therapy:** Articulation, or sound production, exercises involve having the therapist model correct sounds and syllables for a child, often during play activities. The level of play is age-appropriate and related to the child's specific needs. The SLP will physically show the child how to make certain sounds, such as the "r" sound, and may demonstrate how to move the tongue to produce specific sounds.

- **Oral-motor/feeding and swallowing therapy:** The SLP will use a variety of oral exercises—including facial massage and various tongue, lip, and jaw exercises—to strengthen the muscles of the mouth. The SLP also may work with different food textures and temperatures to increase a child's oral awareness during eating and swallowing.

When Is Therapy Needed?

Kids might need speech-language therapy for a variety of reasons, including:

- hearing impairments;
- cognitive (intellectual, thinking) or other developmental delays;
- weak oral muscles;
- excessive drooling;
- chronic hoarseness;
- birth defects such as cleft lip or cleft palate;
- autism;
- motor planning problems;
- respiratory problems (breathing disorders);
- feeding and swallowing disorders;
- traumatic brain injury.

Therapy should begin as soon as possible. Children enrolled in therapy early (before they're five years old) tend to have better outcomes than those who begin therapy later.

This does not mean that older kids can't make progress in therapy; they may progress at a slower rate because they often have learned patterns that need to be changed.

Finding a Therapist

It's important to make sure that the speech-language therapist is certified by ASHA. That certification means the SLP has at least a master's degree in the field and has passed a national examination and successfully completed a supervised clinical fellowship.

Sometimes, speech assistants (who usually have a two-year associate's or four-year bachelor's degree) may assist with speech-language services under the supervision of ASHA-certified SLPs. Your child's SLP should be licensed in your state and have experience working with kids and your child's specific disorder.

You might find a specialist by asking your child's doctor or teacher for a referral or by checking local directories online or in your telephone book. State associations for speech-language pathology and audiology also maintain listings of licensed and certified therapists.

Helping Your Child

Speech-language experts agree that parental involvement is crucial to the success of a child's progress in speech or language therapy.

Parents are an extremely important part of their child's therapy program and help determine whether it is a success. Kids who complete the program quickest and with the longest-lasting results are those whose parents have been involved.

Ask the therapist for suggestions on how you can help your child. For instance, it's important to help your child do the at-home stimulation activities that the SLP suggests to ensure continued progress and carry-over of newly learned skills.

The process of overcoming a speech or language disorder can take some time and effort, so it's important that all family members be patient and understanding with the child.

Section 33.6

Learning Disabilities and the Arts

The arts are more than a fun, superficial way to keep kids occupied. Art activities can help children with learning disabilities begin to overcome the challenges they face in learning in many different ways. Of course, having a learning disability does not necessarily mean that a person has an exceptional artistic talent. However, music, art, crafts, and dance can give students with learning disabilities a chance to express themselves through different media and gain confidence along the way.

Unlocking Confidence

A feeling of self-worth—the knowledge that you can do something—is a critical part of the learning process. Children with learning disabilities often come to think they are incapable of learning because of their ongoing difficulties in school. A paintbrush, a costume, a drum, or paper, scissors, and glue can be new tools for self-expression that boost confidence while providing opportunities for learning and practice.

Learning through Art

The arts can open the world of learning to students who have trouble with traditional teaching methods. The arts are intellectual disciplines—requiring complex thinking and problem solving—that offer students the opportunity to construct their own understanding of the world.

Drawing and painting reinforce motor skills and can also be a way of learning shapes, contrasts, boundaries, spatial relationships, size, and other math concepts.

Music teaches children about rhythm, sound, and pitch. Beats can help children learn rhymes and other features of reading such as phonological awareness. Using repetitive songs to learn academic facts (like the alphabet song or multiplication tables) can make the learning experience easier and more fun.

Dance provides children with a social way to learn about sequencing, rhythm, and following directions. While developing coordination and motor control, students can also learn counting and directionality, which can enhance reading and writing concepts—such as understanding the difference between similar looking letters (like p/b/d/q) and telling left from right.

Performing plays is an opportunity for children to immerse themselves in a theme and learn about it in a profound and personal way. Acting out historical or literary figures and events gives students a sense of ownership about what they've learned, allowing them to acquire a deeper appreciation of the subject matter.

Crafts offer children the opportunity to express themselves in two- and three-dimensional ways. Students can develop vital problem-solving skills without having to rely on areas of expression that may be more challenging.

Arts as a Means of Assessment

Timed tests and take-home reports are traditional means of academic assessment that can be especially difficult for individuals with learning disabilities. Creative projects offer these students the freedom to show what they know without the constraints of printed text. Offering students art projects or multimedia presentations as a way to demonstrate an understanding of material they've learned can be an excellent alternative.

Because a person has difficulty learning through hearing alone or seeing alone does not mean they cannot learn. The arts offer individuals with learning disabilities dynamic ways of learning, and just as importantly, a way to fully discover their own self-worth.

Chapter 34

Coping with
School-Related Challenges

Chapter Contents

Section 34.1

Building a Good Relationship with Your Child's Teacher

Your child is your number one priority, and in a perfect world you could give them everything they need. But let's face it—you cannot do it alone. The best way to support your child's needs is to build and maintain a strong, positive relationship with all the people at school who play a role in educating your child. And, make sure your child knows that this is a team effort—you're all working together to help him or her succeed.

Here are some tips on how you can foster a sense of partnership with the teacher and administration to support your child's education.

Connecting Before the School Year Starts

Begin your relationship with teachers and other school staff members by letting them know that you look forward to working with them as a partner in educating your child.

Exchange email addresses with your child's teacher and agree to keep in touch at least monthly, even if your child is doing well.

Share information about your child that they might not otherwise learn during the course of the school day, such as:

- your child's favorite books, movies, hobbies, and interests;

- learning activities and techniques that seem especially helpful for your child; and

- positive stories and anecdotes about your child, or important events in his or her personal life that may affect how they interact with others.

Maintaining the Connection During the School Year

Stay involved. Make a point to show up and participate in events such as the annual science fair, back-to-school night, and open house.

When your child tells you something they particularly liked or disliked at school (e.g., classmates, activities, etc.), share this information with the teacher.

Be on time, positive, and prepared for school activities and meetings.

Offer to volunteer your time in the classroom or as a chaperone on class trips.

Consider donating classroom supplies or a gift certificate to a store where teachers can purchase materials for the classroom. (You'd be surprised how many supplies teachers buy with their own money.)

Contribute fun extras to the classroom like prizes, disposable cameras, and extra snacks, and look for ways to help the teacher maintain a fun learning environment.

Remembering That the Teacher Is a Person First

Send cards for special events in the teacher's life, such as birthdays or the birth of a child or grandchild.

Don't forget to say "thank you" for both the big things and the little things a teacher does for your child.

Saying "thank you" can be more than just words—give gift certificates, bring a fruit basket, or buy small gifts to give to the teacher "just because."

Respect the teacher's schedule—what might be a good time for you to talk may not be such a good time for the teacher.

Don't forget to acknowledge the teacher's co-workers—classroom aides, lunchroom and playground supervisors, secretaries and school nurses, custodians, and security personnel, bus drivers, and crossing guards—anyone who helps to keep the school running and safe.

Sharing Your Appreciation with Others

Let the administration know how much you appreciate your child's teacher: Stop by the office and speak to the principal or vice principal in person or send a letter to the superintendent, director of special services, special education coordinator, or supervising teacher (with a copy to the teacher).

Nominate your favorite teacher for Teacher of the Year. Many community newspapers offer contests like this. Your teacher may receive a reward.

Ending the School Year on a Positive Note

Volunteer to organize an end-of-the-year art and writing project for students to introduce themselves to their next year's teacher.

Send handwritten notes of thanks to all your child's teachers (and members of the Individualized Education Program [IEP] team), telling them once more how much you appreciated the special attention they gave to your child.

Keep in touch—send a card every now and then to let your child's teacher know the lasting impact they had on your child's future.

When you take your child to school in the morning, you're not dropping them off—you're handing them over to a trusted partner who is dedicated to making sure that your child has everything he or she needs to be successful now and throughout the rest of their educational career. And as with any partnership, communication is the key to success—get involved and stay involved.

Section 34.2

Dealing with Homework

Remember when you couldn't wait to graduate from school because that meant no more homework and studying? Or so you thought. As anyone with children can attest, homework never ends. While many students consider it the toughest part of the school day, homework also can be a painful aspect of parenting—especially for those whose children have learning disabilities (LD), including dyslexia, nonverbal learning disorder (NLD), executive function issues, or attention problems. However, that need not be the case. When homework is a collaborative effort between home and school, with parents and teachers both playing helping roles, it is likely to make the process go more smoothly. Here are some pointers for all involved.

What Parents Can Do

Check in with your child every day: Ask what the homework assignment is and if there's any doubt about the answer, check his assignment book. This lets him know that parents see homework as important.

Make a daily homework plan: At a minimum, it should include a list of what needs to be done and when she plans on doing each assignment. To help her develop time-management skills, have her estimate how much time it will take to complete each assignment (and track this to help her improve the skill). When making a plan, ask about long-term assignments and upcoming tests, so those can be built into the plan.

Provide a clean and quiet workspace: It's also helpful to keep on hand extra supplies such as pencils, markers, scissors, rulers, calculators, etc.

Reward rather than punish: Giving him something he can look forward to when homework is finished may be the incentive he needs to get through it. Saying, "Guess what? You get to do X as soon as you finish your spelling workbook," is more motivating than saying, "If you don't do your homework, X is off-limits."

Supervise, but don't micromanage: The goal is for your child to complete homework independently, but that often depends on maturity, which varies tremendously from child to child. In the early stages, parents often need to sit with children while they work. As they get older, parents can check in frequently, be there for the hard stuff, or just get them started and then leave.

Distinguish between your role and the teacher's role: It's your job to make sure that your child does his homework and puts it in his backpack when complete. It is the teacher's job to make sure it's done right. In most cases it's best to let teachers judge neatness as well (although at times it's effective to let your child know that if you can't read his handwriting, he'll have to redo it).

Reach out for support: If homework battles threaten family functioning, make an appointment with the school. Homework wars should not jeopardize parent-child relationships. If they threaten to do this, then parents and teachers need to put their heads together to come up with alternatives.

What Schools Can Do

When parents and schools each do their part, tensions around homework are significantly reduced. A collaborative effort on the part of you and your child's teachers can help resolve the problems in the short term and put things in perspective. Ways in which your child's school may be willing to collaborate include the following.

Make available end-of-the-day check-ins for students who need it: It's genuinely hard for youngsters with working memory problems to remember everything they have to bring home at the end of the day. Having a teacher or aide check in with the child before she goes home to make sure she's written down all assignments and has the necessary materials solves this problem. To reduce the labor-intensity of this process, some teachers use the last ten minutes of the school day for the whole class to go through the end-of-the-day check-in together.

Post homework assignments on the internet: And keep the postings current and complete. When done consistently, this allows parents to monitor their child's homework. If it's not done right, however, it introduces another crack that a child can slip through.

Make weekly progress reports available for parents who need them: This can be a powerful tool. Letting parents know of any outstanding homework assignments on a Thursday or Friday enables them to structure weekend activities around homework demands.

Be flexible: Kids with attention deficit hyperactivity disorder (ADHD), in particular, often run out of steam by the end of the school day. Medication, too, has often worn off at that point, making homework seem particularly daunting. Some days go more smoothly than others, and when teachers can trust parents to shorten or cut out assignments based on their child's capacity on any given day, this approach can work quite well. Sometimes teachers star the most important assignments, so that parents can ensure that if shortcuts are to be taken, the priority work gets done.

Accept parent involvement: Allowing students with written language problems to dictate homework to parents can significantly reduce parent-child conflicts around homework.

Establish after-school homework clubs: Many students are successful with homework when they're given time either during school or before they leave school at the end of the day. This is because school provides sufficient structure and environmental cues to remind them to stay on task. These same students often experience a letdown in energy and focus when they get home from school that may be difficult to recover from, even after a break for exercise, relaxation, or after-school activities. Whenever passing or failing a course depends on homework, schools need to be willing to offer an in-school alternative so that youngsters whose home life is not conducive to getting the homework done will not be penalized.

Section 34.3

Encouraging Organization

"Organization: A Crucial Executive Skill for Your Child with LD" by Bonnie Z. Goldsmith. Copyright 2012 by National Center for Learning Disabilities, Inc. All rights reserved. Reprinted with permission. For more information, visit LD.org.

- If you'd just get organized!
- How can you find anything in here?
- The report is due tomorrow? And you haven't started it?
- How could you forget to turn in your homework? I helped you with it!

What's one thing that makes for a parent's unhappy day? Getting a phone call or email from school, informing you that your child—who may spend lots of time doing homework—hasn't turned anything in for six weeks. This wake-up call may be your first indication that your child is having trouble in school. The information is doubly disconcerting when you find, buried in your child's heavy backpack, lots of completed homework that was never turned in.

A talk with your child and your child's teacher may reveal that missing homework is only part of the problem. Your child may also be late with assignments, late to class, frequently without necessary supplies, and missing library books. Although your child is intelligent and wants to do well in school, something is getting in the way. Particularly for children with learning disabilities (LD) or attention deficit hyperactivity disorder (ADHD), that "something" is organizational skills.

You Know Your Child

Of all the brain-based habits of thought known as executive skills, organization looms especially large, particularly for children with learning disabilities. Disorganized children with LD or ADHD are often called lazy, unmotivated—even defiant. You may be one of the few people in your child's life who understands that learning disabilities complicate children's development of organizational skills.

All the executive skills are related. The child who doesn't start the report until the night before it's due may have difficulty estimating how long a project will take. Your child may panic when a task seems difficult. Your child may get overwhelmed trying to juggle multiple projects, or simply not know how to plan, begin, and follow through with the steps required to get an assignment done. These are all aspects of organization, that crucial skill that enables us to do what needs doing—whether it's baking a birthday cake, pulling together an agenda for a meeting, or completing a science project.

Your child may well understand the value of being organized but may not have the slightest idea how to get that way. That's where you can provide invaluable assistance and encouragement.

Helping your child learn organizational skills may be quite a challenge for both of you. There is no blueprint for organization. What works one year or for one class will not work for another. Still, if you stay flexible, you can help your child recognize, improve, and work around his or her organizational challenges.

Short-Term Strategies

To help your child, think first of short-term strategies that focus on particular tasks or assignments. When your own project deadlines loom and you have no plan to meet them, you probably feel out of control, maybe even panicky. Disorganized children feel that way too. They may feel helpless in the face of any task that isn't easy and short. As school gets more challenging, these children's frustrations escalate and their self-esteem plummets. Juggling multiple projects becomes so difficult that children may opt out and simply drop everything. You can help your child avoid this destructive pattern.

Begin by convincing your child—through your patience, encouragement, and good example—that organizational skills will help him feel better about himself. No one likes to feel out of control or on a slippery slope to failure. Your child wants to become more independent, wants you to stop nagging about schoolwork, and longs to avoid the fallout from those discouraging parent-teacher conferences. Help your child see that the smallest improvements will make his or her life easier.

Remember that there is only one criterion for an organizational system: it needs to work for your child. It's crucial for you and your child to communicate openly and for you to approach the problem without being critical or blaming. Partnerships between parents and teachers are essential to help children succeed; your partnership with your child is also essential. Even younger children need to take part in finding solutions. No system will work if your child doesn't buy into it.

The Power of Encouragement and Example

Organization is about thinking. What is the most efficient way for me to get this project done on time? What will help me remember to do my homework and turn it in? How can I quickly find the materials I need? Rest assured that you can help your child improve her or his organization with simple, gradual strategies.

You don't need to spend money on a multitude of folders or the latest software. Your most precious asset is your matchless insight into what makes your child tick. Help your child find what will work. Help your child be flexible, since children's preferences change, as do teachers' requirements. Look for quick, easy ways to begin organizing: a simple planner that you and your child check daily, a routine for filling and emptying a backpack, a schedule for daily homework, study, and review.

Show your child the importance of organization in daily life. Encourage planning at home by posting a family calendar and involving your child in keeping it current. Show your child how one family member's obligations affects others in the family. A dental appointment, a school conference, and choir practice can't all happen at the same time without considerable planning. Emphasize how planning saves time. A shopping list gives direction to a trip to the supermarket.

If you're a person who relies on lists, a date book, or a personal digital assistant (PDA), talk with your child about how your personal organizing system works (or falls short). Be honest about your own organizational frustrations, so your child will understand that organization is a skill that many people—even adults—struggle to master.

The Comfort of Routines

All of us develop routines and habits to get us through the day. Your child will benefit greatly from knowing what to expect during a typical school day and week. Keeping track of homework and assignments by writing in a planner every day (or making daily entries on an online calendar) gives your child a visual reminder of what needs doing.

A planner of some kind is vital for organization. You probably know best which kind will work for your child, but discuss it together. If the planner you start with doesn't work, help your child make the necessary changes. Staying organized means creating a system and sticking with it. The system best suited to your child may not be one you could follow, and your child's preferences may change with age.

Your great advantage as a parent is your intimate knowledge of your child's personality, strengths, and challenges. Consider how your child thinks and works. What makes your child feel good or bad? Some children love different-colored file folders and a rainbow of highlighters and sticky notes; others get nervous just looking at them. Getting organized has to make your child feel better.

Turn Big Tasks into Little Steps

Help your child learn to plan by showing how to reduce tasks to their smallest parts. Most teachers provide guidelines for homework and larger projects, usually with interim deadlines. They may distribute checklists so children can check off a step when it's completed. You, however, know your own child best. If the interim steps provided by a teacher are still too big for your child to tackle without extreme stress, help your child simplify and break down each step. If your child needs more deadlines to feel able to progress on a task, add more deadlines to the teacher's list. Guide your child to focus on one task at a time.

Introduce your child to the satisfaction of checking off completed tasks. Help your child break out of the thicket of requirements for a complex project. Together, and with the advice of your child's teachers, set realistic goals. Encourage all positive signs. Don't expect perfection or even consistency. Each movement forward takes away a little anxiety. Reduce your child's stress (and your own) step by step.

Attitude Is Everything

As best you can, stay constructive in your attitude toward your child's organizational difficulties. Don't criticize. Refuse to allow yourself to think of your child as lazy, unmotivated, or incompetent. Give your child some positive things to say to herself:

- I'll get it done.
- I've done my best.
- Good job!
- This is easier than it was last week.

"This is easier than it was last week." Music to your ears. Organizational skills are critical for success in school and in the larger world. Kids with LD need extra support, guidance, and practice as they learn to organize and plan. You are your child's most valuable partner in this endeavor.

Chapter 35

Alternative Educational Options

Chapter Contents

Section 35.1

Home Schooling

It's time to get up! Did you remember to brush your teeth? Please don't forget to pack a snack, and make sure your homework is in your backpack. Call me later if you need to stay after school for a club meeting. Your bus is here. Love you. Bye. Have a good day!

For the vast majority of the almost fifty million children enrolled in public pre-kindergarten through grade twelve programs, this (or some variation thereof) is how each school day morning begins. Students travel from their homes and spend a third or more of the day sharing interactions with dozens of teachers, administrators, coaches, librarians, and specialists, who offer instruction and support in areas such as music, drama, computer technology, speech-language, and reading. At the end of the day, they return home, share time with neighborhood friends and family, and dive into extracurricular activities, homework, and no doubt some screen time before heading off to bed.

For an estimated 1.5 million students, the scenario is quite different. While they may find their way into their neighborhood school building or adjacent sports field for activities and sports, their academics take place in the home. Parents (or others engaged to provide instruction and guidance) are in charge of "teaching." Parents must create opportunities in which their child can master curriculum content they need to meet state graduation requirements and prepare their child for successful transitions from grade to grade, to post-secondary education, and to gainful employment.

Is home schooling (also known as parent-led home-based education) a good option for students with learning disabilities? Read on.

Some Background on Home Schooling

It may be hard to believe, but in 1980, home schooling was illegal in thirty states! It wasn't until 1993 that provisions were set in place to allow for home schooling in every state in the nation. A National Household Education Survey tells us that from 1999 to 2007, there has been a 74 percent increase in the number of students who are homeschooled, more than twelve times the increase of public school enrollment over the same period.

While most sources point to 1.5 million as the number of children currently engaged in home schooling, this number may be subject to question. The 2003 NCES survey (the full 2007 report is not published yet) has a 58 percent refusal rate, suggesting that many home schooling families are strongly opposed to any sort of oversight and are not willing to participate in efforts to gather data documenting their efforts and outcomes.

Even though the numbers of students who are homeschooled is relatively small, there has been concern expressed by education officials that there is no way to assure that these children are receiving the high-quality education they deserve and to which they are entitled by law. For example, according to a 2004 report by the Education Commission of the States, most states do not require parents to obtain any sort of teaching certificate in order to homeschool their children. The report continues to warn that only half the states monitor the educational progress of homeschooled students, and that those that do monitor this progress differ in their requirements for test scores, portfolio assessments, or informal narrative evaluations.

That said, there are many parents who have successfully managed the home schooling process and whose children have graduated high school, gained admission to (and enjoyed success in) selective colleges, enjoyed active social lives, and become contributing members of their school and work communities.

Is Home Schooling Right for You?

Is there a typical profile of a home schooling child or family? Not as far as I can tell. Families who choose to engage in home schooling cross all socioeconomic groups and are represented across all racial, ethnic, religious, cultural backgrounds.

Some reports suggest that a predominance of homeschoolers are from white, middle-class backgrounds, whose families embrace politically conservative values and who describe themselves as religious. Other reports point to the increasing popularity of home schooling among nonwhite groups, with varying levels of income and with levels of parent education ranging from no high school diploma to postgraduate degrees.

There also seems to be a wide range of reasons why parents and children decide upon home schooling for at least some portion of their school day (or school career). Some of the benefits reported are:

- more in-depth learning of content in areas of curriculum that are of greatest interest;

- an opportunity to customize or individualize the learning environment to reduce stress and increase learning progress;

- the ability for children to take responsibility for their learning routines and self-monitor their progress against personal goals and learning objectives;

- the use of teaching approaches (e.g., guided self-discovery, portfolio work) not often available or encouraged in more typical school settings;

- enhanced family relationships between children and parents and among siblings;

- greater oversight of social interactions with peers and adults;

- a safe environment that is free of physical violence and direct exposure to drugs and alcohol;

- limited exposure to social and peer pressures that could lead to activity that is deemed improper and sexually unhealthy;

- the desire to teach a particular set of personal values, beliefs, or worldviews.

Home Schooling for Students with Learning Disabilities?

While home schooling may present many unique opportunities and challenges for all students, parents of children with LD need to weigh a number of other considerations when managing a home schooling program. The following is a sampling of some questions that parents should address to ensure that their child's learning and behavioral needs are being met and that their child is being afforded the best opportunities to make progress toward high school graduation and a successful postsecondary transition:

- Do I really want to take full responsibility for my child's academic learning?

- Will home schooling deny my child the full range of social interactions and experiences with peers and adults that is so important to the development of a well-balanced personality?

- Is there a required curriculum that needs to be taught? If so, where can I get a copy? Are there materials (e.g., textbooks, supplemental worksheets, videos) that can be provided to me? Are these materials available for free, and if not, how much do they cost?

- Are school district personnel available to me to provide assistance in shaping a program of home study? If so, how often can we speak? Can we meet in person on a regular basis?

- What services and supports are available to me given my decision to provide home instruction? Is the Individualized Educational Program (IEP) still a valid document? Will meetings with the school-based child study team or committee on special education still take place?

- Can instructional support (e.g., resource room) and related services (e.g., speech-language therapy) be provided to my child at home?

- Can my child visit the school building for certain classes (e.g., advanced placement science, studio art) but not others? How about participation in sports, chorus, clubs and after-school activities?

- How will my child's progress be officially monitored and reported? Will my child have to take mid-term and final exams? (in school? at home?) Standardized assessments? And will these be given with appropriate accommodations?

- How will my child's grade point average (GPA) be calculated and recorded on the official school transcript?

- Will the decision to home school have an impact on my child's college application process or work application status?

Section 35.2

Choosing a Tutor

Your child with learning disabilities may benefit greatly from the one-on-one attention provided by a qualified tutor. Tutors, working closely with parents and teachers, can help children in various ways: reinforcing specific subject matter, helping with homework, suggesting improvements in organization and other study skills, and serving to bolster a child's self-confidence.

A recommendation that your child might profit from working with a tutor often comes from a teacher or a school's learning specialist or guidance counselor. As a parent, however, you have the deepest insight into your child's needs and may see the need for tutoring before the school does.

Does My Child Need a Tutor?

Children with learning disabilities (LD) or attention deficit hyperactivity disorder (ADHD) almost always need extra assistance in school. A tutor can be a valuable source of help. Ask yourself:

- Is there a particular subject or type of assignment that almost always gives my child trouble?

- Does my child have difficulty studying effectively for tests?

- Does my child have trouble with "executive skills" such as organizing, planning, or seeing a project through to completion?

- Is my child unhappy or anxious about schoolwork?

- Is completing homework a recurring battle in my family?

- Has my child's teacher (or guidance counselor or learning specialist) suggested tutoring?

If the answer to one or more of these questions is yes, investigate the possibility of getting your child a tutor.

What Kind of Learning Support Does My Child Need?

Tutors may or may not have special experience working with children with learning disabilities. For that, you will probably need to employ a learning specialist or educational therapist. These professionals address specific learning disabilities with specialized teaching techniques. Some—but not all—specialists may work within the context of a particular school subject.

Whether or not you turn to a specialist, however, a tutor can be helpful with specific subject matter, particular assignments, and underlying skills such as time management and organization.

What Kind of Tutoring Would Be Best?

There are various kinds of tutoring to choose from. You'll want to think about cost, convenience, and the learning approaches most likely to be effective with your child. Consider your options:

- **Private tutoring:** This is the most common type of tutoring and, perhaps, the most desirable—especially for a child with learning disabilities. A tutor, chosen by you with the assistance of teachers and other experts who know how your child learns best, works with your child one or more times a week. Most tutors are college students or teachers working part-time to help students in particular subjects or with study skills and executive functions. The tutor considers your child's needs and the school's and teacher's expectations. The tutor may come to your home or school, or may prefer that you bring your child to another location.

- **Tutoring centers:** These are companies that employ tutors with various kinds of experience. Some centers use standardized materials and methods. They may offer diagnostic testing to help them develop a learning strategy for your child. Your child will be placed with a tutor for sessions one or more times a week, usually after school or in the evening. Some tutoring centers offer group tutoring, which can be less expensive than individual tutoring. However, you'll need to decide whether your child will work better in a group or one-on-one.

- **Online tutoring:** If you are unable to find a tutor near home, or if your schedule makes attending regular sessions difficult, check out companies that offer one-on-one tutoring online. Online tutoring allows your child to work with a teacher in real time over the internet. Communication between student and online tutor is usually done using headsets. The child's hands are free to type or to write on an electronic pad. Some online programs offer video conferencing, so child and tutor interact face to face. Most programs offered by online tutors are in math and reading. Within those programs, your child can develop more specific skills, such as geometry or writing. But for tutoring to help your child with ninth-grade social studies, you'll probably want to stick with private or school-based tutoring.

- **Tutoring software:** Lots of tutoring software, such as worksheets and educational games, is free. Some programs and online tutorials may charge a subscriber or licensing fee. They do not, of course, offer supervision. You'll need to monitor your child's computer use and ask your child for a certain amount of commitment and discipline. For children who love computers, this can be an attractive option, particularly in combination with private tutoring.

Begin with the School

If your child attends a Title I school that has failed to make Adequate Yearly Progress (AYP) for a third year, he or she may be eligible for free tutoring according to the provisions of the No Child Left Behind (NCLB) Act. Ask school or district administrators if this provision applies to your child. Even if your school isn't required to provide extra help, if your child has performed poorly on your state's required reading or math tests, ask about free or low-cost tutoring. Parent involvement is central to NCLB, so feel free to check this out!

Find out how your child's school handles requests for tutors. Some schools and districts have lists of tutors, including areas of specialization, background, and so forth. However, be sure to inquire about whether the tutors on the list have been interviewed or screened. Some schools and districts compile lists based solely on a tutor's application. You will want references and personal contact before you hire any potential tutor, but particularly with someone who hasn't previously been screened. Your school may also recommend a particular tutoring agency. Many schools also offer after-school homework help from teachers and aides.

Some schools—particularly private schools and schools focused on educating children with LD—have their own tutoring program. Such schools, at a teacher's request, may suggest that your child be tutored. After your consent, they will place your child with the tutor best qualified to help. Schools with their own programs usually provide tutoring during a child's free periods or before or after school. They often have in place a required or suggested communication path between tutor and teacher and between tutor and parent.

You may feel you need more regular communication with your child's tutor than the school provides. You may also want to meet your child's tutor and perhaps observe a session. These are legitimate requests. Discuss them with relevant staff members: the coordinator of tutoring, your child's teacher, perhaps the principal or other administrator. Schools with their own tutoring programs usually can accommodate special requests from parents.

Choosing a Tutor Yourself

The best way to find a good tutor yourself is to get recommendations from other parents. Ask them how they found the tutor, how well the tutor interacted with their child, how successful the tutor was in helping the child, and so forth. It's also good to seek referrals from teachers and other school professionals who know your child.

Check around your area for libraries and community centers that offer tutoring. Use the internet to find private tutoring agencies near you. Look for websites that offer tutor directories.

Finding a tutor for your child with learning disabilities may require some effort. Talk with a potential tutor about your child's learning challenges. Offer your own observations about how your child learns best. See if the tutor has worked with children with similar challenges. Ask the tutor about his or her approaches when beginning to work with a child. How does the tutor get to know the child? How does the tutor get familiar with a child's particular issues? What kind of contact does the tutor generally have with a child's teachers? How does the tutor encourage children and help them feel good about themselves and their work? Does the tutor seem to have a sense of humor?

After you've found a promising tutor, you may find it useful to share all or part of your child's psychoeducational test results. If your child hasn't been tested, or if you're uncomfortable sharing test results, you can still talk with the tutor about your child's learning issues. As a parent, your knowledge of your child is deeper than anyone else's. Make sure the tutor knows what's important.

Include Your Child's Teacher

Even if the idea to seek out tutoring support is yours, be sure to talk with the teacher about your child's needs. Discuss the assignments and skills that should have priority during the sessions. Ask the teacher to collaborate with the tutor and to communicate regularly with you. See if there are any books or materials that the teacher can give you for the tutor to use.

Feel free to ask the teacher to supply the tutor with examples of your child's work or tests. This is an excellent way for the tutor to get a handle on your child's difficulties. It's also extremely helpful for the tutor and teacher to communicate about your child's strengths and weaknesses. The tutor needs to understand the teacher's expectations—as do you and your child. Keep the tutor posted on any feedback you get from teachers about your child's work.

It's extremely helpful if your child and the tutor, in conversations with you and your child's teacher, set several achievable, short-term goals. For example: keeping a planner up to date, setting and meeting interim goals for a bigger project, annotating or taking notes about a book, or proofreading a paper before it is handed in.

Include Your Child

As with any other change you want to make in your child's life, getting his or her buy-in is crucial. Your child may not be thrilled by the idea of working with a tutor, but the process will be much easier if you discuss it in advance. Explain your reasons (and a teacher's reasons) for thinking your child would benefit from tutoring. Discuss the purpose of tutoring and the ways you would expect a tutor to help your child.

If you are hiring a tutor yourself, be sure to allow your child and the prospective tutor to meet and talk together during the interview. Involve your child in the selection process. See how your child and the tutor interact when they first meet. Does this seem like a person who will work well with your child?

It's crucial for your child and the tutor to develop a productive, mutually respectful relationship. Such a relationship takes time, but the essential chemistry between child and tutor needs to be right.

Issues to Consider

When you are selecting a tutor yourself, you'll want to consider various issues that are particularly important to you and your family. For example:

- **Logistics:** Will the tutor come to your home or your school, or will you need to take your child to the tutor's home, a library or other meeting place, or a tutoring center? It's easiest when a tutor comes to your home or school. But if you can provide transportation, consider whether a change of scene may help your child focus. How long will sessions be? How many days of the week? What is the tutor's policy about cancelled sessions?

- **Communication:** Will the tutor commit to being in regular contact with you and your child's teacher, or will you and the teacher be expected to contact the tutor? Is the tutor available to talk with you on the phone or via email? If needed, could the tutor attend school meetings and Individualized Educational Program (IEP) conferences? (For any services beyond the actual tutoring session, ask about extra fees.)

- **Costs:** You may need to comparison shop to find a suitable tutor or tutoring agency with an acceptable hourly rate. Ask about other costs, such as for materials. Find out if you must pay at the end of each session, or if the tutor or agency can bill you. See if the tutor or agency charges for sessions cancelled with short notice.

- **Flexibility:** Is the tutor comfortable with the occasional changed day, time, or length of session, and with adding or subtracting sessions? There may be times—such as before exams or when large projects are assigned—when you'll want your child to have more tutoring than usual. At other times, you may want to reduce the number of sessions.

Talk Regularly with Your Child

Keep the dialogue going after your child begins working with a tutor. Talk through any conflicts or difficulties; ask about what's been fun or helpful about the sessions. Don't overreact if your child complains about the extra time and work involved in tutoring. Monitor your child's relationship with the tutor, but realize that building that relationship will take time. Your child's willingness to continue with tutoring will probably increase as she or he sees improvements or feels less anxiety about school.

Encourage your child to speak up—to ask the tutor questions, request specific help, make suggestions about how tutoring sessions could be improved, and let you know how things are going.

Make clear that you expect your child to cooperate with the tutor, but keep tabs on your child's progress. Make sure your child is comfortable with the tutor.

What to Expect from Tutoring

Tutoring should not be solely about getting better grades. A tutor should help your child improve skills and develop more effective ways to study and to get homework done. A tutor who does your child's homework isn't helping your child be a successful learner.

Resolve to be patient with both your child and the tutor. Your child's progress depends on many things: the number of sessions, a tutor's strategies, your child's cooperation and mood, the assistance of teachers, and the help and support you provide as a parent. With luck, your child will develop a friendly, trusting relationship with a sensitive, flexible adult who can guide your child toward academic independence.

Chapter 36

Transition to High School

Not so very long ago, your child was entering middle school and was tied up in knots worrying about how he would find his way in the huge new school, if he would have any friends, and if the classes would be too tough. Now he's facing high school, and guess what he's worried about? The same things. Plus he knows that now it really counts. He needs to decide if he's aiming for college or the workforce. He definitely must accumulate enough credits to graduate and may need to pass a state-mandated exit exam. And then there's dating, getting a driver license, and his first job.

OK. Slow down, just a bit. High school is a time of great change and numerous "firsts" and transitions. Luckily, you and your student don't have to cope with all of them at once, and certainly not all during his first few weeks as a freshman. So let's take a relaxed look at what is important during the transition from middle school to high school, and what extra concerns may crop up for your child with learning difficulties.

A Sophomore Looks Back

Scott[1], a sixteen-year-old sophomore with learning difficulties, reflects on his early weeks in high school: "I was a little worried about

"Helping Your Middle-Schooler with LD Transition to High School," by Nancy Firchow, M.L.S. Reprinted with permission from GreatSchools.org.© GreatSchools, Inc. All rights reserved. This document can be found online at http://www.great schools.org/special-education/support/982-transition-to-high-school.gs?page=all; accessed June 19, 2011.

finding my way around the new school. But I knew I had managed to get around OK in junior high and I had done the whole locker thing already, so I figured I'd get where I needed to be. After a couple days, it was no problem."

Scott didn't just make the move from junior high to high school, he also transferred from a private school to the local public high school. He credits friends and sports with helping make the transition easier. "I already knew people from my neighborhood and the swim team and seeing familiar faces helped a lot. That made me more comfortable. I met even more people by trying out for water polo."

The classes, on the other hand, were more of a concern. Says Scott: "The workload increased dramatically. Junior high was much more relaxed. In high school, the teachers are stricter and there are more deadlines." He says his parents were (and still are) a great help. "When I get discouraged, they remind me that things will get better and help me to keep going."

Scott's experience confirms formal research findings: Kids moving into high school rely heavily on friends and are, at least at first, caught off guard by the academic workload (Letrello, T., 2002; Mizelle, N., 2000; Akos, P., 2004). This applies to students with learning problems as well as those without. Scott's participation in swimming and water polo probably contributed to his smooth transition. Studies reveal that students who feel they are a part of the school community are more motivated and show higher academic achievement (Isakson and Jarvis, 1999). Parents should also know that the transition period is more than just the first few weeks of school. Many schools treat the transition as a long-term process, beginning in the eighth grade and continuing through the ninth, and provide multiple avenues of support and information to help freshmen settle in socially and academically (ERIC Development Team 2006; Isakson and Jarvis, 1999; National Network of Partnership Schools, 2005).

Choosing Freshman Courses: The First Transition Step

Students know that what happens in high school really counts. Course selection and grades help determine which paths are open immediately after high school. That's a good reason for you and your child to thoroughly understand the choices offered by the high school as you register for freshman classes during eighth grade.

Freshman courses are largely limited to those that meet graduation requirements, without a lot of space for extras. At Scott's school, freshmen had only one class period open for an elective. He and his parents chose to fill that slot with a foreign language, to get that requirement out of the way early. In hindsight, Scott's mother says, that might not have been the best choice. "By including Spanish as his elective, all of Scott's freshman classes were academic. He ended up having to work so hard in every course that it might have been better to have a more creative elective in that spot, to give him a break."

You and your student need to be aware of any flexibility or "tracks" available within the required freshman coursework. For instance, does one version of freshman algebra lead on to trigonometry and calculus, whereas another version fulfills the math requirement but doesn't prepare the student for more advanced courses? Understanding these details allows you to choose the ninth-grade courses most appropriate for your child without inadvertently closing off some academic pathways as he moves through high school.

It's a tricky task for students and parents to choose courses that maximize post–high school options. The average eighth-grader doesn't know for certain if he's headed to college, vocational training, or to a job after high school. That natural uncertainty makes leaving many paths open all the more important. Work with your student's guidance counselor to come up with an appropriate balance of academic and elective courses for your child's freshman year.

Be Prepared to Make Changes

Once the high school workload takes hold, you may find that the study strategies and accommodations that have worked well up to this point are no longer adequate. This is because continued cognitive development means your adolescent is beginning to think more abstractly, use more complex reasoning, and form his own opinions. His schoolwork all through high school reflects this and becomes increasingly demanding.

Scott's mother recalls, "We always knew that Scott had to work twice as hard as other kids to get through his assignments. But not too long into his freshman year it was obvious that sheer hard work and determination weren't going to cut it any more. He was exhausted. I was exhausted. That's when we began meetings with his counselor and started talking about accommodations. Scott now gets extra time on tests and sometimes gets tested separately from the rest of his class. It helps, but he still has to work extraordinarily hard."

Keep a close eye on how well your child is managing his workload.

Help him improve his study skills to meet the demands of high school.

413

Do the increased reading demands warrant the use of digital textbooks and other assistive technology tools?

Would your child be able improve his note-taking and writing by using a laptop computer or other assistive technology tools?

Changing approaches and adding strategies as your child progresses through his first year and beyond will help keep things on track. Stay in touch with his counselor and, if your student has an Individualized Education Program (IEP), review it frequently to make sure it continues to meet his needs.

There's More to High School Than Classes

Extracurricular activities, sports, and social functions are just as much a part of the high school experience as classes. Research shows that involvement in activities makes the high school transition easier for freshmen with learning disabilities as well as for those without (Letrello, T., 2002). And, since the high school years are a remarkable period of self-exploration and identity development, extracurricular activities are a great way for your student to try new things, show off his strengths, and connect with peers with similar interests.

High schools offer many special-interest clubs, such as computers, drama, debate, and photography. There is usually a broader range of sports available than in middle school, and many sports teams need students to help with support functions, such as scorekeeping. Your child can get involved in student government, activity planning (dances, rallies, etc.), leadership, and community volunteering.

Encourage your child to participate. Scott plays water polo and swims on the school team. He knows that he has to maintain a certain grade point average to be on these teams, which is an extra motivator when the going gets tough. He also goes with friends to football games and dances and stays connected to what's going on at school overall. He doesn't let his learning difficulties set him apart from his peers.

Stay Involved

Your involvement in the high school transition is just as important as your child's involvement in school activities. Your student is entering a phase of great change, and support from parents is essential. Scott knows he can count on his parents and acknowledges the critical role their support plays in his schooling. Even if your student seems more likely to push you away than ask for guidance, keep the lines of communication open. Get to know your child's friends. Be aware of school functions and encourage your child to join in. Find out where the school needs parent volunteers.

Your active support and participation will help ensure a successful transition into high school.

Note

1. "Scott" is based on a real-life teenager in the author's extended family. The conversations recounted here, with Scott and his mother, are accurate representations of actual conversations the author had with them.

References

Akos, Patrick. "Middle and High School Transitions as Viewed by Students, Parents, and Teachers." *Professional School Counseling*, April 2004.

ERIC Development Team, "Helping Middle School Students Make the Transition into High School." *ERIC Digest*, ED432411.

Isakson, Kristen, and Jarvis, Patricia. "The Adjustment of Adolescents During the Transition into High School: A Short-term Longitudinal Study." *Journal of Youth and Adolescence*, February 1999.

Letrello, Thesea M. "The Transition from Middle School to High School: Students with and without Learning Disabilities Share their Perceptions." *The Clearing House*, March/April 2002.

Mizelle, Nancy B. "Transition from Middle School into High School." *Middle School Journal*, May 2000.

National Network of Partnership Schools. "Middle and High School Report: Plan to Help Incoming Freshmen and their Parents Transition to High school." *Type 2* Spring 2005, Issue 2.

Chapter 37

Transition to College

Chapter Contents

Section 37.1

How Students with Learning Disabilities Can Prepare for College

Excerpted from "College: You Can Do It! How Students with Disabilities Can Prepare for College." Reprinted with permission from DO-IT (Disabilities, Opportunities, Internetworking, and Technology). © 2012 University of Washington. All rights reserved. DO-IT serves to increase the successful participation of individuals with disabilities in challenging academic programs and careers. Primary funding for DO-IT is provided by the National Science Foundation, the State of Washington, and the U.S. Department of Education. For additional information and resources, visit the DO-IT Center website at http://www.uw.edu/doit.

Some adults with disabilities do not have access to the same academic and career opportunities as their nondisabled peers. Improvements in pre-college education and increased awareness of the rights and abilities of individuals with disabilities has resulted in a growing interest in expanding their postsecondary options. This section addresses issues surrounding the transitions from high school to college and beyond for people with disabilities. It covers three phases:

- Preparing for college while in high school.
- Staying in college, which requires numerous self-management skills.
- Preparing to move beyond college and into a career.

Plan

Getting into college involves thoughtful preparation. It is best to start your planning by your sophomore year in high school.

Entrance Requirements

Participate in college fairs at your school or in your community to meet college representatives in person. Look at the websites or call the institutions that you hope to attend to find out about entrance requirements. Talk with teachers and school counselors. If you find that you are not able to meet specific entrance requirements during high school, consider attending a local community college to earn course credits you are lacking. Starting at a two-year institution can provide a solid foundation for further studies at a four-year college or university.

Establish a Time Line

It is important to establish a time line that includes testing dates and application and student aid deadlines. When offered, consider applying for early-decision admission to colleges in order to have more time to visit potential schools and prepare for the transition to college.

High School Grade Point Average

The grade point average (GPA) you obtain in high school may be an important entrance consideration at your colleges of choice. Work hard to earn grades that are as high as possible.

Pre-College Examinations

Pre-college examination (e.g., SAT, PSAT, ACT) scores may be important for acceptance into your college of choice. Work with a school counselor or teacher to arrange disability-related test-taking accommodations a few months before the test date. Appropriate accommodations can help you demonstrate your abilities to their fullest when taking an exam. If you earn a lower score than you feel capable of, ask if you can re-take the exam. If you provided a list of schools when you applied for the test, your scores may be automatically forwarded to these schools.

Applications

When sending an application to a postsecondary institution, you are essentially sending a portrait of yourself—your grades, coursework, recommendations, personal goals, and abilities. Take time to present a full, positive picture of yourself. Before you submit your application, have someone proofread it and give you suggestions for improvement.

Funding

Life in college is full of expenses that are expected and unexpected. There are resources to assist with and, in some cases, fully cover costs such as tuition, books, rent, lab fees, technology, and application fees.

Start early and talk to teachers, counselors, disability services office, financial aid offices, and undergraduate support programs at institutions you wish to attend.

Support Services

Resources are not the same at each postsecondary institution. Knowing your needs and how they can be met is an important factor when selecting a college. Contact the disability services office at campuses of interest to see if they offer the accommodations and support that you require. Ask what type of disability-related documentation the college requires to provide requested services. Arranging support services can take a lot of time, depending on the services you need and the resources that are available. Be sure to allow enough time before school begins to submit your documentation and accommodation requests.

Transition and Orientation

Ask your high school counselor about transition programs that can prepare you for college. Also, find out if the college you've selected offers summer bridge programs or new student sessions.

Go

Being in college means managing a demanding schedule. It is especially important to develop and use personal skills in the areas of self-advocacy, self-management, and study.

Self-Advocacy Skills

Self-advocacy skills include knowing how to skillfully initiate action and interact with faculty, staff, and other students to obtain support services necessary for your learning needs. You are the one who must recognize your needs, as well as mainstream services and disability-related accommodations that will help you be successful. Make contact with those who can provide support or allow accommodations, follow-up on these contacts, and meet any requirements to receive the services needed.

Self-Management Skills

Take into account your abilities and strengths, as well as your disabilities, when scheduling classes, work, and social activities. If your strength and ability vary daily, allow for flexibility. Self-management skills include maintaining reasonable academic and personal routines on a daily basis.

Study Skills

Study skills involve knowing how you can effectively learn academic content. These skills include strategies for note-taking during lectures and labs, reading, and test-taking. Development of each of these skills is important and leads to effective overall study habits. On many campuses, study skills courses are available to students free of charge. Many campus departments have tutoring, study groups, and open labs to help students be successful. Thoroughly explore the availability of these offerings at your school and take advantage of opportunities available to you.

Support Services

Many students, including individuals with disabilities, find it useful to obtain assistance from campus offices as well as outside resources. A disability services office can be a good place to start. Support services can be long-term or temporary. In many instances, a service that provides assistance requires ongoing attention. For example, to continue receiving some services you may need to provide updates on progress, status reports, and renewal requests. Factoring these requirements into a regular schedule of activities will ensure continuity of services.

Technology

Use of computer and internet resources is often essential in college and work. Assistive technology makes it possible for people with a variety of disabilities to use these powerful tools. Take advantage of opportunities in high school and college to learn about and use computer technologies. Of particular importance is developing skills in word processing and information access for research purposes. Many colleges have computer labs available to students and, in many cases, provide assistive technology. Find out what technology is available at your school and make use of these resources.

Networking

Throughout the process of preparing for and attending college, conversations, interactions, and assistance from a broad range of people will likely take place. Take advantage of networking opportunities through the career center, professional organizations, friends, family, and co-workers because who you know, as well as what you know, can determine your success.

Think Ahead

Working toward a career should begin early in your college life. Making prudent choices academically (e.g., choosing a major, selecting appropriate coursework, engaging in work experiences) can assist you in making your career choices.

Academic and Career Choices

College can prepare you for a specific career as well as provide broad-based preparation for a range of career opportunities. Seek advice from family members, teachers, school counselors, and career guidance counselors when making decisions about choosing a direction that is best for you. Career services offices at your school may offer classes, testing, and consulting in these areas.

Building Your Résumé

To begin building a résumé, make a list of all of your relevant work experiences (paid and volunteer), academic experiences, and other activities. Seek advice from campus career advisors and consult printed and online resources as you select the best style and format for your résumé depending on the type of job for which you are applying.

Work-Based Learning

The career services office at the postsecondary institution you attend may offer employment, cooperative, and internship opportunities. If opportunities are not available, make efforts to obtain other work-based learning experiences for your résumé. These experiences can also help you confirm your area of interest and career path, as well as establish a network of contacts that will be needed for post-college employment.

Community Support Services

For some individuals, the need for support services continues past college graduation. Which support services will need to continue and which ones need to be newly established will depend on specific post-college job requirements. Early awareness of services you need will ease your transition from college life to life on your own and on the job. Work-related accommodations may be supplied by your employer, while personal support services may need to be provided by outside sources. Start planning early as this can be a slow process of research and practice.

Have Fun

Social Activities

A social life is important. Make time in your schedule to socialize and get involved in extracurricular activities. Forming study groups is a good way to tackle challenging classes and meet new people. Joining campus clubs or organizations will help you connect with others who have similar interests.

Helpful Hints

The following helpful hints are offered by participants in DO-IT, most of whom have disabilities and are in college or pursuing careers:

- Research all of your options for college.
- Work with the school you plan on attending ahead of time.
- Seek assistance from student service offices, such as disabled student services, career services, and cooperative education.
- Plan, organize, and evaluate your needs so that support service units can work together to ensure there are no gaps in assistance.
- Communicate with your professors. They are there to help.
- Request accommodations in a timely manner.
- Be realistic about the number of credits you take, especially the first quarter.
- Take some courses that look like fun, as well as more challenging courses.
- Take some time to enjoy the social life on campus. It is a good way to meet new people and make friends.
- Know yourself. Evaluate your strengths, abilities, skills, and values at various times throughout your college experience.

Section 37.2

Practical Advice for College Bound Students with Learning Disabilities

"I'm in, I'm Going, Now What? Practical Advice for College Bound Students with Learning Disabilities," by Renee LeWinter Goldberg, Ed.D., CEP, and Marvin Goldberg, M.S.W. © 2011 Learning Disabilities Worldwide, Inc. All rights reserved. Reprinted with permission from Teresa Allissa Citro, CEO, of Learning Disabilities Worldwide, Inc. For additional information and resources, visit www.ldworldwide.org.

The waiting game is over. You were accepted at the college of your choice, and your parents are off your back (maybe). By now you have helped them understand that you and not they are going to college, and it is you and not they who will study, party, and enter a new stage of your life. Now that you are in, and you have a learning disability, are you ready to go? What knowledge and skills do you need to successfully navigate the college experience? You have been successful in high school, but college is different, very different.

Here are some tips to get you ready for college and advice on how to survive your first semester:

1. You need to understand your learning disability. Simple, maybe, but can you be specific when you describe the nature of your disability? How it affects you? What are your learning strengths and weaknesses? What accommodations do you need or think you need in order to be successful in college? If you have the answers, great; if not, now is the time to reflect upon these questions. In addition, not only think about them, but keep your responses handy so you will be better prepared when you request assistance. You are the one who will ask for help, not your parents or professors.

2. Make sure your documentation is up-to-date. Most colleges want documentation that has been completed within three to five years of college entrance. If assessments for adults have been given, that's fine. If you had assessments normed on children, such as the Wechsler Intelligence Scale for Children, many colleges will

want to see the adult form of this assessment. You should have these assessments completed while still in high school; otherwise, you may discover that you do not qualify for services at college. Review your documentation for timeliness and bring it with you to college; no current documentation, no services.

3. If you want services, you must request them yourself. On every college campus there is an office of disability services. It might be called by a different name, such as student support services or student access office. Be persistent in identifying this office. Then, find out where the office is, gather your current documentation and records, walk over and introduce yourself. Begin the important dialogue that will make your academic life more satisfying. The staff members at these offices are there to assist you with accommodations, organizational and study skill assistance, digitally recorded textbooks, and other tools to make it easier to adapt to college life. Here is where college is radically different from high school. Again, if you want services, you must request them. No one will seek you out. At college, self-advocacy is the name of the game. One of the great things about attending college is a real sense of independence, but with freedom comes responsibility. Some students don't want to be identified as learning disabled. They think they can function well without support. That's fine until there's a problem. Do not expect any significant amount of assistance from your college disability services staff when you have three papers and two exams due in a week, you are way behind, and you rush in deciding to register for services. The key is to anticipate rather than react. So during orientation, reach out to disability services in order to avoid a crisis later. Even if you feel you may not need services, register. You never know.

4. Be consistent. College is an exciting environment, but with it comes all sorts of "interesting" distractions. Early on, find a good place to study, one that is quiet, accessible to restrooms and vending machines, and will allow you an opportunity to study with few distractions. Study in your room only at your own peril. Take advantage of dorm life and try studying with a friend or student from class. Discussing ideas is a great way to reinforce them and helps with memory.

5. Use a planner, personal digital assistant (PDA), or other devices to get organized. Take advantage of technology and become

familiar with these tools, which are very useful and can be adapted to your particular learning style. You certainly can begin using organizational supports in college, but it's better to "hit the ground running" and not lose valuable time getting used to them for the first time. Try some of these tools and see how they work for you before you go to college.

6. If you are taking any medication, be very aware that medications may have serious side effects when combined with alcohol and/or drugs. Just be smart—enough said—no lecturing, I promise!

7. The only way anyone can see your grades, have access to your records, and speak to your professors or college staff is with your written permission—and that includes your parents. This is a major step towards becoming your own person and being responsible for your deeds and actions.

And now for the big finale: College is a big and exciting step in your life. The road to success at college for students with learning disabilities rests on the two pillars of self-awareness and self-advocacy. Once you have made strides in these two areas, a successful transition from high school to college will come as another developmental step. Go off to college, be prepared, follow these tips, and make yourself proud.

Section 37.3

Tips for Scholastic Success in College

Congratulations! You have decided to go to college—excellent decision. A college education can increase your opportunities for success. However, you will find the college learning environment different from that of high school. You will need more self-monitoring skills than you needed in high school. Teachers and parents will be making fewer decisions for you. Be prepared to face an increased level of academic competition and to have less contact with your instructors. You will be more responsible for your learning and for acquiring support services.

If you have a disability this includes dealing with a new and more complex process for securing accommodations you may need for success.

As a student with a disability, it is critical that you understand your disability and how it affects your ability to learn and participate in the college experience. Understanding your rights and, equally important, your responsibilities as a college student with a disability are also critical to your success. The office of disability support services at the college you plan to attend can help you reach these goals. This office can play a key role in your success and will refer you to other areas on campus where support services are available.

Many students believe that if they are interested in college and motivated to learn, they will be successful—this is not enough! You need skills in reading, writing, listening, and studying. Many students, however, have not developed a systematic approach to study skills. In college, your instructors will take for granted that you have these skills, that you can read, write, listen, take notes, and complete exams and assignments effectively. Plan to be a successful student—start college with survival skills!

No two people learn in exactly the same manner. Everyone has unique ways of processing information. It is vital that you understand your own learning style and use this knowledge to create strategies tailored to your personal strengths and information processing skills. Although some techniques may apply to a specific area, it is important to develop strategic problem solving skills that transfer across the curriculum.

Tips for Success

What follows is a list of suggested study skills and strategies that may be helpful to you as you make the transition from high school to college. These tips are paraphrased from interviews of mentors, scholars, and ambassadors in DO-IT (Disabilities, Opportunities, Internetworking, and Technology) programs at the University of Washington. As participants in DO-IT, they are either preparing for college, participating in college, or sharing their past college experiences as youth with disabilities. Consider these suggestions as you build your own study skills inventory:

- Selecting an appropriate set of classes is an important first step. Talk to your academic advisor, disabled student services personnel, faculty members, and other students about classes that you are considering. Ask questions about the class format; class requirements such as amount of reading, papers assigned, type of tests given; and the instructor's teaching style.

- When you are deciding which classes to take remember to take a less demanding class along with more demanding classes each quarter or semester. This will help you balance your workload.

- Complete classes required for graduation early in your program, especially if they are subjects you are not fond of. Don't get stuck in your final year of school needing classes that create scheduling conflicts or are full.

- Try to get a copy of the class syllabus so you can see exactly what the requirements will be for a specific class.

- Purchase your textbooks a couple of weeks before the class starts if possible.

- Organize a study notebook for each class. If your notebook is sloppy and disorganized, visualize your grades in the same vein.

- Attend ALL classes! Don't sign up for a class during a time that you know other activities, such as work, will overlap or encroach upon your study time. Learning how to manage your time lowers the stress you will feel as your coursework increases.

- Buy a calendar and record what you need to do each day. Write in exam dates, when papers are due, reading assignments, and scheduled study times. How much time you will need for each assignment will depend upon the length and difficulty of the assignment. Look at the assignment the day that it is assigned and start breaking it down into manageable chunks. For example, break a research paper assignment down into smaller parts, e.g., library research, read materials, develop outline, create rough draft. Schedule each task on the calendar as a daily assignment that must be completed. Allow extra time in the schedule. That way if you hit a snag you have time to deal with it. Don't procrastinate. Work within your scheduled time frame, and stay ahead of homework assignments.

- Schedule a specific time each day for studying. Plan this time during your "alert" times of the day, not the times when you are ready to go to sleep or are hungry. Study your most difficult or least favorite subject first.

- Take study breaks. Avoid marathon study sessions and cramming.

- Grab stolen moments of time to study or review material. You can read or study flash cards in the waiting room at the doctor's office or while you are on the bus.

- Try to study when you are relaxed and not when you are upset or unable to concentrate on the work you have to do.

- The environment in which you study is important. Choose a location where you feel comfortable, that is quiet, and that is free from distractions. It is often helpful to study in the same conditions in which you will be tested. This means that if you can't eat, drink, or listen to music during the exam, try to study under similar constraints.

- Study groups are great for clarifying some concepts but they should be used to complement personal study time—not replace it. Study groups can digress into discussions about the instructor or other students; try to stay on track. Be sure to read all the necessary material before a study group meeting so that you can contribute to the discussions and maximize your benefit from the meeting.

- Become familiar with the book and begin reading the first chapters before the class starts. This way, when the instructor assigns chapters one through three to be read by the end of the first week you will be ahead of schedule. If you have received a copy of the syllabus early this will help in determining which chapter to begin with as not all texts are read straight through.

- Keep up with the assigned readings, being sure to read the information that will be reviewed in class prior to that class session. By doing this you will be familiar with the vocabulary and the concepts about which the lecturer is speaking, and you can bring up any questions from the reading that the professor may not have addressed during the lecture. Reading ahead will also help you take better notes on the material.

- When you start reading a text, first scan or survey the chapter you are about to read. Look at the pictures, graphs, and headings. Write down vocabulary words that are foreign to you. Look the words up in the glossary or a dictionary before you start reading the chapter. Read the chapter summary and any study questions the author has provided. Ask yourself what you already know about the material to be covered in the chapter.

- When you read a chapter, mark important information as you read. Use a highlighter, underline, or place a check mark in the margins next to the information. If you mark the entire page you are marking too much information; mark just enough to jog your memory.

- Read in short time blocks. You will remember more of what you read than if you undertake marathon reading sessions.

- After you have completed reading and marking the chapter, go back and write concise notes about the material you have marked. Stick with the basic facts and information that was new to you.

- When taking notes in class use short phrases rather than whole sentences. Develop your own set of abbreviations or shorthand. Leave some room in the margins for additional information the lecturer may add later. If you become confused or miss some information mark it with a question mark and ask to have the information clarified then or after class or look up the topic in the text later.

- If you have trouble taking notes, find someone in the class who takes good notes and ask if they would be willing to give you a copy of them. Continue to take your own notes because listening to the lecture and writing notes at the same time helps you remember the information better. Then check them against the other set of notes after class. Look at the information your classmate is recording and use this example to improve your note-taking skills. You may also want to consider tape recording lectures, and then listening to the tapes while reviewing both sets of notes. Be sure to obtain the lecturer's permission before taping a lecture.

- If you need assistance, ask the instructor for help right away, not after you are failing a class.

- Contact the office of disability support services on your campus.

In summary, to maximize your success in college:

1. Develop strategies, study skills, and a network of support!

2. Attend class.

3. Arrive on time, pay attention, and participate in class discussions and activities.

4. Talk to the instructor. Ask questions.

5. Complete and check all work. Turn in neat and clear assignments.

6. Monitor your progress. If you begin to fall behind, ask for help.

7. Stay in contact with the office of disability support services and your professors.

Adapt these tips to fit your unique learning style and needs. Ask friends and classmates about the techniques they use. Never be afraid to try a new method. And, remember that you are ultimately responsible for your success.

Part Five

Living with Learning Disabilities

Chapter 38

Coping with a Learning Disability

The secret to success seems elusive to many people. Is there really a reliable road map to health and happiness? And if you have a learning disability (LD), do you need to take a different course? Not really. Although research has identified several attributes that form the foundation of life success for people with LD, you'll likely recognize the universal relevance of many of these traits, such as perseverance and proactivity. Another is the use of healthy coping strategies, the topic of this chapter.

Here are six things to keep in mind as you teach your child with LD how to navigate the ups and downs of his or her own emotional terrain.

Get your own house in order: If you're anxious about your child's learning disability, if you're fearful about his or her future, if you find yourself tearing your hair out every time you turn around, then you may need to first take a look at your own coping strategies. How do you handle stress? What messages are you sending yourself about your parenting skills? What kind of support system do you have in place?

If you learn to relax and better address your own emotional challenges, you'll be doing yourself and your whole family a big favor. Remember the flight attendant's advice: Put the oxygen mask on yourself before you put it on your child. Doing so helps you to breathe, to accept your child's differences, and to build on his or her strengths. Yes, it's true a child with LD may never be a great reader, but many successful people—from Greg Louganis to Whoopi Goldberg to Richard Branson—have had LD and they've done just fine—in fact, better than fine.

Use and teach a vocabulary of emotions: You want your child to know what it means to have empathy for others or to demonstrate gratitude or to savor nature's beauty. In addition to modeling behaviors like these, name and praise these positive behaviors when you see them in your child. This will help cultivate a sense of emotional awareness and sensitivity.

Likewise, kids need to also know how to name negative emotions. Ask what stress feels like for them, where they notice it in their bodies, and what they think might have caused it. This isn't always an easy exercise, particularly for a child with language-processing issues, says Chris Schnieders, Ph.D., director of teacher training at the Frostig School. It takes some work to figure this all out, and that's where a parent's gentle questioning and calm explanations can make a difference.

Recognize—and trip up—the triggers: The better your child gets at recognizing stress triggers, the more successful he or she will be at handling life's curve balls. Research underscores this point, says Frostig researcher Roberta J. Goldberg, Ph.D. All children in the Frostig success studies[1,2] had been greatly challenged by anxiety or stress—largely as a result of LD, she says. "But the ones who recognized stress triggers, especially of LD, and demonstrated coping strategies were the most successful."

Goldberg admits that it can be difficult to know how to help your child identify his or her own triggers, but with time, he can recognize the signs. Do you know what your child's triggers are? Being asked to turn off the TV? Making transitions from one activity to another? Getting stuck on a math problem? Talk about these with your child and problem-solve ways to "cut them off at the pass"—before your child's stress hormones go into overdrive. If the problem is television or transitions, maybe you agree on five-minute warnings before turning off the TV or you make sure your child has plenty of down time between activities.

What about your child's coping mechanisms? You'd be surprised at how much your child has intuitively figured out. Help support healthy ways of coping. It's idiosyncratic, says Goldberg, so the options are practically unlimited. Is music soothing to your child? Then listening to an iPod may not be an idle activity—even when doing homework. Does your child enjoy texting friends? Well, then those messages—

within limits—might bring a helpful distraction. Or maybe writing in a journal or a walk in the woods has a calming effect on your child.

Look for signs of stress and intervene when your child is unable to do this for herself. If she's been hitting the books for two hours and is starting to unravel, you might want to enforce a trampoline break, or jumping jacks, or at the very least, some deep breathing.

"My son—who's now a mechanical engineer—struggled in school and had meltdowns in college," says Goldberg. "I didn't say, 'Go study.' I'd tell him to go for a run or swim twenty-two laps. I knew those were his coping mechanisms."

And, don't forget to play to your child's strengths. If sports, music, or theatre is his strong suit, then allowing time for these pursuits can greatly enhance self-confidence and positive coping behaviors.

Make coping strategies concrete: If your child struggles with developing specific coping mechanisms, try priming the pump with some questions like these:

- If you were having a problem, who would you talk to?

- What are the fun things or activities that you like to do when you are sad or down?

- What motivates you? In other words, why do you do what you do?

- How do you handle peer pressure? For example, what would you do if a friend or peer asked you to try drugs?

- Who are your role models or people you look up to?

Depending upon your child's age and personality, don't necessarily expect (or request) a direct answer to these questions. You can simply throw these out as food for thought. This may help your child describe and acknowledge—if only to himself—what works best for him. And this will take him a step closer to actually using these concrete strategies.

Learn healthy ways to communicate: Jeff Rice is principal of one of the Briarwood Schools in Houston, Texas, serving students with LD and developmental delays. He reminds parents that the normal teen mentality is to interact as little as possible with adults, especially parents. "It may seem like you've got a stranger living in your home, but trust me, they will come around," says Rice. And, he tells parents they'd be amazed if they knew how often kids identify parents as their "go-to person" in times of trouble.

Rice suggests tips like these for moving toward healthier communication with kids:

- *Ask open-ended questions:* Don't be satisfied with the curtness of a yes-no response from your child. You can get around this by asking open-ended questions like: What was the most surprising thing that happened at school today? Or: What was the school assembly all about? Or: What was something you did to manage your stress? A longer response provides a better opening for give and take. Without lecturing, you're also modeling the art of conversation. Just remember that with open-ended questions, you'll also need to stay open—without judgment—to your child's fears, frustrations, and failures.

- *Be present:* Even more important than questioning is simply being present and listening. When your child is talking with you, don't get distracted by opening bills or checking your phone messages. If you do, you're communicating—without saying a word—that something else is more important. And, though there's a place for "history lessons," don't always cut in with responses like, "Well, when I was a kid . . ." Checking in and displaying empathic listening can often go so much further.

- *Reflect back what your child says:* Restate what your child has said, in his or her own words—not yours. You might say: "What I'm understanding is that you felt bullied today at lunch . . ." Again, this helps your child feel heard and understood.

Seek outside help when needed: Remember that a big part of having a healthy coping strategy is knowing how to find and use support systems. For example, if your child is falling behind in math, a tutor may help in more ways than one—by not only shoring up academic weak links, but also circumventing power struggles over homework. And, if your child struggles with anxiety or depression, seeking outside resources such as counseling may be in order. Remember that you cannot be all things to your child.

Help your child identify both internal and external sources of support for better coping. And, do the same for yourself. This can be critical for developing a healthy approach to emotional challenges—which, as you know, won't disappear with adulthood!

Sources

1. Raskind, M.H. et al. *Learning Disabilities Research and Practice.* 1999; 14(1): 35–49.

2. Goldberg, R.J. et al. *Learning Disabilities Research and Practice.* 2003; 18(4): 222–36.

Chapter 39

Tips for Parenting a Child with a Learning Disability

Has your child recently been diagnosed with a learning disability? Did you immediately begin too worry about school—about all the homework, tests, and projects—and how your kid will make it through? It's only natural as a parent to want the best for your child, and to worry about the challenges he or she is facing. But if you slow down for a second, you may realize that academic success, while important, isn't the end goal.

What you really want for your child is a happy and fulfilling life. With encouragement and support, there's no reason why children with learning disabilities can't succeed and thrive at school and beyond. As a parent, your influence outweighs that of any teacher, tutor, therapist, or counselor. You can help your child build a strong sense of self-confidence and a solid foundation for lifelong success.

When It Comes to Learning Disabilities, Look at the Big Picture

All children need love, encouragement, and support, and for kids with learning disabilities, such positive reinforcement can help ensure

"Helping Children with Learning Disabilities: Practical Parenting Tips for Home and School," by Gina Kemp, M.A., Melinda Smith, M.A., and Jeanne Segal, Ph.D., updated November 2011. © 2011 Helpguide.org. All rights reserved. Reprinted with permission. Helpguide provides a detailed list of references and resources for this article, with links to related Helpguide topics and information from other websites. For a complete list of these resources, including information about support for parents and special education services for children, go to http://www.helpguide.org/mental/learning_disabilities_treatment_help_coping.htm.

that they emerge with a strong sense of self-worth, confidence, and the determination to keep going even when things are tough.

In searching for ways to help children with learning disabilities, remember that you are looking for ways to help them help themselves. Your job as a parent is not to "cure" the learning disability, but to give your child the social and emotional tools he or she needs to work through challenges. In the long run, facing and overcoming a challenge such as a learning disability can help your child grow stronger and more resilient.

Always remember that the way you behave and respond to challenges has a big impact on your child. A good attitude won't solve the problems associated with a learning disability, but it can give your child hope and confidence that things can improve and that he or she will eventually succeed.

Tips for Dealing with Your Child's Learning Disability

- **Keep things in perspective:** A learning disability isn't insurmountable. Remind yourself that everyone faces obstacles. It's up to you as a parent to teach your child how to deal with those obstacles without becoming discouraged or overwhelmed. Don't let the tests, school bureaucracy, and endless paperwork distract you from what's really important—giving your child plenty of emotional and moral support.

- **Become your own expert:** Do your own research and keep abreast of new developments in learning disability programs, therapies, and educational techniques. You may be tempted to look to others—teachers, therapists, doctors—for solutions, especially at first. But you're the foremost expert on your child, so take charge when it comes to finding the tools he or she needs in order to learn.

- **Be an advocate for your child:** You may have to speak up time and time again to get special help for your child. Embrace your role as a proactive parent and work on your communication skills. It may be frustrating at times, but by remaining calm and reasonable, yet firm, you can make a huge difference for your child.

- **Remember that your influence outweighs all others:** Your child will follow your lead. If you approach learning challenges with optimism, hard work, and a sense of humor, your child is likely to embrace your perspective—or at least see the challenges as a speed bump, rather than a roadblock. Focus your energy on learning what works for your child and implementing it the best you can.

Focus on Strengths, Not Just Weaknesses

Your child is not defined by his or her learning disability. A learning disability represents one area of weakness, but there are many more areas of strengths. Focus on your child's gifts and talents. Your child's life—and schedule—shouldn't revolve around the learning disability. Nurture the activities where he or she excels, and make plenty of time for them.

Helping Children with Learning Disabilities Tip 1: Take Charge of Your Child's Education

In this age of endless budget cuts and inadequately funded schools, your role in your child's education is more important than ever. Don't sit back and let someone else be responsible for providing your child with the tools they need to learn. You can and should take an active role in your child's education.

If there is demonstrated educational need, the school is required by law to develop an Individualized Education Program (IEP) that delivers some educational benefit, but not necessarily one that maximizes student achievement. Parents who want the best for their kids may find this standard frustrating. Understanding special education laws and your school's guidelines for services will help you get the best support for your child at school. Your child may be eligible for many kinds of accommodations and support services, but the school might not provide services unless you ask for them.

Tips for Communicating with Your Child's School

Being a vocal advocate for your child can be challenging. You'll need superior communication and negotiation skills, and the confidence to defend your child's right to a proper education:

- **Clarify your goals:** Before meetings, write down what you want to accomplish. Decide what is most important, and what you are willing to negotiate.

- **Be a good listener:** Allow school officials to explain their opinions. If you don't understand what someone is saying, ask for clarification. "What I hear you saying is . . ." can help ensure that both parties understand.

- **Offer new solutions:** You have the advantage of not being a "part of the system," and may have new ideas. Do your research and find examples of what other schools have done.

- **Keep the focus:** The school system is dealing with a large number of children; you are only concerned with your child. Help the meeting stay focused on your child. Mention your child's name frequently, don't drift into generalizations, and resist the urge to fight larger battles.

- **Stay calm, collected, and positive:** Go into the meeting assuming that everyone wants to help. If you say something you regret, simply apologize and try to get back on track.

- **Don't give up easily:** If you're not satisfied with the school's response, try again.

Recognize the Limitations of the School System

Parents sometimes make the mistake of investing all of their time and energy into the school as the primary solution for their child's learning disability. It is better to recognize that the school situation for your child will probably never be perfect. Too many regulations and limited funding mean that the services and accommodations your child receives may not be exactly what you envision for them, and this will probably cause you frustration, anger, and stress.

Try to recognize that the school will be only one part of the solution for your child and leave some of the stress behind. Your attitude (of support, encouragement, and optimism) will have the most lasting impact on your child.

Helping Children with Learning Disabilities Tip 2: Identify How Your Child Learns Best

Everyone—learning disability or not—has their own unique learning style. Some people learn best by seeing or reading, others by listening, and still others by doing. You can help a child with a learning disability by identifying his or her primary learning style.

Is your child a visual learner, an auditory learner, or a kinesthetic learner? Once you've figured out how he or she learns best, you can take steps to make sure that type of learning is reinforced in the classroom and during home study. The following lists will help you determine what type of learner your child is.

Is Your Child a Visual Learner?

If your child is a visual learner, he or she:

- learns best by seeing or reading;
- does well when material is presented and tested visually, not verbally;
- benefits from written notes, directions, diagrams, charts, maps, and pictures;
- may love to draw, read, and write; is probably a good speller.

Is Your Child an Auditory Learner?

If your child is an auditory learner, he or she:

- learns best by listening;
- does well in lecture-based learning environments and on oral reports and tests;
- benefits from classroom discussions, spoken directions, study groups;
- may love music, languages, and being on stage.

Is Your Child a Kinesthetic Learner?

If your child is a kinesthetic learner, he or she:

- learns best by doing and moving;
- does well when he or she can move, touch, explore, and create in order to learn;
- benefits from hands-on activities, lab classes, props, skits, and field trips;
- may love sports, drama, dance, martial arts, and arts and crafts

Studying Tips for Different Types of Learners

Tips for visual learners:

- Use books, videos, computers, visual aids, and flashcards.
- Make detailed, color-coded, or highlighted notes.
- Make outlines, diagrams, and lists.
- Use drawings and illustrations (preferably in color).
- Take detailed notes in class.

Tips for auditory learners:

- Read notes or study materials out loud.
- Use word associations and verbal repetition to memorize.
- Study with other students. Talk things through.
- Listen to books on tape or other audio recordings.
- Use a tape recorder to listen to lectures again later.

Tips for kinesthetic learners:

- Get hands on. Do experiments and take field trips.
- Use activity-based study tools, like role-playing or model building.
- Study in small groups and take frequent breaks.
- Use memory games and flash cards.
- Study with music on in the background.

Helping Children with Learning Disabilities Tip 3: Think Life Success, Rather than School Success

Success means different things to different people, but your hopes and dreams for your child probably extend beyond good report cards. Maybe you hope that your child's future includes a fulfilling job and satisfying relationships, for example, or a happy family and a sense of contentment.

The point is that success in life—rather than just school success—depends, not on academics, but on things like a healthy sense of self, the willingness to ask for and accept help, the determination to keep trying in spite of challenges, the ability to form healthy relationships with others, and other qualities that aren't as easy to quantify as grades and Scholastic Aptitude Test (SAT) scores.

A twenty-year study that followed children with learning disabilities into adulthood identified the following six "life success" attributes. By focusing on these broad skills, you can help give your child a huge leg up in life.

Learning Disabilities and Success #1: Self-Awareness and Self-Confidence

For children with learning disabilities, self-awareness (knowledge about strengths, weaknesses, and special talents) and self-confidence are very important. Struggles in the classroom can cause children to doubt their abilities and question their strengths.

Ask your child to list his or her strengths and weaknesses and talk about your own strengths and weaknesses with your child.

Encourage your child to talk to adults with learning disabilities and to ask about their challenges, as well as their strengths.

Work with your child on activities that are within his or her capabilities. This will help build feelings of success and competency.

Help your child develop his or her strengths and passions. Feeling passionate and skilled in one area may inspire hard work in other areas too.

Learning Disabilities and Success #2: Being Proactive

A proactive person is able to make decisions and take action to resolve problems or achieve goals. For people with learning disabilities, being proactive also involves self-advocacy (for example, asking for a seat at the front of the classroom) and the willingness to take responsibility for choices.

Talk with your learning-disabled child about problem solving and share how you approach problems in your life.

Ask your child how he or she approaches problems. How do problems make him or her feel? How does he or she decide what action to take?

If your child is hesitant to make choices and take action, try to provide some "safe" situations to test the water, like choosing what to make for dinner or thinking of a solution for a scheduling conflict.

Discuss different problems, possible decisions, and outcomes with your child. Have your child pretend to be part of the situation and make his or her own decisions.

Learning Disabilities and Success #3: Perseverance

Perseverance is the drive to keep going despite challenges and failures, and the flexibility to change plans if things aren't working. Children (or adults) with learning disabilities may need to work harder and longer because of their disability.

Talk with your learning-disabled child about times when he or she persevered—why did he or she keep going? Share stories about when you have faced challenges and not given up.

Discuss what it means to keep going even when things aren't easy. Talk about the rewards of hard work, as well as the opportunities missed by giving up.

When your child has worked hard, but failed to achieve his or her goal, discuss different possibilities for moving forward.

Learning Disabilities and Success #4: The Ability to Set Goals

The ability to set realistic and attainable goals is a vital skill for life success. It also involves the flexibility to adapt and adjust goals according to changing circumstances, limitations, or challenges.

Help your child identify a few short- or long-term goals and write down steps and a timeline to achieve the goals. Check in periodically to talk about progress and make adjustments as needed.

Talk about your own short- and long-term goals with your child, as well as what you do when you encounter obstacles.

Celebrate with your child when he or she achieves a goal. If certain goals are proving too hard to achieve, talk about why and how plans or goals might be adjusted to make them possible.

Learning Disabilities and Success #5: Knowing How to Ask for Help

Strong support systems are key for people with learning disabilities. Successful people are able to ask for help when they need it and reach out to others for support.

Help your child nurture and develop good relationships. Model what it means to be a good friend and relative so your child knows what it means to help and support others.

Demonstrate to your child how to ask for help in family situations.

Share examples of people needing help, how they got it, and why it was good to ask for help. Present your child with role-play scenarios that might require help.

Learning Disabilities and Success #6: The Ability to Handle Stress

If children with learning disabilities learn how to regulate stress and calm themselves, they will be much better equipped to overcome challenges.

Use words to identify feelings and help your child learn to recognize specific feelings.

Ask your child what words they would use to describe stress. Does your child recognize when he or she is feeling stressed?

Encourage your child to identify and participate in activities that help reduce stress like sports, games, music, or writing in a journal.

Ask your child to describe activities and situations that make them feel stressed. Break down the scenarios and talk about how overwhelming feelings of stress and frustration might be avoided.

Recognizing Stress in Your Child

It's important to be aware of the different ways in which stress can manifest. Your child may behave very differently than you do when he or she is under stress. Some signs of stress are more obvious: agitation, trouble sleeping, and worries that won't shut off. But some people—children included—shut down, space out, and withdraw when stressed. It's easy to overlook these signs, so be on the look out for any behavior that's out of the ordinary.

Helping Children with Learning Disabilities Tip 4: Emphasize Healthy Lifestyle Habits

It may seem like common sense that learning involves the body as well as the brain, but your child's eating, sleep, and exercise habits may be even more important than you think. If children with learning disabilities are eating right and getting enough sleep and exercise, they will be better able to focus, concentrate, and work hard:

- **Exercise:** Exercise isn't just good for the body, it's good for the mind. Regular physical activity makes a huge difference in mood, energy, and mental clarity. Encourage your learning-disabled child to get outside, move, and play. Rather than tiring out your child and taking away from schoolwork, regular exercise will actually help him or her stay alert and attentive throughout the day. Exercise is also a great antidote to stress and frustration.

- **Diet:** A healthy, nutrient-rich diet will aid your child's growth and development. A diet full of whole grains, fruits, vegetables, and lean protein will help boost mental focus. Be sure your child starts the day with a good breakfast and doesn't go more than four hours between meals or snacks. This will help keep his or her energy levels stable.

- **Sleep:** Learning disability or not, your child is going to have trouble learning if he or she is not well rested. Kids need more sleep than adults do. On average, preschoolers need from eleven to thirteen hours per night, middle school children need about ten to eleven hours, and teens and preteens need from eight and a half to ten hours. You can help make sure your child is getting the sleep he or she needs by enforcing a set bedtime. The type of light emitted by electronic screens (computers, televisions, iPods and iPads, portable video players, etc.) is activating to the brain. So you can also help by powering off all electronics at least an hour or two before lights out.

Encouraging Healthy Emotional Habits

In addition to healthy physical habits, you can also encourage children to have healthy emotional habits. Like you, they may be frustrated by the challenges presented by their learning disability. Try to give them outlets for expressing their anger, frustration, or feelings of discouragement. Listen when they want to talk and create an environment open to expression. Doing so will help them connect with their feelings and, eventually, learn how to calm themselves and regulate their emotions.

Helping Children with Learning Disabilities Tip 5: Take Care of Yourself, Too

Sometimes the hardest part of parenting is remembering to take care of you. It's easy to get caught up in what your child needs, while forgetting your own needs. But if you don't look after yourself, you run the risk of burning out.

It's important to tend to your physical and emotional needs so that you're in a healthy space for your child. You won't be able to help your child if you're stressed out, exhausted, and emotionally depleted. When you're calm and focused, on the other hand, you're better able to connect with your child and help him or her be calm and focused too.

Your spouse, friends, and family members can be helpful teammates if you can find a way to include them and learn to ask for help when you need it.

Tips for Taking Care of Yourself

- Learn how to manage stress in your own life. Make daily time for yourself to relax and decompress.

- Keep the lines of communication open with your spouse, family, and friends. Ask for help when you need it.

- Take care of yourself by eating well, exercising, and getting enough rest.

448

- Join a learning disorder support group. The encouragement and advice you'll get from other parents can be invaluable.

- Enlist teachers, therapists, and tutors whenever possible to share some of responsibility for day-to-day academic responsibilities.

Communicate with Family and Friends about Your Child's Learning Disability

Some parents keep their child's learning disability a secret, which can, even with the best intentions, look like shame or guilt. Without knowing, extended family and friends may not understand the disability or think that your child's behavior is stemming from laziness or hyperactivity. Once they are aware of what's going on, they can support your child's progress.

Within the family, siblings may feel that their brother or sister with a learning disability is getting more attention, less discipline, and preferential treatment. Even if your other children understand that the learning disability creates special challenges, they can easily feel jealous or neglected. Parents can help curb these feelings by reassuring all of their children that they are loved, providing homework help, and by including family members in any special routines for the child with a learning disability.

Chapter 40

Family and Relationship Issues

Chapter Contents

451

Section 40.1

The Impact of Learning Disabilities on Siblings

Excerpted from "Siblings of Kids with Special Needs," http://www.med
.umich.edu/yourchild/topics/specneed.htm, written and compiled by Kyla
Boyse, R.N., reviewed by Brenda Volling, Ph.D., updated July 2009. Content
provided by the University of Michigan Health System, © 2009. All rights
reserved. Reprinted with permission.

What's the upside of growing up with a sibling with special health or developmental needs?

Siblings of children with special needs have special needs themselves. Their sister or brother with special needs will get a bigger share
of attention. While having a special needs sib presents challenges, it
also comes with opportunities. Kids who grow up with a sibling with
special health or developmental needs may have more of a chance to
develop many good qualities, including:

- patience;

- kindness and supportiveness;

- acceptance of differences;

- compassion and helpfulness;

- empathy for others and insight into coping with challenges;

- dependability and loyalty that may come from standing up for
  their brother or sister.

What kinds of difficult feelings might a sibling have?

Your child may, at times, have trouble coping with being the sibling
of a child with special needs. They may have many different and even
conflicting feelings. For example, they may feel:

- worried about their sibling;

- jealous of the attention their brother/sister receives;

- scared that they will lose their sibling;

- angry that no one pays attention to them;

- resentful of having to explain, support, and/or take care of their brother/sister;

- resentful that they are unable to do things or go places because of their sibling;

- embarrassed about their sibling's differences;

- pressure to be or do what their sibling cannot;

- guilty for negative feelings they have toward their sibling or guilty for not having the same problems.

When parents tune in to the individual needs of each child in the family, they can help ease the difficulties.

What are the red flags, or signs that my child needs more help?

Sometimes the feelings can be so intense or disruptive that a child may need professional counseling to help them cope. Meeting and talking with other kids going through the same thing can also be very helpful—even if it's just online.

Talk to your doctor if you see any of these warning signs:

- changes in eating or sleeping (too much or too little);

- physical symptoms like headaches or stomachaches;

- hopelessness;

- perfectionism;

- poor concentration;

- poor self-esteem;

- talk of hurting themselves;

- difficulty separating from parents;

- loss of interest in activities;

- frequent crying or worrying;

- withdrawal.

You can expect some degree of sibling rivalry, even when one child has an illness or developmental disability. But sometimes the rivalry crosses the line into abuse. If there is a chance the sibling relationship has become abusive, you should seek professional help. Talk to your healthcare provider about options.

Some possible signs of sibling abuse are:

- one child always avoids their sibling;

- a child has changes in behavior, sleep patterns, eating habits, or has nightmares;

- a child acts out abuse in play;

- a child acts out sexually in inappropriate ways;

- the children's roles are rigid: one child is always the aggressor, the other, the victim;

- the roughness or violence between siblings is increasing over time.

What are some parenting tips for our family?

You can help your kids better understand what having a sibling with special needs means to your family, and you can also help your kids figure out constructive and appropriate ways to express their feelings and make sure their needs are met.

Caring for a child with special needs along with all the other demands of work and caring for the rest of the family can be very challenging. If the demands and the stress level are high in your family, it is difficult for everyone. Sometimes family counseling helps.

Section 40.2

Dealing with Learning Disabilities in Relationships

Maintaining a long-lasting and satisfying relationship with a spouse or partner is challenging enough. But having a learning disability (LD) may make it even harder. You may want the relationship to be a stronger one, but you don't know how to make that happen. Some of the behaviors associated with your learning disability may annoy your partner, and your partner's criticism of you may cause you to feel dissatisfied with the relationship.

Dependency can be a big issue when it comes to learning disabilities and relationships. You may both have different views about dependency and control. If you are overly dependent on your partner because of your LD, you may both grow tired of the "patient-caregiver" relationship. After a while, you may find that you are no longer emotionally attached to the relationship.

It may make you feel better to know that relationships are hard work for everyone. Maintaining a satisfying, long-term relationship takes daily effort, and both you and your partner/spouse need to be committed to this effort. The following are some tips that you may find useful when building a stronger relationship:

- You should have a good understanding of your strengths as well as your challenges.

- You should understand how your disability affects your behavior and your ability to communicate.

- Your partner/spouse should understand that learning disabilities could interfere with many aspects of everyday life.

- You both should understand that some tasks might take you longer to do than they take other people.

- Be as self-reliant as possible so that your partner does not feel overburdened or in a patient-caregiver relationship.

- Explain to your partner the accommodations you need. For example, if you have trouble following a series of directions and your partner asks you to do three things after dinner, reply with a direct statement, such as "Please write down what you need, or give me the directions one at a time."

- Agree to trade-off household tasks so you handle the ones that you can comfortably do. For example, your partner/spouse may handle such tasks as paying the bills and balancing the checkbook, while you may do the grocery shopping.

- Be open to improving your social skills. Ask your partner/spouse to give you feedback on things you should/should not do.

One of the most important ways you can maintain a healthy and long-lasting relationship is by practicing good, clear, open communication. The following are some pointers for building good communication:

- Be direct and specific about your needs. Ask for what you need from your partner; don't expect him or her to read your mind.

- Avoid criticizing your partner's personality. For example, don't say "You're so messy!" or "You never listen to me!" or "You always think only about yourself!"

- Try not to use "You" statements when there is a conflict. For example: Your partner: "You were going to tidy up the living room, but there's still a bunch of papers and books lying around! Can't you ever finish anything that you start?" You: "You're never satisfied with anything I do!" Instead, use "I" statements, such as the following: Your partner: "When I find the living room cluttered, I feel unsettled. I would appreciate it if you would pick up all the junk mail and books." You: "When you criticize my efforts, I feel bad. I'll be happy to put away the books, but I'll need to know if you want any of these catalogs before I throw them away."

- Look at your partner/spouse when he/she is speaking. Pay attention to the gestures and facial expressions he/she uses. If you are not sure about what your partner/spouse has said, ask for clarification. For the two of you to have open and honest communication, you will both need to be sure that you understand what's being said.

If you and your partner want help in working through your communication problems and building a stronger relationship, you may consider seeing a family or marriage counselor. It is important to select a counselor who understands how learning disabilities can affect relationships.

Section 40.3

Parenting Issues for Adults with Learning Disabilities

For adults with reading, writing, or math learning disabilities, or those who have trouble staying organized and remembering things, parenthood can mean facing your learning challenges in a new way. Your struggle with these problems may affect your home life and even your child's behavior.

Parenting is an ever-changing role that challenges most adults, but the challenges you face as a result of your learning disability may affect your ability to manage your family's schedule, keep appointments, and relax enough to give your children your full attention.

Creating family routines and guidelines can help make everyday activities more manageable. For example, late afternoon and early evening can be particularly stressful times. This is the time when each family member is eager to share his or her thoughts and feelings from the school day or workday. This is also the time when homework, sports, music lessons, and other activities place demands on parents' time. Setting and keeping to a pattern or routine can make things easier on you. Here are some tips than can help you and your family.

If you struggle with memory and organization:

- Make sure your family has one calendar displayed in a central place like the kitchen:

  - Place all family members' important dates and appointments on this one calendar.

- Make sure someone checks the calendar every day. Color-coding the appointments can help: assign each family member a color to help identify who has something scheduled each day.

- Placing dates on the calendar can happen at the same time each day, such as after dinner or before bedtime. Put reminders in notebooks to help your children remember to give you important notices from school. Keep the house (especially areas used for schoolwork) as organized as possible.

- Teach your children to be responsible for their belongings and to stick to a plan for staying organized.

- If your family has difficulty getting out of the house in the morning (and since mornings are rough for most people), do what you can to get belongings for school and everything needed for the morning routine organized the night before. For example, children can put their homework and anything they need for after-school activities in their backpacks and also pick out their clothes the night before.

These simple routines may help to reduce stress for all family members and leave more time to find ways to help your child develop his or her special interests and talents one of the real joys of parenthood.

All parents struggle to find ways to help children grow up to be happy and feel successful. Support groups can give parents an opportunity to share their concerns and learn positive parenting strategies. Local organizations like the YMCA or groups associated with your children's school often run parenting classes or parent support sessions that you can join. The key is knowing what causes your problems and then finding simple strategies to help you and your children get through the day successfully.

Chapter 41

Educating Others about Your Child with a Learning Disability

Once you understand your child's learning disabilities, it's crucial to share his profile with everyone who significantly impacts his life and even some who play a minor role. But before you engage the town crier to broadcast the details of your child's learning style, use the following guide to help evaluate who needs to know what.

Knowledge providers (teachers, tutors, aides, extracurricular instructors, coaches, scout leaders, playground monitors, religious instructors, camp counselors): People who guide your child's acquisition of knowledge have enormous power over his self-esteem and cognitive development. Be thorough, persistent, and considerate when filling them in. Talk to them individually about all aspects of his learning. Share the results of testing and interventions. Encourage a positive attitude by describing his strengths and talents. Likewise, when you describe situations that might confuse or frustrate him, give examples of approaches that work to ease the situation.

Healthcare providers (physicians, school nurses, social workers, psychological, occupational, and physical therapists, social skills facilitators): Everyone who helps safeguard your child's health should know how her learning disability might affect her well-being. Acquaint each provider with her history and any issues that specifically impact her care. For example, children with sensory processing disorders may benefit from the dentist knowing what triggers reactive behavior and what engenders trust. Children with attention deficit hyperactivity disorder (ADHD) may respond better when appointments are kept short. If your child has difficulty expressing herself, suggest ways for the professional to elicit substantive responses. And innocuous as it may seem, recognize that children with reading problems may be aggravated by all the publications cluttering the typical waiting room.

Random people (store clerks, service providers, bus drivers, airline seatmates): When you bring your child into a situation that might trigger impulsive or defensive behaviors, anticipate problems and intervene ahead of time. Explain to a sales associate that it's best not to bring out fifteen pairs of shoes at one time. Alert the bus driver to possible triggers for disruption or bullying. When someone interferes with your child's unobjectionable activities on a bus, train, or plane, explain in firm, positive tones that your child prefers listening to a book on tape while simultaneously reading the text. Be upbeat when you tell travel mates that walking up and down the aisle is actually a positive behavior.

Social acquaintances (peers, parents of peers, family friends): Most parents would not leave a child with impaired vision at a friend's home without explaining that some activities might be challenging. Yet parents of children with invisible disabilities often think that if they don't mention difficulties, none will be noticed. Nothing could be farther from the truth.

When children know that people in their social world accept the accommodations they need, they feel comfortable and productive. You can elicit trust and even respect for your child's uniqueness if you explain how he responds to stimuli. A child who has difficulty processing auditory information might need several reminders before following directions. Make sure that parents and friends don't misinterpret such behavior as oppositional. Explain that a child who fidgets might simply be seeking reinforcement to maintain alertness.

Family members: A child's learning disabilities will definitely cause ripples throughout the immediate and extended family, but proactive parents can minimize difficulty while maximizing potential.

In easy-to-understand language explain your child's learning and living profile to all family members. Never use learning disabilities as an excuse for your child to avoid homework, appropriate behavior, or chores done by other siblings. Instead, find ways that she can contribute at levels that correspond with others. More important, never expect other children to assume responsibility for the needs of their sibling with LD.

When explaining something that might be more difficult for your child with LD, also stress the skills and positive qualities she possesses. Make sure that all family members respect diversity.

Finally, support your child's interests, defend her against people and processes that undermine her self-esteem, and provide her with the tools to succeed academically and socially. Love her unconditionally, and never miss an opportunity to tell her and show her that you do.

Chapter 42

Bullying and Learning Disabilities: What Parents Need to Know

Students with learning disabilities and/or attention disorders are at a greater risk for being bullied or of becoming a bully. The purpose of this chapter is to help parents become aware of signs of bullying, to give some suggestions on how to work with the school system to create a safe environment for children, and to promote zero tolerance programs for bullying.

Every day in our nation's schools, children are threatened, teased, taunted, and tormented by schoolyard bullies. For some children, bullying is a fact of life that they are told to accept as a part of growing up. Those who fail to recognize and stop bullying practices as they occur actually promote violence, sending the message to children that might indeed makes right. Bullying often leads to greater and prolonged violence. Not only does it harm its intended victims, but it also negatively affects the climate of schools and the opportunities for all students to learn and achieve in school.

So begins the 11/3/1998 US Department of Education report, *Preventing Bullying—A Manual for Schools and Communities.*

Bullying can take different forms. Bullying can be physical, verbal, emotional, or sexual. The American Medical Association defines bullying as a pattern of repeated aggression; with deliberate intent to harm or disturb a victim despite apparent victim distress; and a real or perceived imbalance of power (e.g., due to age, strength, size), with the more powerful child or group attacking a physically or psychologically vulnerable victim.

Who Gets Bullied?

Although there are many characteristics or behaviors that might lead to a child becoming the target of a bully, the following represent a fairly comprehensive list:

- Kids who are different or perceived as different
- Students who are overweight, shorter, or taller than their peers
- Students whose interests differ markedly from those of their peers
- Those who are not good at or not interested in sports
- Special needs students or those with disabilities
- Students sexually stereotyped as effeminate or masculine
- Bright students who are perceived as nerdy

Evidence of Bullying

The warning signs of a child being bullied are many. Without intervention by a caring adult, there are often tragic results. Parents and school staff need to be aware of what to look for if they think a child has become the victim of a bully (Beane 1999):

- Frequent illness
- Sudden changes in behavior
- Anxiety, fearfulness, moodiness
- Reluctance to attend school
- Changes walking route to school
- Wants to change buses
- Possessions are often lost or damaged
- Needs extra money for lunch and supplies

- Talks about or attempts to run away
- Talks about or attempts suicide
- Carries or wants to carry protection such as a kitchen knife, a gun, or a box opener
- Has started bullying or is aggressive to other children and younger siblings

Victims of Bullying

There are two types of victims:

- Passive victims who appear as anxious, sensitive loners who give off victim signals, lack self-defense skills, don't think quickly on their feet, and have few friends to support them
- Provocative victims who are easily aroused, impulsive, kids that tease or taunt bullies, egg them on, and make themselves targets but can't defend themselves (Beane 1999)

Many children with learning disorders (LD) or attention deficit hyperactivity disorder (ADHD) fit into one of these two categories.

What Parents Can Do If Their Child Has Been Bullied

If you suspect that your child has been bullied, or has witnessed bullying at school, talk with your child and listen to his or her concerns. Listening gives your child a feeling of value. Let your child know it is not his or her fault and does not deserve to be treated in that manner. Tell your child that you will make sure he or she is protected and you will work with the school to get the issue resolved. Frequently children who witness bullying have the same reactions as the victim, feeling powerless and scared. They may also wonder if they will be the next victim.

Teach your child strategies and behaviors that will help to deal with bullies like avoiding the bully, spending more time with supportive friends, always being with a group, and learning how to verbally respond to the bullies. However, telling the bully to back off or stop should be done when surrounded by friends, as there is strength and safety in numbers. Role-playing with the child can help him or her remember what to say and what to do. Some parents have found that participation in sports or martial arts classes have helped children build self-esteem, confidence, and the ability to defend themselves. Reaffirm to your child that you will do all that is possible to ensure safety at school, on the way home from school, and in the neighborhood. Talk to your child's teacher, the school counselor or social worker, and principal and ask for their help. All schools should have written anti-bullying policies in place. Become familiar with those policies and the forms of discipline, both positive interventions and negative consequences, used to carry out those policies. This information should give you a clear understanding of how the school is going to help your child and how school personnel will work with the bully to put a stop to the behavior.

What Schools Are Doing to Stop Bullying

The harassment of students with disabilities became so obvious that in July 2000 a joint letter was issued from the Office of Civil Rights and the Office of Special Education and Rehabilitative Services, U.S. Department of Education. The letter was sent to principals in every school in United States to "develop greater awareness of the issue, to remind interested persons of the legal and educational responsibilities that institutions have to prevent and appropriately respond to disability harassment, and to suggest measures that school officials should take to address this very serious problem."

Research has shown that the school climate is directly attributable to the educational leadership in a school, whether the vision for that school has been forged by the principal, or by the principal acting in concert with the teaching staff (Weiss 1995). School administrators across the country have responded to the call for safe schools by promoting zero tolerance for bullying and violence and are upholding the practice of consistent enforcement of the anti-bullying rules. Some states require each school to have a detailed emergency response plan to situations that weren't even thought about ten years ago.

Schoolwide anti-bullying programs can be built into the curriculum and carried out on a daily basis. For example:

- posters featuring the importance of respecting differences and helping others can decorate the halls;
- in lower elementary school teachers can incorporate understanding and appreciation of differences and the importance of using kind words and treating each other with respect;
- in third and fourth grade learning how to be assertive; how to talk and how to say stop to someone who is being a bully;
- fifth-graders are at a good age to learn the art of mediating disagreements.

However, it is important to know that in the case of bullying, peer mediation tends not to be effective because of the power the bully holds over the child who is a victim.

Teachers are receiving training on how to handle bullying and the different forms of bullying, from mild teasing to constant harassing. Bullying behavior gives feelings of power and control to the bully by creating feelings of fear and intimidation in the victim. The best way to stop bullying is to have an adult quickly step into the situation, letting the bully know that behavior is not acceptable and will not be tolerated.

The school plan should contain the follow-up steps which might include reassuring the victim in private, talking to students who witnessed the incident, and reinforcing the importance of bringing an adult into the situation. One very important part of the plan is how the school staff is going to work with the bully and the bully's parents to change the behavior.

Ten years ago bullying was treated like a part of life, that if ignored would go away. Thanks to public concern and research on this topic, there is now a national awareness about bullying and the disastrous lifelong effects that this behavior can have on children who are bullied, and on those children who are bullies. This awareness has resulted in the development of many excellent anti-bullying programs that are now available to help community agencies, school systems, and families work together to get the message across that bullying is no longer considered to be a part of growing up.

References and Resources

American Medical Association, Report 1 of the Council on Scientific Affairs, 2002, www.ama-assn.org.

Beane, A. L., (1999). *The Bully Free Classroom*. Minneapolis, MN: Free Spirit Publishing, Inc.

Dwyer, K., Osher, D., and Warger, C. (1998). National Education Association, National Bullying Awareness Campaign, www.nea.org/school-safety/bullying.html.

The Public Schools Parent's Network: An Information Source and Resource Guide for Parents, www.paparents.net Article: Bullying in Public Schools, Date: 01, Feb, 2004. This website is an excellent resource for parents covering a variety of subject matters.

U.S. Department of Education. (2000, July 25). Letter on harassment based on disability. Washington, DC: Office of Civil Rights and Office of Special Education and Rehabilitative Services. The U.S. Department of

Education. A manual: *Early Warning, Timely Response: A Guide to Safe Schools,* to assist schools in the development of strategies and plans to deal with violence or threats of violence. The twenty-nine-page manual is available online at http://cecp.air.org/guide/guidetext.htm.

Weiss, C. H. (1995). The Four 'I's' of School Reform: how interests, ideology, information and institution affect teachers and principals. *Harvard Educational Review*, 65, 571–92.

Chapter 43

Social Skills: A Difficult Area for Many with Learning Disabilities

Chapter Contents

Section 43.1

Learning Difficulties and Social Skills: What's the Connection?

Most of us understand that kids who have learning difficulties struggle with academics. What many parents and educators don't realize is that having a learning problem can also impair a child's social skills and prevent him from having successful relationships with family members, peers, and other adults. The extent and impact on social skills varies with the child, depending on his basic temperament and the nature of his learning problem. Getting along with others is as important as getting along in school, so it's critical for kids with learning issues to develop good social skills (social competence).

What Is Social Competence?

Social competence refers to a person's interpersonal skills with family, friends, acquaintances, and authority figures, such as teachers and coaches. Here's how two noted learning experts describe social competence:

> Social competence refers to those skills necessary for effective interpersonal functioning. They include both verbal and nonverbal behaviors that are socially valued and are likely to elicit a positive response from others. —Betty Osman, Ph.D.

> Social skills are all the things that we should say and do when we interact with people. They are specific abilities that allow a person to perform competently at particular social tasks. —Michele Novatni, Ph.D.

How Do Learning Difficulties Affect Social Competence?

If a child has a learning problem, such as a language processing disorder, he may have difficulty understanding what another person says or means. He might also have trouble expressing his ideas in speech. Either of these problems can interfere with interpersonal communication.

A child who has attention deficit hyperactivity disorder (ADHD) may be inattentive, impulsive, hyperactive—or any combination of these. If he's inattentive, he may have a hard time paying close attention to other people's speech and behavior; his mind may wander, or his attention will be drawn to something else going on nearby. If he's impulsive and/or hyperactive, he may interrupt others when they're speaking and may find it difficult to wait his turn. While such a child doesn't behave this way on purpose, others will likely be frustrated or offended by his behavior.

The Three Elements of Social Interaction

Before you assess your own child's social skills, it's helpful to think of social interaction as consisting of three basic elements:

- **Social intake:** Noticing and understanding other people's speech, vocal inflection, body language, eye contact, and even cultural behaviors.

- **Internal process:** Interpreting what others communicate to you as well as recognizing and managing your own emotions and reactions.

- **Social output:** How a person communicates with and reacts to others, through speech, gestures, and body language.

Social Intake: Reading Social Cues

Social interactions require a child to interpret, or "read," what other people communicate. Picking up on spoken and unspoken cues is a complex process. A child with learning problems may misread the meaning or moods of others. Janet Giler, Ph.D., outlines three potential problem areas for such kids:

- Inability to read facial expressions or body language (kinesis)

- Misinterpreting the use and meaning of pitch (vocalics)

- Misunderstanding the use of personal space (proxemics)

471

If your child struggles with these issues, ask yourself if his particular learning difficulty could be causing the problem. Is he inattentive or easily distracted when dealing with others? Does he have a hard time grasping what other people say to him?

Internal Process: Making Sense of It All

Having read another person's social cues, a child must next process the information, extract meaning, and decide how to respond effectively. Thomas Brown, Ph.D., calls this ability "emotional intelligence," which, he explains, "is a form of social intelligence that involves the ability to monitor feelings and emotions in self and others; discriminate among feelings; and use this information to guide thinking and action."

If your child misses or misinterprets another person's words, meaning, or mood, he'll end up processing incorrect or incomplete information. This can lead him to inaccurate conclusions and inappropriate reactions. And if your child is impulsive, he may react before processing all the social cues and deciding on an appropriate response.

It's difficult to observe exactly how your own child processes social cues internally. But if you're concerned about how his internal "gears" process social data, you might gently probe by asking him how and why he decided to respond to someone in a particular manner.

Social Output: Responding to Others

After a child interprets and internalizes social cues from other people, he then responds. This behavior, social output, is easy to observe. But it can be painful or frustrating to watch if the child's response isn't appropriate.

Inappropriate responses can take many forms. If the child didn't understand a question or comment, his response may seem silly (such as nervous giggling) or unintelligent (an irrelevant answer). Another child may overreact with angry words or actions. Finally, if a child has really tuned out, he might not react at all, even when a response is required or expected from him. Understandably, such responses can cause problems and confusion with family members, friends, classmates, and teachers.

Teaching Social Skills: How Parents Can Help

If you realize your child's learning difficulty is hampering his social interactions, there are many ways you can guide him toward better social skills. Try practicing the three Rs: Provide social skills instruction that is relevant, deals with real-life, and is delivered in real-time. That means watching for teachable moments to coach your child in his interactions with others and doing so right away (or soon after). Focus on specific behaviors. Offer prompts before your child acts, and praise him for positive interactions. Additional suggestions:

- Model appropriate behavior when you interact with your child and other people.

- Encourage role-playing. Help your child rehearse his behavior in "pretend" situations. With your guidance, he can practice and improve specific social skills. He'll then be better prepared to apply those skills in real-life situations.

- Promote generalization. Help your child learn how and when to apply specific social skills to different situations. For example, once he learns to take turns playing a game with his sister, help him relate that to waiting his turn in line at the ice cream store.

Social Competence Builds Confidence

Kids with learning problems are at risk for low self-esteem. Helping them become socially competent can go a long way to bolster their self-confidence. Furthermore, a child with good social skills will have an easier time advocating for himself—whether he's asking a teacher for specific help or deflecting teasing from a classmate. We all face social situations around the clock—at home, at school, and in other settings. Helping your child overcome his social challenges is a gift he will benefit from throughout his life.

Section 43.2

Nurturing Social Competence in a Child with Learning Disabilities

"Nurturing Social Competence in a Child with Learning Disabilities," by Betty Osman, Ph.D. Reprinted with permission from www.GreatSchools.org. © GreatSchools, Inc. All rights reserved. Reviewed by David A. Cooke, M.D., FACP, February 2012.

Research has indicated that children with learning disabilities (LD) have more difficulty making and keeping friends than young people without these problems. Adolescents with LD have been shown to be less involved in recreational activities and to derive less satisfaction from their social interactions than their peers without LD. In this section, Betty Osman, Ph.D., discusses the nature of these social disabilities among children with LD, and what, if anything, can parents do to help their children and adolescents "fit in."

Learning to successfully interact with others is one of the most important aspects of a child's development, with far-reaching implications. Although most children acquire social skills by example, and possibly osmosis, research clearly suggests children with learning disabilities (LD) may have difficulty making and keeping friends. Adolescents with LD have also been shown to interact less with their peers and to spend more leisure time alone, addicted to TV, computer games, and the internet.

Parents devote much time and effort trying to impart the information and values they consider important. Yet, the development of children's social skills frequently is taken for granted. It goes without saying that it is painful for parents to see a child rejected by peers. In a sense, it becomes their rejection. Some parents relive their own unhappy social experiences as children, while others have expectations or dreams for their children that, not realized, become a source of disappointment and frustration.

Certainly not all young people with learning disabilities experience social problems. Typically, the good athlete, class comedian, resident artist, or owner of the most magic cards is likely to be accepted regardless of his learning issues. Then, too, some children, with or without LD, seem born to make life easy for parents—and for themselves as well. They appear to develop social awareness early in life and, as they grow, display innately good "people skills"—a sense of humor, a positive attitude toward life, and empathy for others, qualities guaranteed to win friends.

But for many children and adolescents with LD, the lack of peer acceptance can become the most painful of their problems. Computers and calculators can help children with writing and arithmetic, but there is no similar technology to help them handle a lonely recess at school, a family outing, or a date. These require social competence.

"Social competence" in this context refers to those skills necessary for effective interpersonal functioning. They include both verbal and nonverbal behaviors that are socially valued and are likely to elicit a positive response from others.

Lack of these behaviors, though, does not represent a simple or unilateral problem. Rather, social disabilities might be conceptualized as occurring on three levels:

- The first is a cognitive deficit, i.e., lack of knowledge of how to act in a given social situation—knowing not to shout out in church, or when it is appropriate to offer assistance to a stranger. Intervention on this level consists of teaching the requisite skill in much the same way as a new math concept or social studies lesson might be presented.

- The second might be referred to as a "performance deficit" and can be seen in children or adolescents who understand both appropriate behavior and what is expected, but their own needs interfere with their cognitions. Some children who understand the concept of fair play and know they shouldn't cheat, simply can't tolerate losing, so they cheat to make sure that they win. The children have the skills but are unable to apply them.

- Still others with social difficulties know how to act and can suppress their needs appropriately, but they lack the ability to evaluate their own or others' behavior. They don't understand the effect of their actions and, therefore, have no means of monitoring what they do or say. Each experience is a new one, with little transfer or generalization taking place. Anticipation and cause and effect are nonexistent.

In sum, young people with social disabilities frequently are less able than others their age to figure out how to behave in social situations and less aware of how others respond to them. Therefore, they act without knowledge or regard for social consequences. Most, though, tend to be unaware of their role, perceiving themselves as the victims of others' mistreatment. Therefore, they take little responsibility for their actions, blaming others or simply "bad luck" for events in their lives. What they do feel, though, is an overdose of criticism from peers and adults alike.

To help young people with social problems, it is important to understand on what level they are having trouble and how their social disabilities relate to their learning disabilities. The immaturity of many children with LD transcends academic areas, affecting their social adjustment as well. Communication skills, both verbal and nonverbal, also have social implications. Children who don't "read" body language and facial expressions well are likely to miss important signals in life that are apparent to others.

Parents cannot afford to ignore their children's social difficulties. The consequences are too great for the child and the family. I view the social domain, along with academic instruction, as within the realm of educational responsibility at home and at school. Education, after all, is not confined to the classroom but occurs in all aspects of life.

To help children and adolescents develop social skills and promote social acceptance, parents might consider these techniques:

- Listen to children with the "third ear," i.e., active listening, not only to the words they say but the feelings they are expressing.

- Initiate and practice pro-social skills at home, including:

  - how to initiate, maintain, and end a conversation;

  - the art of negotiation—how to get what you want appropriately;

  - how to be appropriately assertive without being overly aggressive;

  - how to give and receive compliments;

  - row to respond to teasing by peers.

- Practice how to accept constructive criticism.

If there is a social support group in your area, encourage your child to participate. Sharing concerns, problems, and social experiences can facilitate social skills and peer acceptance.

Although not all children and adolescents with learning disabilities incur social difficulties, those who do require special understanding, not only in terms of their current functioning but for the people they are capable of becoming. Although each young person is unique, all have the same needs—acceptance, approval, and a sense of belonging. To truly help them, we must go beyond the 3 Rs to include the 4th R—relationships.

Chapter 44

Self-Esteem Issues and Children with Learning Disabilities

Chapter Contents

Section 44.1

Self-Esteem Risks and Learning Disabilities

"Self-Esteem and Learning Disabilities," by Aoife Lyons, Ph.D. (www.draoifelyons.com), © 2004. All rights reserved. Reprinted with permission. Reviewed by David A. Cooke, M.D., FACP, February 2012.

There is much research that shows that children who have learning disabilities are at risk for having lower self-esteem and self-worth than that of their peers. From an early age, children compare themselves with others in areas such as academics, the ability to make and keep friends, and athletic prowess. For younger children the comparisons and subsequent self-judgment can be rather simplistic or "black and white."

Children with learning disabilities may judge themselves as "stupid," "slow," or "dumb," based on academic comparisons with other children. These self-judgments are often global in nature such that children who are having difficulty at school may perceive themselves negatively in all areas of their development.

Children who are diagnosed with learning disabilities have likely been having difficulty in school for many years before the actual diagnosis. Because the diagnosis of a learning disability is often based on a discrepancy between a child's academic competence and his or her measured IQ score, it is more difficult to diagnose children before first or second grade simply because expectations for academic achievement are not that high. Subsequently, children with learning disabilities may have endured many years of negatively comparing themselves to their peers and developing lowered self-esteem and self-worth before being formally diagnosed.

After a diagnosis is made, children and families need help understanding the diagnosis and label. For some children and families, the diagnosis can bring relief, as they now have a label to help explain the academic difficulties. For other children and families, the label may be stigmatizing and can lead to more negative appraisal of a child's abilities.

As professionals who work with children with learning disabilities, we have important roles in helping these children recognize both their areas of difficulty and their areas of strength. We also need to educate children and families about the nature of learning disabilities. Families need to hear that children with learning disabilities are bright; they just have a deficit in a particular area of learning. The message that learning-disabled children have average or even above-average IQ is one that bears repeating often, to children as well as families.

Learning-disabled children have often spent many years struggling in school and feeling "stupid." They have likely felt confused, discouraged, and hopeless as their efforts do not produce a desired result. Some learning-disabled children become immobilized by failure and develop "learned helplessness," and an attitude of "why bother when I always fail?" It is our job to help children undo these negative self-evaluations and see themselves in a realistic light.

Learning-disabled children often need support around assimilating both positive and negative characteristics in to their self-image. While much time is spent helping learning-disabled children master academic skills, we should also be working on improving self-esteem through recognition and appreciation of their areas of strength.

Some ideas for parents, educators, and others who work with LD children: Help the child feel special and appreciated. There is research that shows that the presence of at least one adult who makes a child feel special and appreciated leads to greater resilience and hopefulness in the child. Children feel special when their efforts are appreciated, when adults notice what makes them different in a positive light and when adults carve out special time to spend with the child.

Help the child with problem-solving and decision-making skills. Solid problem-solving skills have been linked to higher self-esteem. Instead of providing a child with the solution to his or her difficulty (whether academically, socially etc.), help the child brainstorm possible solutions and the possible consequences of different decisions. Avoid judgmental comments and praise the effort children put into their work. Often children with learning disabilities are putting effort into their work but still struggle. Help the child around finding new strategies for learning that will help him or her feel more successful. Be empathic around the child's special learning needs and his or her level of frustration when learning. Don't compare learning-disabled children with peers or siblings. Highlight a child's strengths in non-academic areas, whether in music, art, athletics, etc., or highlight the strengths of his or her personality (kindness, tenacity, helpfulness, sense of humor, etc.). Provide opportunities for a child to help.

Helping others helps a child show that they have something to offer his or her family and community. Children often enjoy participating in volunteer activities with their friends and family. Helping others bolsters self-esteem. Have realistic expectations. If we have realistic expectations about a child's performance it will help the child develop a sense of control. By working together, professionals and parents should help the learning -disabled child overcome both academic difficulties and the subsequent self-esteem difficulties that often arise. If we can appreciate the learning-disabled child in a holistic manner, the child should also learn to appreciate his or her own unique strengths.

Section 44.2

Tips for Developing Healthy Self-Esteem in Your Child

"Developing Your Child's Self-Esteem," November 2008, reprinted with permission from www.kidshealth.org. Copyright © 2008 The Nemours Foundation. This information was provided by KidsHealth, one of the largest resources online for medically reviewed health information written for parents, kids, and teens. For more articles like this one, visit www.KidsHealth. org, or www.TeensHealth.org.

Healthy self-esteem is a child's armor against the challenges of the world. Kids who feel good about themselves seem to have an easier time handling conflicts and resisting negative pressures. They tend to smile more readily and enjoy life. These kids are realistic and generally optimistic.

In contrast, kids with low self-esteem can find challenges to be sources of major anxiety and frustration. Those who think poorly of themselves have a hard time finding solutions to problems. If given to self-critical thoughts such as "I'm no good" or "I can't do anything right," they may become passive, withdrawn, or depressed. Faced with a new challenge, their immediate response is "I can't."

Here's how you can play important role in promoting healthy self-esteem in your child.

What Is Self-Esteem?

Self-esteem is the collection of beliefs or feelings we have about ourselves, our "self-perceptions." How we define ourselves influences our motivations, attitudes, and behaviors and affects our emotional adjustment.

Patterns of self-esteem start very early in life. For example, a toddler who reaches a milestone experiences a sense of accomplishment that bolsters self-esteem. Learning to roll over after dozens of unsuccessful attempts teaches a baby a "can-do" attitude.

The concept of success following persistence starts early. As kids try, fail, try again, fail again, and then finally succeed, they develop ideas about their own capabilities. At the same time, they're creating a self-concept based on interactions with other people. This is why parental involvement is key to helping kids form accurate, healthy self-perceptions.

Self-esteem also can be defined as feelings of capability combined with feelings of being loved. A child who is happy with an achievement but does not feel loved may eventually experience low self-esteem. Likewise, a child who feels loved but is hesitant about his or her own abilities can also end up with low self-esteem. Healthy self-esteem comes when the right balance is reached.

Signs of Unhealthy and Healthy Self-Esteem

Self-esteem fluctuates as kids grow. It's frequently changed and fine-tuned, because it is affected by a child's experiences and new perceptions. So it helps to be aware of the signs of both healthy and unhealthy self-esteem.

Kids with low self-esteem may not want to try new things, and may frequently speak negatively about themselves: "I'm stupid," "I'll never learn how to do this," or "What's the point? Nobody cares about me anyway." They may exhibit a low tolerance for frustration, giving up easily or waiting for somebody else to take over. They tend to be overly critical of and easily disappointed in themselves. Kids with low self-esteem see temporary setbacks as permanent, intolerable conditions, and a sense of pessimism predominates.

Kids with healthy self-esteem tend to enjoy interacting with others. They're comfortable in social settings and enjoy group activities as well as independent pursuits. When challenges arise, they can work toward finding solutions and voice discontent without belittling themselves or others. For example, rather than saying, "I'm an idiot," a child with healthy self-esteem says, "I don't understand this." They know their strengths and weaknesses, and accept them. A sense of optimism prevails.

How Parents Can Help

How can a parent help to foster healthy self-esteem in a child? These tips can make a big difference:

- **Watch what you say:** Kids are very sensitive to parents' words. Remember to praise your child not only for a job well done, but also for effort. But be truthful. For example, if your child doesn't make the soccer team, avoid saying something like, "Well, next time you'll work harder and make it." Instead, try "Well, you didn't make the team, but I'm really proud of the effort you put into it." Reward effort and completion instead of outcome.

- **Be a positive role model:** If you're excessively harsh on yourself, pessimistic, or unrealistic about your abilities and limitations, your child may eventually mirror you. Nurture your own self-esteem, and your child will have a great role model.

- **Identify and redirect your child's inaccurate beliefs:** It's important for parents to identify kids' irrational beliefs about themselves, whether they're about perfection, attractiveness, ability, or anything else. Helping kids set more accurate standards and be more realistic in evaluating themselves will help them have a healthy self-concept. Inaccurate perceptions of self can take root and become reality to kids. For example, a child who does very well in school but struggles with math may say, "I can't do math. I'm a bad student." Not only is this a false generalization, it's also a belief that will set the child up for failure. Encourage kids to see a situation in its true light. A helpful response might be: "You are a good student. You do great in school. Math is just a subject that you need to spend more time on. We'll work on it together."

- **Be spontaneous and affectionate:** Your love will go a long way to boost your child's self-esteem. Give hugs and tell kids you're proud of them. Pop a note in your child's lunchbox that reads, "I think you're terrific!" Give praise frequently and honestly, without overdoing it. Kids can tell whether something comes from the heart.

- **Give positive, accurate feedback:** Comments like "You always work yourself up into such a frenzy!" will make kids feel like they have no control over their outbursts. A better statement is, "You were really mad at your brother. But I appreciate that you didn't yell at him or hit him." This acknowledges a child's feelings, rewards the choice made, and encourages the child to make the right choice again next time.

- **Create a safe, loving home environment:** Kids who don't feel safe or are abused at home will suffer immensely from low self-esteem. A child who is exposed to parents who fight and argue repeatedly may become depressed and withdrawn. Also watch for signs of abuse by others, problems in school, trouble with peers, and other factors that may affect kids' self-esteem. Deal with these issues sensitively but swiftly. And always remember to respect your kids.

- **Help kids become involved in constructive experiences:** Activities that encourage cooperation rather than competition are especially helpful in fostering self-esteem. For example, mentoring programs in which an older child helps a younger one learn to read can do wonders for both kids.

Finding Professional Help

If you suspect your child has low self-esteem, consider professional help. Family and child counselors can work to uncover underlying issues that prevent a child from feeling good about himself or herself.

Therapy can help kids learn to view themselves and the world positively. When kids see themselves in a more realistic light, they can accept who they truly are.

With a little help, every child can develop healthy self-esteem for a happier, more fulfilling life.

Chapter 45

Coping Skills for Teens and Young Adults with Learning Disabilities

Chapter Contents

Section 45.1

Grocery Shopping and Meal Preparation

"Tablespoons and Teaspoons: Teaching Teens with LD the Art of Meal Preparation," by Arlyn Roffman, Ph.D. Reprinted with permission from www.GreatSchools.org. © GreatSchools, Inc. All rights reserved. This document can be found online at http://www.greatschools.org/special-eduction/ health/926-tablespoons-and-teaspoons-teaching-teens-with-ld-the-art-of -meal-preparation.gs?page=all; accessed May 14, 2011.

The multi-step process of planning and preparing a meal is a daunting prospect for many young adults. For individuals with learning disabilities (LD) and/or attention deficit hyperactivity disorder (ADHD), even organizing a trip to the grocery store can be trying, as it requires putting together a grocery list, locating house and/or car keys, and finding one's checkbook, debit card, or enough cash to pay for purchases.

This section will explain how the characteristics of LD and ADHD may present challenges for kids who are learning to plan and prepare meals. I will also offer strategies for teaching your child the various skills involved in meal preparation, from planning a menu through kitchen cleanup.

Meal Planning

Some people enjoy planning a meal; others find it a chore. The process of planning a balanced and tasty meal requires imagination, a basic understanding of nutrition, a sense of whether the meal being planned is within the limits of one's budget, and the ability to obtain the necessary ingredients.

Table 45.1 illustrates some of the ways various characteristics of LD and ADHD can result in challenges to meal planning.

Grocery Shopping

The chaotic environment of a grocery store can be overwhelming, and working one's way through the aisles and the checkout line can be very stressful. The process of shopping for food is complicated by specific deficits associated with LD and ADHD.

Table 45.1. Meal Planning Challenges

Learning or Attention Problem	Challenges When Planning a Meal
Reading	Trouble reading through cookbooks for recipes
Receptive language (understanding written or spoken language)	Problems understanding common meal planning terms, such as "appetizer" or "main course"
Math	Trouble adjusting recipe ingredients to suit the number of people to be served (e.g., "doubling" a recipe)
Writing	Problems making a list of items to be purchased for the meal
Distractibility	Difficulty staying focused during the meal-planning process (e.g., while making up a shopping list of groceries needed to prepare the meal)

Table 45.2 illustrates how various types of learning and attention problems can result in challenges at the grocery store.

Table 45.2. Grocery Shopping Challenges

Learning or Attention Problem	Challenges When Shopping
Reading	Trouble deciphering aisle signs and food labels
Math	Difficulty understanding unit pricing, calculating the cost of sale items, and tracking the accumulating costs as items are selected and placed in the shopping cart
Visual memory	Remembering the layout of the store and which aisle to go to for certain items
Visual figure-ground discrimination (trouble focusing one's vision on a single item within a "busy" visual background)	Trouble finding a specific brand of bread or cereal among the dozens of choices on the shelves
Distractibility	Trouble staying focused and on task while shopping
Impulsivity	Difficulty controlling "impulse buying" of items that are not on the shopping list

Meal Preparation

Once food is purchased, it must be prepared. Cooking presents a number of challenges to individuals with LD and/or ADHD, as outlined in Table 45.3.

Table 45.3. Meal Preparation Challenges

Learning or Attention Problem	Challenges When Preparing Meals
Executive function (organizing, prioritizing)	Difficulty planning the preparation of several different items so they can all be served at the appropriate time during the meal
Receptive language (understanding written or spoken language)	Problems understanding common cooking terms, such as "sauté" or "dice"
Reading	Difficulty decoding (reading the words in) recipes
Math	Trouble measuring ingredients
Visual discrimination	Problems telling the difference between look-alikes (e.g., a teaspoon and a tablespoon)
Fine-motor coordination (ability to use one's hands and fingers effectively)	Difficulty peeling, slicing, and chopping
Temporal perception (sense of time)	Trouble planning enough time for various parts of a meal to cook, resulting in burnt or undercooked food
Distractibility	Difficulty maintaining focus and following all of the steps involved in preparing a meal

Serving and Cleaning up after a Meal

Serving a meal—and cleaning up afterward—requires coordination. It entails choosing appropriate serving dishes and utensils, providing any necessary condiments, and socializing during the meal. Once the meal is over, the dishes must be cleared and washed, any leftovers safely stored, and the table and kitchen cleaned up.

LD and ADHD can present challenges in these aspects of meal preparation, as described in Table 45.4.

Table 45.4. Serving and Cleanup Challenges

Learning or Attention Problem	Challenges in Serving a Meal and Cleaning Up
Executive function (organizing, prioritizing)	Difficulty deciding the order in which food should be served
Spatial perception	Trouble choosing appropriate serving dishes for the quantity/type of food prepared; difficulty washing dishes and pans thoroughly and wiping down the counters and table
Social skills	Difficulty demonstrating good table manners and conversation skills during the meal

Tips for Teaching Your Teen Meal Preparation Skills

Meal preparation can be introduced very early, with children as young as toddlers getting involved in baking and making simple sandwiches. As your child with LD or ADHD matures, you should gradually involve him more in the food preparation process.

As you practice the following strategies, keep in mind that it is very helpful for children to hear "think alouds" from adults, as they reveal their thought process. While teaching your child to plan and prepare meals, try to model your decision making by actually saying what you're thinking as you make your choices. For example, you might explain, "We're having company to dinner, so I'll buy the big box of rice instead of the small one that we usually buy just for the three of us." Thinking aloud about each step of the meal planning and preparation process will help your child learn steps that might seem obvious to you.

Here are strategies for teaching meal planning and preparation skills during your child's middle and high school years.

At the Grocery Store

- Point out the categories of foods and household items and the layout of the aisles. Note, for example, that all the breads are grouped and that spaghetti and sauce and other food items that tend to be used together are placed in close proximity. As your child catches on, take the next step and ask him to help you locate items throughout the store.

- Explain unit pricing and how you make decisions about purchases with unit prices in mind (e.g., "The big box is cheapest, but we rarely eat this, and it'll just get stale, so I'll spend a little more per unit and buy the smaller size.").

- Have your teen use a calculator to track the accumulating cost of the food being placed in the cart. Explain that particularly for those shopping within a budget, tracking purchases when shopping is a very helpful habit.

- Point out the differences among the various checkout lines. Explain when it is appropriate to use the express lane versus and the regular line.

- Explain how to use coupons and store membership or discount cards to save money.

In the Kitchen

- Ask your child to be your cooking assistant. Give him increasing responsibility for unwrapping, slicing, and measuring as he grows old enough to tackle these aspects of the process. Read through recipes together and explain cooking terms (e.g., "chop" versus "slice") as they are introduced in recipes.

- Teach your child how to use kitchen knives safely. Supervise as he practices slicing and chopping until he's comfortable handling and using knives for various food preparation techniques.

- Show your child how to use the appliances needed for basic cooking. Introduce one appliance at a time (e.g., oven, stovetop, microwave oven) and let him practice using it until he can do so safely and comfortably, without your coaching. If he has difficulty remembering the steps involved in using an appliance, write them neatly in a notebook or on a Post-it note near the appliance for him to refer to as long as he needs the extra support.

- Use cookbooks with photographs and step-by-step diagrams. Novice cooks with LD and/or ADHD benefit from step-by-step diagrams that show how a recipe should be prepared as well as photographs that show how the recipes they are preparing will look when they are completed.

- Color-code measuring spoons and cups. Marking the quarter teaspoon and quarter cup with red, the half teaspoon and half cup with blue, etc. provides an additional visual clue to help differentiate similar-looking items while cooking.

- Model with think-alouds as you cook, walking your child through the process of planning the timing of different parts of the meal. Be sure to mention any ancillary needs (e.g., "Since we're having burgers, we'll need ketchup and mustard too."). Planning ahead exactly when each part should be prepared and cooked and creating a chart that outlines the entire process eliminates the need for on-the-spot decision making, which can be very stressful for any new cook, particularly those with LD and/or ADHD.

- Give guidelines for storing leftover food. Discuss how long foods can safely be stored in the refrigerator and how to properly store leftovers in aluminum foil, plastic wrap, or food containers. Demonstrate how to label and date leftovers to be refrigerated. As foods go bad, show your child how they look and smell before you throw them out.

- By the time your teen is nearing completion of high school, you might assign him to cook one meal per week for the family. Many teens find it helpful to verbally walk through the full meal planning process beforehand with a parent and make lists of all steps, from shopping to cooking to setting the table to cleaning up. The need for your supervision will taper off as he becomes more experienced and comfortable in the kitchen.

- Collect your child's favorite recipes in a file box to take along when he moves out on his own!

Recipe for Success in the Kitchen

Planning and preparing a meal is a complex process that requires a broad range of skills. Your teen with LD and/or ADHD will benefit from explicit instruction in each step of the process as he develops the skills and confidence to tackle this crucial aspect of daily living.

Section 45.2

Money Management

"Dollars and Sense: Financial Skills for Teens with Learning Disabilities" by Arlyn Roffman, Ph.D. Reprinted with permission from GreatSchools.org. © GreatSchools, Inc. All rights reserved. This document can be found online at http://www.greatschools.org/special-eduction/health/928-financial-skills -for-teens.gs?page=all; accessed May 14, 2011.

Becoming a responsible consumer is essential for adjusting to adult life, yet many adults with learning disabilities (LD) rank handling money and banking as the most difficult among the problems they encounter. Problems in this area are often tied to specific characteristics of LD or attention deficit hyperactivity disorder (ADHD). This section describes common pitfalls and offers parents strategies for providing teens with LD or ADHD a foundation of money management know-how necessary for independent living.

Table 45.5 illustrates some of the ways various characteristics of LD and ADHD can result in financial challenges.

Table 45.5. Money Management Challenges for Those with LD and ADHD

Learning or Attention Problem	Challenges When Managing Money
Impulsivity	Problems with impulse buying beyond the limit of one's budget
Memory problems	Difficulty remembering to record bank transactions (for example, automated teller machine [ATM] cash withdrawals)
Temporal problems	Issues with remembering to pay bills on time
Organizational problems	Difficulty gathering all the items (monthly statement, check register, calculator, etc.) necessary to balance one's checkbook
Distractibility	Trouble maintaining concentration during the process of reviewing one's checking account
Visual discrimination	Tendency to make errors in calculation due to number inversions (for example, writing "61" or "19" instead of "16")
Spatial issues	Tendency to misalign numbers in the check register columns, leading to computation errors
Visual figure-ground problems (focusing on one image against a busy background)	Problems focusing on individual lines of the monthly bank statement
Reading	Trouble reading store signs (or price tags), notices from the bank, and contracts (for instance, for membership to a gym)
Spelling	Difficulty spelling numbers correctly when writing out checks
Math	Problems performing mental math (estimating how much an item on sale at 25 percent off will cost, for instance, or knowing how much change to expect when making purchases); difficulty performing calculations involved in reconciling a checking account

Teaching Your Teen Financial Skills

Money management skills can be introduced very early, with children in the lower elementary school grades learning the value of the coins and currency they save in their piggybanks and having your guidance when deciding how to spend their savings. As your child with LD or ADHD matures, you should gradually introduce more complex skills, such as budgeting and managing a checking account.

Here are some strategies for teaching consumer skills and money management during your child's middle and high school years.

Consumer Skills

- Orient your child to a variety of types of stores, such as the drug-store, grocery store, and department store. In each store, note the layout and the groupings of items. Point out the aisle signs and conduct "think alouds" as you shop (for example, "We need some Band-Aids, so I'm going to the aisle that says first aid. If I can't find them there, I can ask the clerk at the cash register where they are.") By middle school your child should be able to find items she commonly uses (school supplies, hair products, etc). By the end of high school, she should be able to shop on her own at any of these stores for basic items.

- Help your child learn the sizes of the shoes and clothing she wears. Too many parents of middle and even high school students with LD and ADHD continue to choose their children's clothing well beyond the point when this type of control is appropriate. By middle school, your child should be able to choose her own clothing, within guidelines you have set. This is one way you can foster the self-determination necessary for successful adjustment to adult life.

- Discuss tipping with your teen. List the kinds of people she might tip (waiters, bellhops, etc.) and how to determine the tip for each person based on the quality of service and the going rate. When you dine out together, have your teen calculate the tip using a tip chart (available in most stationery stores).

- Counsel her about credit cards. Explain how credit cards work as well as the associated dangers of using them. When your teen reaches age eighteen, numerous banks will start sending her invitations to apply for credit cards. Choose one reputable bank, and have her apply for a card with a credit limit of $500 or less. Discuss with her what may be charged, and walk her through the process of paying the monthly bills—preferably in full to avoid paying interest while still establishing her credit history.

- Teach your teen about basic contracts, such as rental leases, gym memberships, cell phone agreements, and internet service contracts. Warn her about high-pressure sales tactics that offer a special price "only if you sign up today."

Money Management

- Establish a basic budget early in the teen years. Have your teen list all of her anticipated expenses, including school lunches, entertainment, clothing, and miscellaneous items (for example, compact discs [CDs] or snacks) and establish a weekly budget to manage her allowance and earnings from any jobs she may have.

- Encourage her to use a "budget envelopes" book, an inexpensive and handy tool, available in most stationery stores, which has separate envelopes for each specific budget category. She should place enough cash for her various budget categories in each envelope at the beginning of every week and make a commitment to spend the allotted funds only for the stated purposes. This is a very concrete way to develop the concept of budgeting and is a highly recommended first step in the process of learning how to manage money.

- Toward the end of high school, teens need to learn how to manage a checkbook and pay bills. Opening her own checking account is the best vehicle for learning this skill. Many youths with LD or ADHD prefer carbon checks, which help ensure that transactions are recorded. After teaching your teen how to write a check, slip an example of a completed check into her checkbook to remind her of how it's done. Provide a crib sheet with correctly spelled numbers to be kept in her checkbook for easy reference when writing checks.

- Help your teen set up a home office at a desk table where she can keep all the items needed for successful money management and bill paying, including: supplies (paper, pens and pencils, tape, a ruler, paper clips, a stapler, stamps, and a calculator); an accordion file, where important papers may be filed under separate headings, such as "bank statements" or "unpaid bills"; a budget book to record expenditures and realistically estimate future expenses; a calendar, which can be used to note the receipt of monthly bills and to record when each is due (Posthill and Roffman, 1991).

The Role of Technology in Managing Money

Teens who are comfortable with technology may find budgeting software like Quicken and online banking services helpful in managing their money. If your teen has access to her checking and savings accounts online, she can check her transactions and balance—and transfer money between accounts—without having to wait for the monthly statement to arrive by mail.

Building a Foundation for Your Teen's Financial Future

Parents who make a point of teaching their teens with LD or ADHD consumer skills and money management skills will help them avoid many of the problems that surface for adults in this population. When your teen prepares to leave home after high school, assure her that you will continue to be available for support and advice as she puts her new money management skills to practice.

References

Posthill, S. and Roffman, A. (1991). The impact of a transitional training program for young adults with learning disabilities. *Journal of Learning Disabilities*, 24(3), 619–29.

Roffman, A. Herzog, J. and Wershba, P. (1994). Helping young adults understand their learning disabilities. *Journal of Learning Disabilities*, 27 (7), 413–14.

Section 45.3

Travel and Transportation

"On the Right Track: Teaching Your Teen with LD to Manage Travel and Transportation," by Arlyn Roffman, Ph.D. Reprinted with permission from www .GreatSchools.org. © GreatSchools, Inc. All rights reserved. This document can be found online at http://www.greatschools.org/special-education/health/929-ld -manage-travel-and-transportation.gs?page=all; accessed June 20, 2011

People with learning disabilities (LD) and/or Attention Deficit Hyperactivity Disorder (ADHD) often have difficulty getting from one location to another. They frequently lose their way, have trouble using public transportation, and struggle with driving-related issues. Contributing factors may include poor time management, problems with spatial and visual perception, and difficulties with eye-hand coordination. Diane Swonk, a successful economist who has dyslexia, admits, "Every time I get off the elevator in the place that I've worked for seventeen years, I'm still lost. I still can't get on the right train going home from work unless I try really hard. Going from Point A to Point B is just not easy for me."

This section will explain many of the challenges individuals with LD and ADHD face in travel and transportation. It will offer a variety of strategies for teaching your teenager how to get around effectively, which will further prepare him to function independently as a young adult.

Table 45.6 illustrates how various characteristics of LD and ADHD can result in challenges to getting around.

Driving Presents Special Challenges

As I explain in my book, *Meeting the Challenge of Learning Disabilities in Adulthood*, driving presents its own set of challenges:

With all of its complexities, driving can be of particular concern to individuals with LD and AD/HD. Difficulties vary and can develop for a multitude of reasons. For example, people may find it difficult to train their right foot to recognize the difference between the accelerator and the brake and, on standard [manual] transmission vehicles, to train their left foot to simultaneously work the clutch. They may find it challenging to develop a working understanding of the reactivity of the steering wheel, which must turn only so much to pass another car but must turn even more when it is time to round a corner. They may struggle to interpret what they are seeing in the rearview mirror. On cars with manual [standard] transmission, they may have difficulty moving from one gear to another, particularly to reverse, which generally requires an additional thrust. Further, they may have considerable difficulty learning how to parallel park. Indeed, many find it difficult to meld the many separate aspects of car handling into one coordinated driving experience. (Roffman, 2000, p. 191)

Table 45.6. Travel and Transportation Challenges

Learning or Attention Problem	Challenges in Travel and Transportation
Reading	Difficulty reading road signs
Temporal perception (sense of time)	Problems planning enough time to get where one wants to go
Attention	Tendency to get sidetracked on the way to a destination
Spatial perception	Tendency to become disoriented easily; have trouble following maps; have problems navigating around new, unfamiliar areas
Directionality	Difficulty distinguishing east from west and right from left and a subsequent tendency to follow directions inaccurately
Depth perception	Problems gauging how fast cars are coming, when crossing a street as a pedestrian or when driving through an intersection
Receptive language	Difficulty understanding spoken directions
Auditory processing	Difficulty following the steps or sequence of spoken directions
Auditory figure-ground (focusing on one sound against a noisy background)	Problems "tuning in" to messages delivered over public address systems in noisy bus depots, train stations, and airports
Visual memory	Trouble remembering landmarks along a familiar route
Visual figure-ground (focusing on one object in a crowded visual field)	Difficulty reading maps; problems reading departure and arrival boards at airports, train stations, and bus depots; trouble finding one's car in a large parking lot or one's suitcase on an airport baggage carousel

Tips for Teaching Your Teen to Manage Travel and Transportation

The following strategies may be used during your child's middle and high school years to help him learn to get around safely and on track.

Planning Your Trip

- Practice reading maps with your child. Start by discussing simple routes; gradually make the hypothetical journey more complex. Teach him how to use online mapping tools, such as Mapquest.com, which offer written directions as well as maps between any two addresses. When he understands how to read a map, have him plan a short trip or two, first with your supervision and then on his own.

- Teach your teen how to read transportation schedules. If you live in a town with a local bus route, review the schedule together, pointing out the departure and arrival columns, the weekday versus weekend schedules, and any other pertinent information. If there's a map of the route, suggest marking the way from one location to another with a colored marker. Ask him travel-related questions until it's clear that he understands how to use the schedule. Send him on a short trip that requires him to practice both his ability to read transit schedules as well as his newly acquired map-reading skills.

- Discuss how to estimate the travel time between two places. Many factors can cause delays, including traffic jams and mass transit problems. For important appointments, such as job interviews, encourage him to take a "dry run," to travel there beforehand in order to gauge how much travel time to set aside on the actual day. Suggest that he build in at least a ten-minute cushion of time for unexpected travel delays.

- Teach strategies that will help your child avoid getting lost. Many people who are prone to disorientation in new places write down simple directions (e.g., how to get from the front door of the medical building to his doctor's office or, when traveling, how to go from the elevator to the family's hotel room). Use a "think-aloud" to demonstrate taking note of where you've left the car when you go to a crowded parking lot (e.g., "Okay, we're in row 19, right in line with the main entrance to the mall").

- If your teen carries a cell phone, help him program frequently called phone numbers (e.g., parents, friends, emergency roadside assistance) into his phone's directory. If he finds himself lost or in an emergency situation, he may be nervous, so being able to call for assistance at the touch of a button will be a tremendous help.

On the Way to Your Destination

- Explain how to read Departure and Arrival boards in train stations and airports. By the time your child is in upper elementary school, you can teach lessons during your family trips, talking through the steps of traveling from door to door. For example, you might explain, "Now that we're at this busy airport, we're going to hold on tight to our bags and wallets. The first step is to check in. We're flying on X Airlines. You tell me where the check-in counters are for our airline." Talk your way through checking the Departure board for your gate, going through security, etc. Point out who your resources are (e.g., employees behind the counters, people in airline uniforms). If you don't travel regularly, take your teen on a "field trip" to the airport.

- Model tying a colorful item to the handle of your suitcase when you check your baggage on family trips, and explain that practicing this strategy will make it easy for him to spot his own luggage in the baggage claim area when he travels on his own.

- Discuss the importance of identifying appropriate resources in certain situations. "Think alouds" will help him understand your thought process. For example, you might say, "Okay, we aren't sure where the train station is. There's a policeman; I'll ask him if we're headed in the right direction." Explain to your teen that we all get lost or disoriented at times, and that asking for help is a sign of resourcefulness rather than weakness. If he has memory problems, suggest that he repeat the directions back or, better yet, carry a notepad and pen so he can write down the directions he hears.

- Review safe pedestrian habits, particularly if your child has a problem with depth perception and may not be able to judge the speed of oncoming vehicles. Remind him that it's safest to use crosswalks and obey traffic signals to get from one side of a street to the other.

Special Advice for Drivers

- If your child would like to learn to drive but you're afraid that he might not be able to master the necessary skills due to the

499

severity of his LD or ADHD, contact a large hospital rehabilitation center in your area for an assessment. By using simulators to test his reaction time, depth perception, and other related skills, professionals there can determine whether the disability is severe enough to prohibit him from getting his license. If he is found to have the potential to become a safe driver but in need of extra support as he learns, the rehabilitation center should be able to recommend a local driving school attuned to the needs of those who would benefit from special instruction due to disabilities.

- If your teen does get a driver's license, teach him that there are both low-tech and high-tech ways to avoid problems. One high-tech item, a geographical positioning system (GPS), can help him avoid getting lost while on the road. A colorful cloth tied to the car's radio antenna is a low-tech aide that can help him locate a parked car.

- Explain the importance of concentrating fully on driving at all times. Talking on cell phones or changing compact discs (CDs) while driving are dangerous risks and illegal activities in an increasing number of states. Model safe behavior by pulling over when you need to talk on your cell phone or when you want to find a particular CD.

- Keeping a directions file in the car is very useful, particularly if directions both to and from the destination are explicitly spelled out. A folder of directions can be stored in the glove compartment.

On the Road to Independence

Perhaps no one activity more clearly represents independence than being able to travel around on one's own. Although there are many complex skills involved in travel and transportation, most teens with learning disabilities and ADHD are able to learn them if they're given explicit training and support.

Section 45.4

Learning to Drive

"Teaching Kids with LD to Drive: A Complex Family Matter," by Melinda Sacks. Reprinted with permission from www.GreatSchools.org. © GreatSchools, Inc. All rights reserved. This document can be found online at http://www.great schools.org/special-education/support/892-teaching-kids-with-ld-to-drive-a -complex-family-matter.gs?page=all; accessed August 3, 2011.

All parents worry when their children reach driving age and blurt out the inevitable question, "When can I get my license?"

But for those of us whose children are distractible, hyperactive, impulsive, or learning disabled (LD), the question is much more complex. Not only is it worrisome to think of the impact of these qualities on mastering the driver's education manual on the rules of the road, and the written test covering copious material that must be memorized, but the idea of a new driver with any sort of disability that impacts concentration taking to the road in a two-ton vehicle can be downright frightening.

This spring, we joined the ranks of concerned parents as our son Alex turned sixteen and announced he wanted to learn to drive. As a fan of racing video games, and the owner of a life-sized steering wheel and gas pedal that attach to our home computer, our son figured he was ready to go. After all, he asked, how much harder could real driving be than his favorite game, "Crazy Taxi"? (The game's name says a lot about our fears.)

For the months preceding Alex's sixteenth birthday we circumvented the question of driving by telling him he had to make the call to sign himself up for driver's education at the local driving school. For whatever reason, he never seemed to get around to it. And we were secretly relieved.

But now that it's summer and his friends are taking driving classes, we can no longer dodge the issue.

Driver's Education Isn't Easy for Teens with LD

While most kids find the driver's education course to be long (six hours a day for four days in California), most don't consider it particularly difficult. Not so for kids with LD, who, like Alex, may find the in-class reading and frequent tests a significant struggle. And peer pressure, performance anxiety, and the group setting is, for many, far from ideal.

Thankfully an increasing number of programs are offering online driver's education, which is a great solution if you have a child like ours who enjoys the computer, needs to take his time digesting material, and feels pressured and uncomfortable in big groups.

If you don't have a computer or don't want your child online, many of these programs offer printed booklets that contain the same content.

Beware, though, that the at-home course isn't always a complete solution. When I went online and searched for online driving schools, there were myriad choices but I had a hard time telling how they differed. Once I chose a course and registered Alex, he wanted to start right away. But within twenty minutes he had given up, discouraged by the first chapter, which was so text-heavy that he was exhausted after reading just a few pages of small print.

Shop Around Before Enrolling Your Teen in Driver's Ed

Before you embark on the driver's education road with your teen, be sure to check the requirements for the state where you live. Surprisingly, there is a fair amount of variation. Thirty-six states require teens to have a driving permit, twenty-three of them require the permit be held for at least six months before they can apply for a driver's license. Graduated licenses—those that allow a new driver incremental privileges to drive alone or carry passengers under age twenty-one—are increasingly common and also differ from one state to another. Even the age at which you can obtain a permit or driver's license differs across the country. Your local Department of Motor Vehicles can provide the specifics for where you live.

Driving schools also vary in approach and curriculum, although all are required to cover the same material in their final exams. Some courses, we found, are much more "friendly" to kids with LD, providing more interactive materials and experiences, including videos, computer simulations, and group work. Some contain just one final exam that encompasses the entire course curriculum, while others are broken into chapter tests.

You can also decide to conduct the driving lessons yourself, but we felt it was worth the cost to give Alex a professional introduction to driving.

Know Your Child and Stay Involved

As is true with many issues around parenting a child with LD, staying involved and applying what you know about your teen's strengths and weaknesses factor heavily into how you can help him learn to drive.

Knowing our son loves video games that glorify speeding, and in some cases, even crashing, we had long ago embarked on a heavy campaign to talk about driver safety. The fact that I had been in a serious car accident before I was married gave us plenty of ammunition for our discussions. On the road, we tried to point out mistakes other drivers made, and potential hazards such as kids on bikes, dogs near the road, and cars running red lights. Real driving, we said over and over, bears no resemblance to a video game.

We also repeatedly recited one line from Alex's driver education book describing driving a car: "Dangerous as a loaded gun if not operated properly."

Because Alex is such a weak reader, we were also concerned about how much he would digest from the home study driver's education booklet we chose. The 154-page soft cover book has fairly big print, which was a plus, but like all the home study books, it is quite text heavy.

Even though we knew it would take forever, we decided we would read the book aloud with Alex. Taking turns with the reading, then doing the chapter quizzes together, gave my husband and me a first-hand look at how well Alex understood the material. When he seemed to glaze over, we'd stop. We broke the lessons into small segments and did just a little at a time. We told stories about our own experiences as we read, hoping the real-life scenarios would help impress certain points upon him.

My brother, who has a dyslexic daughter, found that for her, an online course produced by www.penschool.com was ideal because there was no big final test, just small quizzes along the way. The thirty-day completion policy requiring students to complete the course within thirty days of when they started was great incentive for her to finish.

At our house I was in no hurry to put Alex behind the wheel, so the fact that there was no time limit and we could go at our own pace was a huge plus.

Getting Behind the Wheel . . . of a Golf Cart

No matter how long you stall, the day will come when your teen slides into the driver's seat and you give up control of the car. This is a day I was not looking forward to, so I was delighted when we happened upon an interim solution that eased the way.

It turns out that starting out in a golf cart is a great way to give a new driver the feeling of operating a moving vehicle with two pedals. It is a relief to introduce the challenges of negotiating parking spaces, tight turns, and oncoming traffic in a small, battery-powered vehicle that won't exceed five to ten miles an hour.

With Alex behind the wheel of the little electric golf cart we borrowed, we set off on paved paths that were mostly unpopulated for our practice.

At first, his driving was jerky, and my nonstop instructions punctuated every second of our short trips, leaving us both exhausted.

- "You're too close to the curb!"

- "Slow down!"

- "Watch out for that bump!"

- "Stay on your side of the road!"

- And, "Do you see that bicycle?"

But little by little, Alex learned to watch for obstacles, smoothed his acceleration and braking, figured out how to make a three-cornered turn, and even parallel parked. Thankfully it was all done at about five miles per hour.

It turns out that behind the wheel, Alex is far more conservative than I expected, and he is in fact overly concerned with kids, pedestrians, and other cars, often stopping to wait for them when they were far, far away.

"But You Didn't Make My Sister Wait!"

One problem we didn't anticipate was the sibling rivalry that occurred when Alex realized we were stalling letting him drive, something we had not done with his older sister (who does not have LD). No amount of explanation or justification seemed to satisfy him.

The only approach we could take was to be honest. We revisited our reasons for taking it slow, and offered to drive him anywhere he needed to go. He wasn't pleased when it involved outings such as going to the movies with a girl, but we pointed out numerous times that due to our graduated licensing laws, even if he had his license, he wouldn't be allowed to drive other teens for six months.

Practice, Practice, Practice

The fact that in our state parents are required by law to spend fifty hours with their teen driving was a plus for our family. We figured the more time Alex spent practicing driving in a very controlled situation, the better.

I decided long ago that teaching our kids to drive was my husband's job, since he tends to be unflappable, a word that does not describe me. And while many parents let their new driver get behind the wheel with the entire family in the car, we did not go this route with Alex. The less distraction and the fewer people around, the better, so he and his dad are going to be spending a lot of quality time together.

It is still unclear when, exactly, Alex will be ready to get his license. But we are determined that by the time he goes to take the test, we will be sure he will not be a hazard on the road—to others or to himself.

Some things just can't be hurried, and learning to drive is one of them.

Chapter 46

After High School: Learning Disabilities and the Law

Do the legal rights of students with learning disabilities continue after high school?

Legal rights may continue. It depends upon the facts in the individual case. Children with learning disabilities who receive services under the Individuals with Disabilities Education Act (IDEA) or the Rehabilitation Act of 1973 (Rehabilitation Act) in public elementary and secondary school may continue to have legal rights under federal laws in college programs and in employment. When students graduate from high school or reach age twenty-one, their rights under the IDEA come to an end.

The rights that may continue are those under the Rehabilitation Act and the Americans with Disabilities Act of 1990 (ADA). To understand which rights continue, it is important to understand the three basic federal statutes that confer rights on people with disabilities.

The IDEA, initially enacted in 1975, provides for special education and related services for children with disabilities who need such education and services by reason of their disabilities. The IDEA provides for a free appropriate public education (FAPE) and for an Individualized Education Program (IEP).

The Rehabilitation Act, most notably Section 504, prohibits discrimination against children and adults with disabilities. The Rehabilitation Act applies to public and private elementary and secondary schools and colleges that receive federal funding. It also applies to employers that receive federal funding.

The ADA prohibits discrimination against children and adults with disabilities and applies to all public and most private schools and colleges, to testing entities, and to licensing authorities, regardless of federal funding. Religiously controlled educational institutions are exempt from coverage. The ADA applies to private employers with fifteen or more employees and to state and local governments.

It may help to consider an example of how rights may continue over many years. Jeff has a reading disorder. For a long time he wanted to become a lawyer, and now he is in law school. He received special education and related services under the IDEA during public elementary school. He went to a small private religious high school and received accommodations under Section 504 of the Rehabilitation Act. He received extra test time on the Scholastic Aptitude Test (SAT), during college, on the law school admission test (LSAT), and in law school. Under the ADA, he will be entitled to extra test time on the Bar Examination.

Do all people with learning disabilities have legal rights under the Rehabilitation Act and ADA?

No. Many have legal rights, but some do not. Under the Rehabilitation Act and ADA, a disability is an impairment that substantially limits a major life activity, such as learning. Children and adults with learning disabilities, in many cases, have been found to have an impairment that substantially limits learning. That substantial limitation means that these individuals have a disability under the Rehabilitation Act and ADA and are protected under these laws.

Let's look at an example. Jim was diagnosed with a reading disorder and math disorder when he was six years old. He received special education under the IDEA for most of elementary school to assist with reading and math. By the time he entered high school, his reading comprehension and speed tested as average, but he continued to receive services under the IDEA for his math disorder through the end of high school. After graduation, Jim enrolled in art school. The art school required one math course as a requirement for graduation, but had a policy allowing course substitutions for the math requirement for students with disabilities that interfered with math. Jim disclosed his math disorder, requested a course substitution for math, and submitted good professional documentation of his disability and his need for accommodation. Since he had largely compensated for his reading disorder and tested in the average range, he was not substantially limited in reading. Thus, his reading disorder was not a disability under the law. He did not disclose his reading disorder and did not seek any accommodations for it.

What rights do I have under the Rehabilitation Act and ADA as a person with a disability?

Basically you have the right to be free from discrimination on the basis of a disability. In the early school years, a child may be found ineligible under the IDEA but eligible under Section 504 and the ADA. The child would then receive services and accommodations under these anti-discrimination laws. In college, the Rehabilitation Act and ADA provide a right to accommodations for qualified persons with disabilities, so that courses, examinations, and activities will be accessible. These laws also require reasonable accommodations in the workplace for qualified individuals with disabilities.

Notice that the protections of these laws are for qualified persons with disabilities. This means you must be qualified to do the college program or job in order to be protected under the law. You may have to prove you are qualified. This is different from public elementary and secondary school, where you were presumed to be qualified to be educated.

An example will illustrate this point. Karen had a reading disorder, auditory processing and memory retrieval problems. She received special education throughout public school. She had extra time on the SAT and did well enough to get into a college social work program. She disclosed her disabilities, requested the accommodation of extra test time and a reader for examinations, and provided supporting professional documentation. She received the requested accommodations, but failed essay tests anyway. She was dismissed from the social work program. She then sought to set aside the dismissal on the ground that she couldn't take essay tests on such complex material because of her memory retrieval problem. In the end, the finding was that the school had provided all requested accommodations, that the school had done nothing improper, and that Karen was not qualified for the program.

What accommodations would I be entitled to in college?

College accommodations depend upon your particular disabilities and how they impact on you in the college setting. Accommodations might include: course accommodations (e.g., taped textbooks, use of a tape recorder, instructions orally and in writing, note taker, and priority seating) and examination accommodations (e.g., extended test time, reader, and quiet room).

What accommodations would I be entitled to in my job?

Workplace accommodations depend upon your particular disabilities and how they impact on performing the essential functions of your job. Accommodations might include: instructions orally and in writing, frequent and specific feedback from supervisors, quiet workspace, and training course accommodations.

What about attention deficit disorder (ADD)? Is it covered under the law?

Yes, if it meets the criteria of the particular law. ADD, while not expressly listed, may be covered by the IDEA under one of three categories: other health impairments, specific learning disabilities, and serious emotional disturbance. ADD has been found to be an impairment under the Rehabilitation Act and ADA and, like learning disabilities, is a disability if it substantially limits a major life activity, such as learning.

How do I assert my rights in college?

You need to disclose your disability to the college, request specific accommodations, and supply supporting professional documentation. In public school, the school system has a duty to identify students with disabilities. This is not so in college. The student has the responsibility to disclose the disability and to request accommodations. You must be specific about the accommodations that you need because of your disability. It is not enough to say that you have learning disabilities, so the college must help you.

Let's look at an example. Sarah is taking courses at the community college. She has a reading disorder, expressive writing disorder, and ADD. She requested one and one-half time on tests, separate room for tests, a reader to read exam questions to her, and a scribe to take down her answers. She provided good professional documentation to support her request and was granted the requested accommodations.

There are student requests that the college is not obligated to grant. For example, if you did not request an accommodation on a test and failed it, generally you may not require the college to eliminate the failure from your record.

Should I disclose my disability at work?

It depends. If you do not need accommodations in the application process, generally it is best to wait until after you have the job. Once on the job, if you see that a part of your job is a problem for you and believe you need an accommodation, it is best to act promptly and not allow a long period of poor performance. Also, at the time you disclose your disability, request the specific reasonable accommodations that will enable you to do your job.

Let's consider an example. Carlos has problems with expressive writing, spelling, and fine motor coordination. After high school, he was hired as a security guard. On the job, he began to have problems with the reports he had to write. The reports were messy, had spelling errors, and were often submitted late. He sensed that his boss was becoming annoyed. Carlos disclosed his disabilities and requested that he be able to dictate his reports into his tape recorder and then type them up on one of the computers (with spell check) at the main office at the end of each day. His request was granted.

How should I disclose my disability?

Disclose the disability in writing. Be confident and positive. Combine the disclosure with a request for accommodations that will enable you to perform the job. Provide professional documentation of your disability and need for accommodations.

What documentation of my disability and need for accommodations do I have to provide?

You need to provide documentation that establishes that you have a disability and that you need the accommodations you have requested. This might be a letter or report for the college or employer from the professional who has evaluated you. It should state the diagnosis and tests and methods used in the diagnostic process, evaluate how the impairment impacts on you, and recommend reasonable accommodations.

What if I find out I have a learning disability during college or even later?

A late diagnosis of learning disabilities may be questioned more than an early diagnosis. It is important to have excellent documentation of the disability. It may be important to explain why the disability was not evident earlier. For example, Janet was diagnosed during her first year of college with a reading disorder. There were reasons why the problem had not shown up earlier. She had done well in the elementary and secondary school because she went to schools that did not have timed tests. She put in the extra time needed to successfully complete her coursework and her tests. In college, timed tests posed a major problem for her and led her to seek a thorough evaluation. She was able to document her reading disorder and her need for extra test time in college and medical school.

What if I take medication for ADD? Do I still have rights?

Yes. The existence of a disability ordinarily must be judged without reference to the possible beneficial effects of medication. The taking of prescription medication for ADD does not result in loss of disability status under the Rehabilitation Act and ADA or in loss of reasonable accommodations.

Can learning disabilities or ADD cause a person to be rejected for service in the Armed Forces?

It depends. Many individuals with learning disabilities or ADD join the Armed Forces and report that the structure and clear expectations help them to do well. However, these conditions may prevent some individuals from obtaining the required score on the Armed Forces Qualifying Test. The Armed Forces are not required to grant accommodations, such as extended test time, on the qualifying test. Further, military regulations provide that academic skills deficits that interfere with school or work after the age of twelve may be a cause for rejection for service in the Armed Forces. These regulations also provide that current use of medication, such as Ritalin or Dexedrine, to improve academic skills is disqualifying for military service.

Can I be fired from my job or dismissed from college even if I establish that I have a disability?

Yes. Having a disability does not create absolute entitlement to a job or college education. The purpose of the anti-discrimination laws is to make sure you have equal opportunity. For example, if you have math disorder and cannot pass a required math course (with no substitutions permitted) for an engineering program, then you would not be qualified for the engineering program.

What about confidentiality of disability records I file with a college or an employer?

Colleges generally have confidentiality policies with respect to disability material. The employment provisions of the ADA contain confidentiality provisions. However, these provisions are not as strong as the IDEA provision that provides for a right to delete disability records contained in your public school files.

For example, Ruth's parents submitted professional documentation of her learning disabilities and depression to her public high school. Ruth submitted the same documentation to her first employer when she disclosed her disabilities and requested job accommodations. After leaving her first job and being hired by a new employer, Ruth decided that she did not need accommodations in the new job. She also decided to request deletion of her disability information from prior files, while retaining copies in her own files in case she would need the records later. The public high school complied with her request. Her first employer informed her that the disability information could not be deleted but was kept in a separate, confidential file.

If I don't get what I ask for, should I sue?

A lawsuit is not the first step. First, you must evaluate your own position. It may be wise to consult with a lawyer to review the strong points and weak points in your case. If your case has merit, and you wish to pursue it, then follow these steps: communicate to the college or employer the basic facts and the reasons why you are entitled to what you have requested, negotiate by marshaling the facts that support your request, consider alternative dispute resolution (e.g., mediation and arbitration), and finally consider formal proceedings, such as litigation in the courts.

Remember, even if you have a strong case, it does not mean you must take legal action. You may decide that you wish to put your energy into moving on to a new college program or job rather than disputing events at the prior program or job.

Chapter 47

Preparing for Adulthood: Tips for Adolescents with Learning Disabilities

Life is full of transitions, and one of the more remarkable ones occurs when we get ready to leave high school and go out in the world as young adults. When the student has a disability, it's especially helpful to plan ahead for that transition. In fact, the Individuals with Disabilities Education Act (IDEA) requires it.

A Quick Summary of Transition

- Transition services are intended to prepare students to move from the world of school to the world of adulthood.

- Transition planning begins during high school at the latest.

- IDEA requires that transition planning start by the time the student reaches age sixteen.

- Transition planning may start earlier (when the student is younger than sixteen) if the Individualized Education Program (IEP) team decides it would be appropriate to do so.

- Transition planning takes place as part of developing the student's IEP.

- The IEP team (which includes the student and the parents) develops the transition plan.

"Transition to Adulthood," National Dissemination Center for Children with Disabilities, September 2009.

- The student must be invited to any IEP meeting where postsecondary goals and transition services needed to reach those goals will be considered.

- In transition planning, the IEP team considers areas such as postsecondary education or vocational training, employment, independent living, and community participation.

- Transition services must be a coordinated set of activities oriented toward producing results.

- Transition services are based on the student's needs and must take into account his or her preferences and interests.

Not enough detail? We can fix that! Keep reading...

IDEA's Definition of Transition Services

Any discussion of transition services must begin with its definition in law. IDEA's definition of transition services appears at §300.43. It's rather long but see it in its entirety first, and then we'll discuss it in parts.

§300.43 Transition services.

(a) *Transition services* means a coordinated set of activities for a child with a disability that—

(1) Is designed to be within a results-oriented process, that is focused on improving the academic and functional achievement of the child with a disability to facilitate the child's movement from school to post-school activities, including postsecondary education, vocational education, integrated employment (including supported employment), continuing and adult education, adult services, independent living, or community participation;

(2) Is based on the individual child's needs, taking into account the child's strengths, preferences, and interests; and includes—

(i) Instruction;

(ii) Related services;

(iii) Community experiences;

(iv) The development of employment and other post-school adult living objectives; and

(v) If appropriate, acquisition of daily living skills and provision of a functional vocational evaluation.

(b) Transition services for children with disabilities may be special education, if provided as specially designed instruction, or a related service, if required to assist a child with a disability to benefit from special education.

Considering the Definition

A number of key words in the definition above capture important concepts about transition services:

- Activities need to be *coordinated* with each other.

- The process focuses on *results*.

- Activities must address the child's *academic and functional achievement*.

- Activities are intended to smooth the young person's movement into the post-school world.

You can also see that the definition mentions the domains of independent and adult living. The community, employment, adult services, daily living skills, vocational, postsecondary education. This clearly acknowledges that adulthood involves a wide range of skills areas and activities. It also makes clear that preparing a child with a disability to perform functionally across this spectrum of areas and activities may involve considerable planning, attention, and focused, coordinated services.

Note that word—*coordinated*. We italicized it above because it's very important. Transition activities should not be haphazard or scattershot. Services are to be planned as in sync with one another in order to drive toward a result.

What result might that be? From a federal perspective, the result being sought can be found in the very first finding of Congress in IDEA, which refers to "our national policy of ensuring equality of opportunity, full participation, independent living, and economic self-sufficiency for individuals with disabilities" [20 U.S.C. 1400(c)(1)]. Preparing children with disabilities to "lead productive and independent adult lives, to the maximum extent possible" is one of IDEA's stated objectives. [20 U.S.C. 1400(c)(5)(A)(ii)].

Students at the Heart of Planning Their Transition

For the students themselves, transition activities are personally defined. This means that the postsecondary goals that are developed for a student must take into account his or her interests, preferences, needs, and strengths. To make sure of this, the school:

- must invite the youth with a disability to attend IEP team meeting "if a purpose of the meeting will be the consideration of the postsecondary goals for the child and the transition services needed to assist the child in reaching those goals under §300.320(b)," and

- "must take other steps to ensure that the child's preferences and interests are considered" if the child is not able to attend [§300.321(b)].

When Must Transition Services Be Included in the IEP?

What's not apparent in IDEA's definition of transition services but nonetheless critical to mention is the timing of transition-related planning and services: When must transition planning begin?

The answer lies in a different provision related to the content of the IEP. From §300.320(b):

(b) *Transition services.* Beginning not later than the first IEP to be in effect when the child turns sixteen, or younger if determined appropriate by the IEP Team, and updated annually, thereafter, the IEP must include—

(1) Appropriate measurable postsecondary goals based upon age appropriate transition assessments related to training, education, employment, and, where appropriate, independent living skills; and

(2) The transition services (including courses of study) needed to assist the child in reaching those goals.

So, the IEP must include transition goals by the time the student is sixteen. That age frame, though, is not cast in concrete. Note that, in keeping with the individualized nature of the IEP, the IEP team has the authority to begin transition-related considerations earlier in a student's life, if team members (which include the parent and the student with a disability) think it is appropriate, given the student's needs and preferences.

A Closer Look at What to Include in the IEP

Breaking the provisions at §300.320(b) into their component parts is a useful way to see what needs to be included, transition-wise, in the student's IEP. This is also where the rubber meets the road, so to speak, because what's included in the IEP must:

- state the student's postsecondary goals (what he or she hopes to achieve after leaving high school);

- be broken down into IEP goals that represent the steps along the way that the student needs to take while still in high school to get ready for achieving the postsecondary goals after high school; and

- detail the transition services that the student will receive to support his or her achieving the IEP goals.

The Domains of Adulthood to Consider

The definition of transition services mentions specific domains of adulthood to be addressed during transition planning. To recap, these are:

- postsecondary education;

- vocational education;

- integrated employment (including supported employment);

- continuing and adult education;

- adult services;

- independent living; or

- community participation.

These are the areas to be explored by the IEP team to determine what types of transition-related support and services a student with a disability needs. It's easy to see how planning ahead in each of these areas, and developing goal statements and corresponding services for the student, can greatly assist that student in preparing for life after high school.

Types of Activities to Consider

Remember that IDEA's definition of transition services states that these are a "coordinated set of activities" designed within a results-oriented process? Specific activities are also mentioned, which gives the IEP team insight into the range of activities to be considered in each of the domains above:

- Instruction
- Related services
- Community experiences
- The development of employment and other post-school adult living objectives
- If appropriate, acquisition of daily living skills and provision of a functional vocational evaluation. [§300.43(a)(2)]

Confused by all these lists? Putting them together, what we have is this: The IEP team must discuss and decide whether the student needs transition services and activities (e.g., instruction, related services, community experiences, etc.) to prepare for the different domains of adulthood (postsecondary education, vocational education, employment, adult services, independent living, etc.) That's a lot of ground to cover!

But it's essential ground, if the student's transition to the adult world is to be facilitated. A spectrum of adult activities is evident here, from community to employment, from being able to take care of oneself (e.g., daily living skills) to considering other adult objectives and undertakings.

Chapter 48

Employment Issues for People with Learning Disabilities

Chapter Contents

Section 48.1

Transitioning from College to Work

Transitioning from college to work, like transitioning through secondary education, is a process. Students must begin this process early and transfer their knowledge of the disability into the world of employment. Students should consider the following:

- What is the impact of the learning disability (LD) on job performance?

- How or when does one disclose a disability?

- What are typical accommodations made in the workforce?

- What kinds of social demands and interactions are needed?

Students must recognize the disability's impact on both educational and career choices. An important variable in relation to job satisfaction is a clear understanding of one's disability. Knowledge of one's disability and how it affects work are critical to satisfying employment. In addition to clearly understanding their disability, students need to identify their goals. They must analyze vocational goals in relation to their disability. What kind of tasks will the job entail? What will be the interaction between the job tasks and the disability? When answering these questions, the individual should evaluate the work environment, the type and amount of colleague interaction, specific tasks one must perform, and how one is evaluated.

At the College Level

Choosing a Major/Career

Choosing a major, and the career that ensues, is a difficult and anxiety-provoking task for most students. Students can seek help with this process by doing the following:

- Read the catalog and course descriptions carefully.

- Work with your academic adviser and discuss the requirements for different majors.

- Make an appointment with faculty members in the departments that interest you. Learn what kinds of jobs people who have graduated from these programs have gotten.

- Investigate whether your school has any job shadowing or mentoring programs.

- Consider doing an internship.

- Meet with the disability service provider and discuss how your disability might be an issue in the work setting.

Skill Development

Students strengthen the likelihood for successful, satisfying employment by developing their basic skills and learning strategies. It is important for students to take advantage of reading and writing laboratories, and any other academic resources to enhance skills. One of the most important areas to develop is an understanding of available technologies. Many facets of the employment world rely on technology. The new technologies also offer many advances that can be useful accommodations for some individuals.

The Laws That Govern Employment

It is important for students to learn about the laws that recognize their rights to equal access and nondiscrimination. They should clearly understand the aspects of the Americans With Disabilities Act (ADA) and the Rehabilitation Act of 1973, Section 504, which assure equal access and nondiscrimination. It is not enough to merely know one's legal rights. Students must recognize how equal access applies to them individually, within that particular setting, and in relation to the disability. They need to ask themselves the following questions:

- Is it necessary for me to disclose my disability in order to perform more efficiently?

- To whom do I disclose?

- How do I disclose?

- When do I disclose?

- How do I negotiate accommodations?

Being able to articulate the effect of the disability in relation to the work environment is central to successful employment.

Steps to Successful Employment

Develop a History of Work Experience

Look for opportunities to gain work experience. Some examples include:

- campus leadership opportunities, i.e. student government, mentoring programs, organization involvement, etc.;
- work study positions on campus;
- internships;
- off-campus jobs that may be listed in the college career center;
- summer jobs;
- talk to family and friends about job opportunities.

Understand the Job Culture

Every company or organization has its own unique culture. The culture consists of company rules, values, and beliefs, which are widely held but often unspoken:

- Observe your co-workers.
- Know what is expected of you.
- Watch how others communicate and interact.

Job Accommodations

Match job tasks with individual strengths and weaknesses to identify specific accommodations that will enhance job performance. Accommodations that may be used in the workplace include:

- tape recorders;
- taped materials;
- dictation;
- written instructions;
- demonstration of tasks/assignments;
- diagrams to explain an assignment;

- extended time on projects;

- separate work space;

- spelling and grammar check software for computers;

- a word processor;

- color coding of files;

- talking computers or spell checkers.

Identify and Tap into Your Support System

Family, loved ones, friends, and co-workers can be a critical variable to successful employment:

- Devise an Individualized Plan for Employment (IPE).

- Clients of the Office of Vocational Rehabilitation (OVR—in some states called Rehabilitative Services Administration, or RSA) can work with counselors to design an individualized plan regarding employment, assessments, and services related to employment.

Develop Job Skills

- Job shadowing

- Coaching/mentoring

Section 48.2

Helping Your Child Choose a Career and Find a Job

Parents of children with learning disabilities should be involved in helping their children think about work and explore careers. Academic achievement is important, but it should not be considered the most important part of the child's life. It is a means to an end. The end is a satisfying adulthood where your child can make a contribution.

During adolescence, your child should be developing his strengths. He might be athletic, academic, attractive, good with his hands, talented in technology, or socially adept. Whatever the strengths, effort and encouragement can help them to grow.

His career choice will be based on his strengths, and you should encourage him to think about future jobs. Can he fix items so they can work? Can he wash small, delicate items without breaking them? Coordination and mechanical ability is useful in many careers from car mechanic to dentist. Is he the one the family turns to when they can't figure out a computer problem? Today, technology skills are in high demand. Has he always been expert at knowing which parent to approach first to get what he wants? Can he charm grades out of his teachers? These skills are also important for many jobs from salesperson to diplomat.

It's not easy to determine which career uses your child's strengths. Many books about job hunting have practical exercises to help your child make that match. Private job placement firms can administer tests and advise adolescents. Vocational rehabilitation counselors can also help. Vocational skills tests can serve as a valuable guide, but they are not accurate for everyone. Some school systems offer career education, systematically exposing the students to the world of work. If your child's school doesn't have such a course, perhaps you could recommend establishing one. After the teenager thinks of a potentially interesting job, he should learn more about it and try to talk to people doing that job. If possible, he should visit the actual office, factory, or worksite. He should use social networking to connect with adults who are working in the field. Volunteering, internships, apprenticeships, and part-time jobs will enable him to experience the work and find out if he can do it well and enjoy it.

Careful career exploration is especially important to learning-disabled youth since they must be careful to avoid their areas of disability. For example, Carla, who is talkative and friendly, thought she might want to be a telemarketer who would sell over the phone. She volunteered to help a community group set up appointments to pick up furniture for sale in a thrift store. She found that she couldn't do the job, because it required staying in the same seat for hours at a time. She was hyperactive and needed to move more than the job allowed. James wanted to enter the field of television production. He became an intern at a neighborhood cable TV station and found that the mechanical aspects of production were difficult for him. Now he is thinking about scriptwriting.

Your child should know about his disabilities. It will help him avoid his weak areas. Without clear information on his disabilities, he may still think of himself as stupid, lazy, crazy, or personally weak. These explanations lead to a low self-image and paralyze the desire to improve. Tell your child what you know. If you feel uncomfortable about this, ask a professional to talk to him. Let him know the exact nature of the learning disability and how it affects him. Teach him the scientific words. Be sure he knows about what he has to overcome. Improvement should be ascribed to his efforts, not to "outgrowing it," upbringing, or treatment. Most learning-disabled people feel relieved when they find out about their disabilities, although some initially deny them.

They deserve to be proud of what they have overcome, a pride that will make them feel good about themselves. A strong and realistic self-image is one of the most important qualities in success. It will be vital during the time your child is looking for work.

Looking for Work

Looking for work is difficult for everyone, especially when high unemployment allows extreme selectivity among job applicants. Chances are strong that your child will face this challenge while living at your home. How can you make your home a supportive place for job hunting? Here are some ideas:

- **Insist your child actively look for work:** Do not let him spend extensive time watching TV, playing video games, social networking, or being with friends. If necessary, tell him that looking for work is a full-time job, which he must do in order to earn your financial support. Help him by not overloading him with chores during working hours on the weekdays when employers are in. Help him overcome his failures, but do not accept lack of effort.

- **Help him to organize himself:** Some learning-disabled people do not know how to look for work. There are many books about job-hunting, each with a slightly different approach. Together, you might decide on a plan of action. Or help might be needed with the fine points of planning and scheduling. You could remind him of necessary follow-up activities.

- **Be a good listener:** Ask him how the day went. Listen carefully to his adventures. Let him express his feelings of frustration, anger, and nervousness. Emphasize his actions and behavior, rather than the results. If he is actively seeking work, he deserves your respect and praise, even if he does not succeed in finding work. For example, praise your child if he does a good job of describing his qualifications at an interview, even if he is not selected for the opening.

- **Help with reading and writing:** If your child needs it, assure he has computer software that allows him to listen to text on the screen. You may need to help with online job applications, as they are impossible for some people with learning disabilities. Consider offering to look at their e-mails and proof them before they send them.

- **Help with transportation, if necessary:** If your child does not know how to drive, help them to learn and pass the examination to get a license. If you transport your child to an interview, do not go with them.

- **Grooming is important:** Learning-disabled people with visual perceptual problems are often unaware of tears and stains on their clothing, sloppy hair, or dirt on their hands. It helps if someone looks them over before an interview.

- **Talk to people you know to help your child find work:** Talk to your friends, co-workers, and other parents of learning-disabled children. Tell them about your child. Stress your child's positive qualities and describe her as a capable worker. Don't spend a lot of time describing her learning disability. Ask her to follow up any leads that you discover.

- **Be aware of community resources:** Know the applicable civil rights laws. Consider government programs such as vocational rehabilitation and job service. If you know of other parents whose children are job hunting, you may want to form a support group for yourselves and/or your children.

With your help, your child will be able to locate a satisfying job. However, this is only half the battle. Your child will have to work hard in order to keep that work. Be sure your child gets a complete job description and check for problem areas. If your child might have difficulty with any task because of his disability, he may want to consider trading that task with a co-worker in return for a task that he can do. Technology helps solve many problems. A learning-disabled person should not accept a job that includes many tasks in his area of disability.

Social skills are important to job success. Help your child to understand the point of view of co-workers and to adjust to the many hidden rules of the organization.

Many learning-disabled adults are successful. Learning-disabled people work in every conceivable job—salesperson, optometrist, pilot, doctor, psychologist, computer programmer, video-game designer, janitor, and waiter. Remember to pay as much attention to your child's abilities as to his disabilities. Teach him to feel pride in his achievements. Help him to select an interesting career that does not emphasize his area of disability. And support him as he hunts for a job. With your help and your clear belief that your child can succeed, he can "make it." Good luck!

Section 48.3

Essential Elements of an Effective Job Search

Reprinted from the Office of Disability Employment Policy, U.S. Department of Labor, November 7, 2004. Despite the date of this document, the information provided here is still relevant for readers seeking guidance in making a job search.

What Job Seekers with Disabilities Need to Know

Whether you are entering the workforce for the first time, returning to the job market, or seeking advancement, the challenges of a job search are similar. Your goal is to find the position that best meets your needs. You must be qualified and able to sell yourself as the best applicant for the job(s) for which you apply. Here are some tips that can help you in meeting your job search goal.

Know Thyself

Have a strong sense of who you are. Know your assets and how to market them to employers.

Commit to Lifelong Change

Follow job trends. Take the initiative to maintain cutting-edge skills that match changing employer requirements.

Be Computer Literate

Increasing your technical computer skills increases your marketability in the job market. Conduct online job searches. Visit employer webpages and key job sites such as the following:

- CareerPath: http://www.careerpath.com

- Monster Board: http://www.monster.com

- CareerBuilder: http://www.careerbuilder.com

Update Your Resume Often

Customize your resume to reflect the assets you bring to each job. Use key words that can be electronically scanned by potential employers to positions you want. Reflect continuous employment in your skill area. Summer employment should support your field of interest. Volunteer or obtain temporary jobs if you are unemployed. Select a resume format that minimizes any gaps in employment.

Be Your Best

Locating a job is a full-time endeavor. Give full attention to all that you do. Errors will knock you out of the running.

Be Organized

Have a written personal plan for vertical and lateral growth opportunities. Know what you must do each day to move closer to your goal. Stay focused.

Expand Your Network

Maintain and continuously strive to broaden your network. If you are working, network inside the company. Join professional groups.

Research Job Trends and Companies

Select targets of opportunity that match your skill areas. Request and study annual reports of select companies. Reflect each company's image in all communications with each company's representatives. Make good use of library resources. Read trade journals and business publications.

Have a Positive Attitude

A pleasant personality is a necessary asset. Your eagerness to adapt and to be a team player is essential. Show that you are flexible. A sense of humor and positive attitude are pluses.

Disclose a Disability Only as Needed

The only reason to disclose a disability is if you require an accommodation for an interview or to perform the essential functions of a particular job. Your resume and cover letter should focus on the abilities you bring to the job, not on your disability.

Be Prepared to Conduct an Effective Interview

Look your best from head to toe. Dress conservatively. Be brief and to the point when answering interview questions. Maintain a demeanor of success and reflect the company image when you respond. Have full confidence in what you bring to the employer and show how your skills meet the company's specific hiring needs. Ask thoughtful questions about the job and the company. *Never* say anything negative. Follow up immediately with a thank you letter or e-mail transmission.

Remember

Push yourself to go the extra mile in your job search and you will find the opportunity you are seeking.

Section 48.4

Handling the Job Interview

Excerpted from "Finding a Job That Is Right for You: A Practical Approach to Looking for a Job as a Person with a Disability—Step 3: Are You Prepared for the Job Interview?" Job Accommodation Network. The full text of this document is available online at http://askjan.org/job/Step3.htm; accessed June 20, 2011.

What should be my first step in looking for a job?

First, be sure that you are prepared. It is important to know the job market—what jobs are out there and where—as well as to know yourself, your skills, abilities, knowledge, and experience.

If I know where the jobs are and what jobs are available, now what?

Next, develop a resume presenting your qualifications to an employer. Remember, a resume is usually what the employer sees first.

How do I develop a resume?

A resume provides the employer with the skills, abilities, knowledge, and experience you have developed to date. So, if you have not already created a list of these, now is the time.

What else do I need to prepare beside the resume?

A good cover letter is essential to submitting your resume to an employer. Again, the cover letter and resume give the employer a first impression of you so you want both to be perfect.

If I have my cover letter and resume complete, what is next?

You will need to scan the newspaper "want ads" and job bank websites. Be sure you also let your friends, teachers, community members, church members, and others know that you are looking for a job. Many positions are filled with people the employer knows. Telling everyone you know that you are job hunting may open a job opportunity through this informal network.

What if an employer I am interested in working for is not currently hiring?

If you know an employer that you would like to work for but the employer is not currently hiring, ask for an informational interview so you can be considered for employer's future job openings. This informational interview can be the start of a relationship leading to a future job.

If I found a job opening that I am qualified for, it is in the area I want to live, the pay is enough to support me, I have sent my cover letter and resume, and I have been called for the job, how should I prepare?

Being prepared shows an employer you are motivated. Because some employers require a completed application before hiring, gather all the information typically needed to fill out a job application. Much of the information will be found in your resume, but some may not. For example, you may be asked to provide all of your education, even from elementary school, including addresses.

Then, research the company offering you an interview. Learn what the company does, who the company's customers are, and who is involved with the company. If you know someone who has worked for or is still working for the company, talk to them in person. Search the internet for the company name to get additional information. By knowing this information, you will be better able to tell the employer what you can do for the company. You will also be able to ask relevant questions about the company and the job during the interview.

Should I have references available at the interview?

Many recruiting professionals suggest having your references ready to provide to the interviewer. Most of the time three references will be sufficient. References should include people who can provide positive feedback about your work history or your character. Remember to ask permission from the people you want to use as references before giving the list to a potential employer. This will prevent your references from being surprised by a call from the employer and give your references time to prepare accordingly.

The day of the interview, what is expected of me and what should I expect?

Generally, the company will explain the procedure before your interview so you will have time to prepare. Remember, preparation is the most important thing. Plan ahead for what you will say and take the time to present your qualifications in a professional manner.

Being on time for an interview is very important. If late, it will reflect badly on how the interviewer sees you. Few excuses will work if you are late. However, if you plan ahead and scout the interview location before, check traffic reports, check bus or train schedules, and follow weather reports, lateness will not be a problem. If you find that you are going to be late, call the employer and explain that you have been delayed. While this is not the best situation, a call may show you are responsible and determined to meet your commitments.

You will face different types of interviews during your job search. At times you will be part of a short interview called a screening interview. During this interview, the employer is checking to see if you have the qualifications the employer needs and what you say in the interview is consistent with your resume. If you meet the employer's requirements, you may be invited to a longer interview. These interviews may be one-on-one or by a group of people. But whether the interview is with one person or a few, be prepared to discuss why you should be hired.

Finally, first impressions are very important. An employer can make a snap judgment about you even before you have a chance to say anything. Therefore, personal grooming is very important on the day of the interview. A fresh shower, a clean shave (for men), brushed teeth, and brushed or combed hair are all good grooming habits. Applicants are urged not to wear any perfume products including after shave cologne as many individuals have allergies and find scented products offensive. The person interviewing you may be one of these individuals.

Always remember interviewers will see a messy person as someone who may not be able to handle the job. Personal grooming takes little time, but it can make a lasting impression. Also keep good eye contact for the greeting. You want to present yourself as a strong person who can work individually and as a team member. Remember to smile when you first greet anyone. You are happy for this opportunity to show an employer that you are the right person for the job.

If I have an obvious disability, how can I positively address this in the interview?

How you present yourself at an interview helps an interviewer decide whether to hire you. For example, how you sit or how you walk promotes to the interviewer a perception of the kind of person you are. If, because of an obvious disability, you walk with a limp or are unable to sit straight, you may want to develop a positive strategy for addressing your limitations. For example, an individual without arms shared that when he was interviewing he would ask the interviewer if it was appropriate to take notes. He would then pull his notepad and pen out of his pocket with his foot and start writing with his toes. It was not as important to the applicant to take specific notes as it was to let the interviewer see him taking the notes.

Another suggestion, if you use a piece of assistive technology, would be to bring the equipment into the interview. For example, if you have a vision impairment and use a screen reading software, bring in the software on a laptop to show the interviewer the notes used to prepare for the interview.

Are there questions an interviewer should not ask?

Questions are the main part of the interview and are one of the main ways the interviewer can know if a candidate is right for the job. You can expect lots of different questions, from discussion about your education to your last job. However, there are questions that an interviewer cannot legally ask. An employer may not ask or require a job applicant to take a medical examination before making a job offer. An interviewer cannot make any pre-employment inquiry about a disability or the nature or severity of a disability. However, during the post-offer, pre-employment stage of the process, an employer can ask medical questions not related to the job as long as everyone going into the position is asked the questions. An employer may, however, ask questions about the ability to perform specific job functions and may, with certain limitations, ask an individual with an obvious disability to describe or demonstrate how s/he would perform a specific function.

How do I explain recent gaps in my work history because of my disability?

One of the questions often asked of candidates is their work history from most recent to first experience. Individuals can be asked to explain gaps in employment history. While there is not a perfect answer, JAN consultants suggest that "The best way to handle difficult questions during the interview is to be prepared for them. Make a list of the questions you know you are going to have trouble with and formulate an answer, then practice your delivery of these answers so you will be ready from them." For example, "I see that there is a two-year gap in your work history. What have you been doing during this time?" This is an opportunity to talk about what you have been doing, not what you have not been doing. Think about valuable life experiences that you have gained during this time. Have you been taking care of children or a parent, going to school, taking art classes, or volunteering? This question may prompt you to disclose your disability if you have not already done so. Be sure to do it in a way that shows how you have dealt with a difficult situation in a positive manner. Remember to keep the past in the past, stating that you are ready to move forward and are qualified and able to do the job you want. If and when this question arises, it is also wise to have researched the position for which you have applied as well as the organization's focus, mission, and history. Using the information you found during the research, you can transition the conversation back to why an employer should hire you.

Can an employer require medical examinations or ask questions about a disability?

If you are applying for a job, an employer cannot ask you if you are disabled or ask about the nature or severity of your disability. An employer can ask if you can perform the duties of the job with or without reasonable accommodation. An employer can also ask you to describe or to demonstrate how, with or without a reasonable accommodation, you will perform the job duties.

An employer cannot require you to take a medical examination before you are offered a job. Following a job offer, an employer can condition the offer on your passing a required medical examination, but only if all entering employees for the job category have to take the examination. However, an employer cannot reject you because of information about your disability revealed by the medical examination, unless the reasons for rejection are job-related and necessary for the conduct of the employer's business. The employer will also have to consider reasonable accommodation, barring an undue hardship, to allow an applicant the ability to perform the essential functions of the job up to the expectations of anyone entering the position. Finally, the results of all medical examinations must be kept confidential and maintained in separate medical files.

At this point, do I tell the employer I may have a disability?

Disclosing a disability is voluntary during the application and interview stages of the employment process. Some individuals decide to disclose to a potential employer at that time. Disclosure during the application or interview stage may be because the disability is not hidden or the individual decides this is the right time. Many, including the U.S. Department of Labor's Office of Disability Employment Policy (ODEP), suggest a positive approach to disclosing before a job offer has been made. This approach would anticipate the concerns of the employer, have innovative accommodation suggestions available, practice demonstrating how you would perform difficult functions, and keep the focus on your abilities. This approach should send a message to the interviewer that you are an innovative individual who can anticipate job changes.

JAN Consultants suggest that if you need to disclose during an interview, "remember to talk about your abilities, not your disabilities. Employers need qualified, capable individuals to fill positions. Find a way to show that you are that person. Sell them on what you can do, not on what you cannot do and the interview will go better than you expect. Be positive about yourself and be honest."

John Williams, an award-winning columnist, who has been writing about disability issues for twenty-two years wrote in a 2001 National Organization on Disability article, "It is your choice whether or not to mention your disability; by law, interviewers cannot ask candidates disability-related questions. And it is best not to discuss specific medical problems during your interview. However, if you use assistive technology, describing what you use and how it helps your performance can make a positive impression on the interviewer. This indicates problem-solving ability and self-confidence. Remind the person interviewing you that any purchase of assistive technology products is a capital investment."

Job candidates should be aware that once disclosure of a disability or an accommodation request is made, employers may ask the employee about the limitations related to the job and are permitted to make medical inquiries.

Disclosing a disability requires a lot of thought and planning. Candidates with disabilities should plan how they will disclose and assess the consequences of sharing this intimate information with a prospective employer. Ultimately, the job candidate must decide the time, place, and degree of information to share with others.

How do I ask for help when filling out the application and for the interview?

If you think you will need assistance in order to participate in the application and hiring process, you should inform the employer. Assistance needed to reduce the barrier a disability creates is called reasonable accommodation. Employers are required to provide reasonable accommodation only for the known physical or mental limitations of a qualified individual with a disability. Generally, you, as the applicant, have the responsibility to request an accommodation from the employer.

I have submitted a request for accommodation and the employer is asking for medical records. What do I do?

In asking for help, you are disclosing to the employer that you have an impairment. When a job applicant requests help, or a reasonable accommodation, an employer may require that the employee provide medical documentation to establish whether the employee has an Americans with Disability Act (ADA) disability and needs the requested accommodation.

After the interview, are there things that I should do?

After the interview, don't forget to send a thank you letter to the interviewer. If you have not heard from a company from ten days to two weeks after you sent your thank you letter, you can follow up with a phone call. During this call, state your name, the date of the interview, and the position. Let the employer know you are still interested in the position and ask if there is a timetable for making a decision. Generally, an interviewer will tell you when the decision will be made.

Another thing that should be done is your self-evaluation of the interview. How did you do? Do you know? Can you take a step back and evaluate yourself on how you did during the interview? You should take some time and review what happened at the interview. Did you take notes? If you did, they are a good sign you were paying attention. Do you remember if you stumbled over your words? Did you delay answering a question? Did you sit up straight and ask appropriate questions? Did you give the interviewer the extra resume asked for? If you felt you did something wrong, what was it? How would you handle it differently? Think of corrections and if you do not get the job, be better prepared for your next interview. In addition, by reviewing the interview you may discover additional questions for the employer you can ask during your follow-up call or second interview.

Should I wait to hear back after an interview before considering other jobs?

While you are waiting for word from the employer about the job, you can be getting ready for other interviews or continue searching for other positions. You should not wait until you hear back from an employer. If you wait and do not get the position, you will have wasted valuable search and possible interview time.

Effective interviewing is essential to getting the job. Job openings occur every day. Being prepared for these opportunities and being at the right place at the right time, often makes the difference in who is hired.

What should I do if I feel the interviewer has asked an illegal question?

Should you be asked an illegal question, you do not have to answer it. However, you do not want to point out to the interviewer the question is illegal and possibly ruin your chances to be hired. You can change the subject or politely explain that you are not comfortable answering the question. Also, do not dwell on the interviewer's mistake. This may be just a mistake and will have nothing to do with your being hired.

Section 48.5

Do's and Don'ts of Disclosure

Reprinted from the Job Accommodation Network, March 24, 2010.

Disclosing a disability may be a consideration when starting a new job; transitioning from school, another job, or unemployment; or retaining a job after acquiring a disability. For individuals who may still be struggling with accepting their medical condition, making the decision to disclose can be overwhelming. Because some impairments are not visible, individuals may face such challenges as understanding their impairments and determining what types of accommodations are available. As with any new experience, preparation is vital. The following provides an overview of the do's and don'ts of disclosure. Note that disclosing is a very personal decision, but some of the following tips may be helpful in making that decision.

Do Disclose When You Need an Accommodation

Deciding when to disclose can be a difficult choice for a person with a disability. If you have a hidden disability such as brain injury or post-traumatic stress disorder, knowing when to disclose your condition can be a real dilemma.

Under the Americans with Disability Act (ADA) you can request an accommodation at any time during the application process or while you are employed. You can request an accommodation even if you did not ask for one when applying for a job or after receiving a job offer. So when should you disclose that you have disability? In general, you should disclose your disability when you need to request a reasonable accommodation—when you know that there is a workplace barrier that is preventing you, due to a disability, from competing for a job, performing a job, or gaining equal access to a benefit of employment like an employee lunch room or employee parking.

Do Know Who to Disclose To

This can be tricky. Many employers have their own in-house procedures that detail how they handle accommodation requests. Check your employee handbook or your company's intranet for this information. Also, if you have an Equal Employment Opportunity (EEO) office or a human resources department, they can assist you. The other option is to talk to your manager or supervisor directly.

Do Know How to Disclose

According to the Equal Employment Opportunity Commission (EEOC), you only have to let your employer know that you need an adjustment or change at work for a reason related to a medical condition. You can use "plain English" to make your request and you do not have to mention the ADA or use the phrase "reasonable accommodation." Once you disclose, then the interactive process should begin. At this point, your employer can ask for limited information about your disability and your need for accommodations.

Don't Disclose Too Soon

Many people with hidden disabilities may feel that they are not being completely honest with an employer if they do not tell everything about their disability up front at the time of their interview. Just remember that you are not obligated to do so. When you disclose, just provide basic information about your condition, your limitations, and what accommodations you may need.

Don't Disclose Too Late

Don't wait to disclose until after you begin to experience work performance problems. It is better to disclose your disability and request accommodations before job performance suffers or conduct problems occur. Employers do not have to rescind discipline that occurred before they knew about the disability, nor do they have to lower performance standards as a reasonable accommodation. Remember, the purpose of an accommodation is to enable a qualified person with a disability to perform the essential functions of the job. So, disclose when you first realize you are having difficulties.

Don't Disclose to Everyone

Remember that you have a right to keep information about your disability private. It is not necessary to inform co-workers and colleagues about your disability or your need for accommodations. While they may be aware of the accommodations, especially if you are allowed to take extra breaks or you have a flexible starting time, they are not entitled to know why. Your employer is required by the ADA to keep your disability and medical information confidential and to give it to managers and supervisors only on a need-to-know basis.

Most Importantly, Do Your Homework

No one knows more about your disability than you do, so tell your employer what you think you need, but also research other accommodations options such as flexible start time or working from home part of the time.

Section 48.6

Tips for Self-Advocacy in the Workplace

"Tips for Self-Advocacy in the Workplace," copyright 2008 Dale S. Brown. All rights reserved. Reprinted with permission.

Here are some tips for obtaining the help that you need to get the job done. Many people with learning disabilities find it challenging to get accommodation and this section is designed to help you succeed in your request.

Setting the Stage

Be Productive

Bosses and co-workers are more likely to accede to accommodation requests from people who are perceived as high performers than from those who are not considered essential to the organizational mission. Of course, being productive is hard without reasonable accommodation! You can end up in a Catch 22 situation. But do your personal best at all times.

Market Your Work to Your Bosses and Co-workers

You need to be perceived as productive. This often is different from your actual productivity. Each organization has its own signals that show you are a hard worker. Common expectations include wearing clean, well-fitted clothes; arriving at work on time; staying at your desk; keeping connected to the office through e-mail if you are working at home; and keeping conversations with co-workers related to the job. Marketing your work to your supervisors may mean asking their advice, keeping them posted, writing memoranda, and representing yourself well with internal reports. For sales jobs, talk up your successful sales. Of course, you should not carry this too far and risk being considered a braggart.

Be Helpful

When you are asked to do something, see it as an opportunity to serve. The more people who feel supported by you, the more likely they are to give you the support you need when you ask.

Determining the Accommodation You Need

Know Your Legal Rights as a Person with a Disability

Study the Americans with Disabilities Act. However, as you research your rights, remember that the best accommodations are those that are won without resorting to complaints and lawsuits. However, knowing that the law is on your side will give you tremendous confidence. If you are in a unionized workplace, meet your union steward or other union officials before you need them to represent you. In order to receive accommodation as your legal right, you must disclose your disability.

Study Yourself Doing Your Job

Determine where you need accommodation. As part of that survey, see if there are things that can be done on your own. Consider:

- **Your work space:** Can you find everything you need? Does it support your productivity? How well does your computer or other machinery help you do the job?

- **How you communicate with others:** Does your supervisor insist on writing you e-mails rather than talking to you? Are you familiar with your voice mail system and can you use it to send messages to groups? What is the procedure for handing off your assignments to co-workers and turning them in for production? Does the system work for you? How do you give and get instructions?

- **The tasks themselves:** Are there some tasks which are not that important to your job but are challenging to you because of your dyslexia? Many employees have successfully received help with reading through the use of clerical aid, text-to-speech software, and other technical solutions. In other cases, tasks have been assigned to other employees. For example, in one team, members took turns filling in the forms of a talented salesperson who is unable to complete them.

Research the Range of Accommodation Options and Choose One

Information on accommodations is available through learning disabilities organizations. The Job Accommodation Network (JAN) has qualified people able to help you find the best accommodation solutions. Call them at 800-526-7234 and be ready with a clear definition of your problem before you pick up the phone.

Making Your Request

Consider a Productivity or Quality Argument

If you do not wish to disclose your disability or prefer to stay away from legal discussions, productivity and quality improvement are good reasons for the employer to meet your disability-related needs. Explain what you want in positive terms. Here are some examples:

- If you let me work more flexible hours, I could work in the evening when I do my best work and complete more jobs.

- I need Mary to proof my work before you see it. That way we can both pay more attention to the content and not worry about the way it's typed.

- On important matters, I'll probably write you an e-mail and ask you to read it to be sure I understand. That way we'll both have something to refer to and not have to rely on our memories.

Tell Them about Your Disability and Ask Them for What You Need to Work Around It

If you decide to ask for accommodation on the basis of disability, first talk to your supervisor. If you believe your supervisor may not be supportive and you work for a large company, visit your human resources department. If you work within a self-managed work team, your accommodation might be an issue for consideration by the entire team. In that case, talk to the team leader or bring it up at a team meeting.

Although you do not need to submit medical documentation of your disability at the time you first make your accommodation request, you should have this documentation available to you. Your employer can demand proof of your disability prior to providing an accommodation.

Have a clear description of your disability, the accommodation(s) needed, and the modifications needed in the work environment to ensure that you meet with success in approaching your job tasks. The Americans with Disabilities Act allows employers to legally turn down accommodation requests if they can prove they constitute "an undue hardship." For this reason, propose the least costly and time-consuming accommodations that will enable you to do your job well.

Follow Up With a Written Request

Make the request brief; include relevant information about your disability and the need for accommodation. Explain how it will help you meet your employer's goals. Of course, should that fail, the next step is a written complaint under the Americans with Disabilities Act.

Following Up

Assess the Results of Your Request

If you are able to obtain reasonable accommodation, be sure to use it well. Be productive and helpful to your co-workers and your supervisors. Make them glad that they granted the accommodation to you. This will make it easier for the next person seeking accommodations. Thank those who supported you. If the accommodation does not help restart the process at studying yourself doing your job.

Section 48.7

Job Accommodation for Employees with Learning Disabilities

Excerpted from "Accommodation and Compliance Series: Employees with Learning Disabilities," Job Accommodation Network, February 3, 2010.

Information about Learning Disabilities

What Are Learning Disabilities?

According to the National Institute of Neurological Disorders and Stroke (2007), learning disabilities are disorders that affect the ability to understand or use spoken or written language, do mathematical calculations, coordinate movements, or direct attention. Although learning disabilities occur in very young children, the disorders are usually not recognized until the child reaches school age. Learning disabilities are a lifelong condition; they are not outgrown or cured, though many people develop coping techniques through special education, tutoring, medication, therapy, personal development, or adaptation of learning skills. Approximately fifteen million children, adolescents, and adults have learning disabilities in the United States (National Center for Learning, 2006b).

What Causes Learning Disabilities?

Experts have not been able to pinpoint specific medical causes for learning disabilities. Learning disabilities are not caused by economic disadvantage, environmental factors, or cultural differences. In fact, according to the National Center for Learning Disabilities (2009a), there is frequently no apparent cause for learning disabilities. However, much research points to heredity, problems during the mother's pregnancy, or incidents after birth such as head injuries, nutritional deprivation, and exposure to toxic substances.

Only qualified professionals who have been trained to identify learning disabilities can perform a formal evaluation to diagnose learning disabilities. Such professionals may be clinical or educational psychologists, school psychologists, neuropsychologists, or learning disabilities specialists. Adults who suspect they have learning disabilities should seek out professionals who have training or direct experience working with and evaluating adults with learning disabilities (National Center for Learning, 2006b).

Learning Disabilities and the Americans with Disabilities Act

Is a Learning Disability a Disability under the Americans with Disabilities Act (ADA)?

The ADA does not contain a list of medical conditions that constitute disabilities. Instead, the ADA has a general definition of disability that each person must meet (EEOC, 1992). Therefore, some people with learning disabilities will have a disability under the ADA and some will not.

A person has a disability if he/she has a physical or mental impairment that substantially limits one or more major life activities, a record of such an impairment, or is regarded as having such an impairment (EEOC, 1992).

Accommodating Employees with Learning Disabilities

Note: Employees with learning disabilities may experience some of the limitations discussed below, but seldom experience all of them. Also, the degree of limitation will vary among individuals. Be aware that not all people with learning disabilities need accommodations to perform their jobs and many others may only need a few accommodations. The following is only a sample of the accommodation possibilities available. Numerous other accommodation solutions may exist.

Questions to Consider

1. What limitations is the employee with the learning disability experiencing?

2. How do these limitations affect the employee and the employee's job performance?

3. What specific job tasks are problematic as a result of these limitations?

4. What accommodations are available to reduce or eliminate these problems? Are all possible resources being used to determine possible accommodations?

5. Has the employee with the learning disability been consulted regarding possible accommodations?

6. Once accommodations are in place, would it be useful to meet with the employee with the learning disability to evaluate the effectiveness of the accommodations and to determine whether additional accommodations are needed?

7. Do supervisory personnel and employees need training regarding learning disabilities?

Accommodation Ideas

Reading: People with learning disabilities may have limitations that make it difficult to read text. Because it can be difficult to visually discern letters and numbers, these characters may appear jumbled or reversed. Entire words or strings of letters may be unrecognizable.

Accommodations to help when reading from a paper copy:

- Convert text to audio
- Provide larger print
- Double space the text of print material
- Use color overlays (Irlen lenses) to help make the text easier to read
- Provide materials that are typewritten, in a font that is not italicized; if handwritten material must be provided, use print, not cursive
- Have someone read the document aloud to the employee
- Scan the documents into a computer and use optical character recognition (OCR), which will read the information aloud
- Use a reading pen, which is a portable device that scans a word and provides auditory feedback

Accommodations to help when reading from a computer screen:

- Use voice output software, also called screen reading software, which highlights and reads aloud the information from the computer screen
- Use manual or electric line guide to help an employee "keep his/her place" on the computer monitor
- Alter color scheme on computer screen to suit the employee's visual preferences

- Adjust the font on computer screen to suit the employee's visual preferences

Spelling: Employees with learning disabilities might have difficulty spelling, which can manifest itself in letter reversals, letter transposition, omission of letters or words, or illegible handwriting. Accommodations to help with spelling:

- Allow use of reference materials such as dictionary or thesaurus
- Provide electronic and talking dictionaries
- Use word prediction software that displays a list of words that typically follow the word that was entered in a document
- Use word completion software that displays sample words after someone starts typing part of a word
- Allow buddy, co-worker, or supervisor to proofread written material

Writing: Employees with learning disabilities might have difficulty with the cognitive or the physical process of writing.

Employees with learning disabilities involving the cognitive process of writing might have difficulty organizing a written project, identifying themes or ideas, structuring sentences or paragraphs, or identifying and/or correcting grammar errors.

Accommodations to help with the cognitive process of writing:

- Use Inspiration software, a computerized graphic organizer
- Use Texthelp Read & Write Gold, a software program assisting with spelling, reading, and grammar
- Provide electronic/talking dictionaries and spellcheckers
- Create written forms to prompt the employee for information needed
- Allow the employee to create a verbal response instead of a written response
- Permit use of reference books such as a thesaurus or dictionary

Employees with learning difficulties involving the physical process of writing may find it difficult to fill in blanks, bubble in dots, or line up numbers or words in a column, on a line, or within a margin. Handwriting may be illegible.

Accommodations to help with the physical process of writing:

- Provide writing aids
- Use line guides and column guides
- Supply bold line paper
- Permit typewritten response instead of handwritten response
- Allow use of personal computers, including Alpha Smart, Palm, tablet PC, and Blackberry
- Use Inspiration software, a computerized graphic organizer
- Use speech recognition software that recognizes the user's voice and changes it to text on the computer screen

Mathematics: An employee with a learning disability could have difficulty recognizing or identifying numbers, remembering sequencing of numbers, understanding the mathematical sign or function (whether symbol or word), or performing mathematical calculations accurately and efficiently.

Accommodations to help with mathematics:

- Use scratch paper to work out math problems
- Permit use of fractional, decimal, statistical, or scientific calculators
- Provide talking calculator
- Use calculators or adding machines with large display screens
- Use construction calculator, such as Jobber 6
- Provide talking tape measure
- Use talking scales
- Use pre-measurement guides or jigs
- Post mathematical tables at desk or in work area

Speaking/communicating: Employees with learning disabilities may have difficulty communicating with co-workers or supervisors. For employees with learning disabilities, poor communication may be the result of underdeveloped social skills, lack of experience/exposure in the workforce, shyness, intimidation, behavior disorders, or low self-esteem.

Accommodations to help with speaking and communicating:

- To help facilitate communication, provide advance notice of topics to be discussed in meetings

- To reduce or eliminate anxiety, provide advance notice of date of meetings when employee is required to speak

- Allow employee to provide written response in lieu of verbal response

- To reduce or eliminate the feeling of intimidation, allow employee to have a friend or co-worker attend meeting

Organizational skills: An employee with a learning disability may have difficulty getting organized or staying organized.
Accommodations to help with organization:

- Help employee reduce clutter in work area

- Hire a professional organizer or job coach

- Use color-code system to label or identify materials

- Use calendars (paper, electronic, or both) to remind employee of deadlines, meetings, and upcoming tasks

- Build organization skills by attending time management workshops, like those offered by Franklin Covey

- Build organization skills through self-education at sites like mindtools.com

- Build "catch up" time into work week or work day

Memory: An employee with a learning disability could have memory deficits that affect the ability to recall something that is seen or heard. This may result in an inability to recall facts, names, passwords, and telephone numbers, even if such information is used regularly.
Accommodations to help with memory:

- Provide checklists to help employee remember job tasks

- Use flowchart to describe steps to a complicated task (such as powering up a system, closing down the facility, logging into a computer, etc)

- Safely and securely maintain paper lists of crucial information such as passwords

- Prompt employee with verbal or written cues

- Allow employee to use voice-activated recorder to record verbal instructions

- Provide additional training time on new information or tasks

- Provide refresher training as needed

Time Management: An employee with a learning disability may have difficulty managing time. This can affect the employee's ability to organize or prioritize tasks, adhere to deadlines, maintain productivity standards, or work efficiently.

Accommodations to help with time management:

- Make to-do lists and check items off as they are completed

- Use calendars to mark important meetings or deadlines

- Divide large assignments into smaller tasks and goals

- Remind employee verbally of important tasks or deadlines

Social Skills: Employees with learning disabilities may have difficulty exhibiting appropriate social skills on the job. This may be the result of underdeveloped social skills, lack of experience/exposure in the workforce, shyness, intimidation, behavior disorders, or low self-esteem. This can affect the employee's ability to adhere to conduct standards, work effectively with supervisors, or interact with co-workers or customers.

Accommodations to help behavior on the job:

- To reduce incidents of inappropriate behavior, thoroughly review conduct policy with employee

- Provide concrete examples to explain inappropriate behavior

- Provide concrete examples to explain consequences in a disciplinary action

- To reinforce appropriate behavior, recognize and reward appropriate behavior

Accommodations to help employee in working effectively with supervisors:

- Provide detailed day-to-day guidance and feedback

- Offer positive reinforcement

- Provide clear expectations and the consequences of not meeting expectations

- Give assignments verbally, in writing, or both, depending on what would be most beneficial to the employee

- Establish long-term and short-term goals for employee

- Adjust supervisory method by modifying the manner in which conversations take place, meetings are conducted, or discipline is addressed

Accommodations to help employee in interacting with co-workers:

- Provide sensitivity training to promote disability awareness
- If feasible, allow employee to work from home
- Help employee "learn the ropes" by providing a mentor
- Make employee attendance at social functions optional
- Allow employee to transfer to another workgroup, shift, or department

Situations and Solutions

A new-hire telemarketer had deficits in reading comprehension. He participated in CBT (computer-based training), which included watching a customer service tutorial, then completing timed quizzes on the computer. To accommodate this employee, the employer adjusted the color scheme, resolution, and font size of the computer screen, making the appearance of material easier to view. The employee held a ruler to the computer screen to "stay on the line" when reading test questions. The employee was allowed to watch the tutorial over again, and was given extra time to complete quizzes.

A teacher with a learning disability had difficulty spelling words correctly on the chalkboard. The employer provided an overhead projector with plenty of blank overhead sheets. In advance of class, the teacher wrote words, phrases, or sentences on the overhead sheets, which were double-checked by her mentor for accuracy. This helped the teacher display correctly spelled information to her students.

A researcher in a technology company had expressive writing disorder. The employee's job tasks included gathering information for written reports. To accommodate this employee, Inspiration software was provided to help organize, prioritize, and then outline the information for reports. The employer also provided a hard copy dictionary and thesaurus.

An employee who works in a manufacturing environment had a learning disability. The employee had difficulty remembering task sequences of the job. The supervisor provided written instructions, whereby each major task was broken down into smaller, sequential subparts. Each subpart was color-coded for easy reference (green means start, red means stop).

An employee who had expressive language disorder had difficulty communicating with the supervisor. This employee preferred to read communication, then, respond in writing. The supervisor adjusted the method of supervision, whereby communication with this employee occurred through email instead of face to face.

A building contractor with dyscalculia was inefficient when creating job quotes. To ensure the mathematical calculations were accurate, the employee spent extra time "figuring" and "double-checking" the numbers. The site supervisor purchased the Jobber 6 contractor's calculator to help the employee "figure" fractions, triangles, circles, area (and more) efficiently and accurately.

A clerical worker with auditory processing disorder worked for a large employer where different work assignments were handed out daily. To ensure the job assignment was accurate, the employee used a voice recorder to capture information about the work assignment, such as the job location, the supervisor's name, and tasks to be completed. To refresh his memory, the employee was able to listen to this recorded information whenever necessary, sometimes several times each day.

References

Equal Employment Opportunity Commission. (1992). A technical assistance manual on the employment provisions (title I) of the Americans with Disabilities Act. Retrieved January 13, 2010, from http://askjan .org/links/ADAtam1.html.

National Center for Learning Disabilities. (2006a). Fact sheet: LD at a glance. Retrieved January 13, 2010, from http://www.ncld.org/ld-basics/ ld-explained/basic-facts/learning-disabilities-at-a-glance.

National Center for Learning Disabilities. (2006b). Fact sheet: Learning Disabilities In Adulthood. Retrieved January 13, 2010, from http:// www.ncld.org/ld-basics/ld-explained/ld-across-the-lifespan/learning -disabilities-in-adulthood-the-struggle-continues.

National Institute of Neurological Disorders and Stroke. (2007). NINDS learning disabilities information page. Retrieved January 13, 2010, from http://www.ninds.nih.gov/disorders/learningdisabilities/ learningdisabilities.htm.

Chapter 49

Coaching: A Supportive Tool for Adults with Learning Disabilities

Chapter Contents

Section 49.1

Coaching Adults with Learning Disabilities: The Basics

What is coaching?

Coaching is an ongoing, collaborative relationship that begins by helping you clarify important personal or professional goals. Coaches then support you as you take action steps toward realizing your goals—similar to mentors whose only desire is to see you succeed.

How is coaching different from psychotherapy?

Coaching and psychotherapy are distinctly different, but complementary services. Consider the analogy of physical conditioning. A coach, like a personal trainer, collaborates with you and provides support and encouragement so that you can reach higher levels of performance and satisfaction in life. A psychologist, like a physical therapist, approaches a working relationship by focusing on "problems" which prevent you from feeling better or behaving in healthy ways. The goal of coaching is to facilitate positive change by focusing on human strengths and the widest available range of resources. Together we clarify your most important personal and professional goals and work as partners until they have been achieved.

Who needs a coach? Do learning style differences limit your success at work? Do you have difficulty communicating or advocating for yourself on the job or at home? Many young adults need assistance in making the transition from school to work. Other adults find that they work harder than friends or colleagues to blend in socially or adapt to changes on the job. Is it especially challenging to learn new or complex information? Would you benefit from learning effective strategies for succeeding in professional or social settings? Can you picture lifestyle changes which would make you happier and healthier? Would you like to live the life that you've always dreamed of . . . *now*?

Of course you do! Many adults continue to develop strategies for success in adulthood. Don't just dream about a more fulfilling life— decide to live it! Coaching can help you identify and achieve goals which will result in feeling successful, enthusiastic, and energized.

What are some sample areas for coaching?

- Job search
- Organizational skills
- Communication skills
- Self-advocacy
- Pragmatic and social skills
- Reading and writing skills

How does coaching work?

Coaching relationships are completely confidential and flexible. Clients can choose to work in person or by telephone. Clients and coaches meet regularly to stay focused and motivated, either on a weekly or bi-weekly basis. Coaching fees and frequency of meetings are determined by the needs of each client.

Section 49.2

Special Concerns in Coaching Adults with Attention Deficit Hyperactivity Disorder

When you have attention deficit hyperactivity disorder (ADHD), making certain changes, following through on projects, managing your time, accomplishing your goals, and even getting to work on time can be difficult. Symptoms such as inattention, distractibility, and restlessness cause you to get stuck—on a regular basis. But a coach who specializes in ADHD can help.

Sandy Maynard, MS, a veteran ADHD coach who operates Catalytic Coaching, discusses how ADHD coaches can—and can't—help clients, and how readers can find the right coach for them.

What ADHD Coaches Do

According to Maynard, ADHD coaches "help clients clarify what's problematic." They break down problems into definable goals and steps the client can take.

They have a unique understanding of how ADHD affects their clients and the challenges that ADHD creates. That means that they're able to "adjust strategies to help with ADD challenges [such as] impulsivity, inattention, or whatever the aspect of the problem is." This helps clients learn to better cope with their ADHD.

Coaches also keep clients accountable and provide support. The cheerleading component, Maynard said, is especially valuable because people without ADHD aren't able to appreciate how difficult it is to do things like make it to work on time. Maynard "helps clients tap themselves on the back for accomplishing something that others without ADD happen to do so easily."

What Coaches Don't Do

It's often hard for people to distinguish the difference between coaches and therapists. Maynard noted that "coaches don't deal with traumatic, emotional, and psychological difficulties and roadblocks." And of course they can't diagnose a person with attention deficit disorder or any other disorder. Only a licensed mental health professional is empowered to treat someone with a mental disorder—which is what attention deficit disorder is. Coaches can help with life problems as a result of the disorder, but they can't treat the disorder itself.

Here's one way to see the distinction: Maynard's client was having issues with her family. They expected her to do a lot of work because she didn't have a job; however, she did have a dissertation that left her little time for anything else. While Maynard didn't help the client resolve her family issues—this is a therapist's territory—she did help her set boundaries and find strategies to get her work done.

It's common for people with ADHD to struggle with other disorders, and these can interfere with coaching. Not surprisingly, a client with untreated depression won't get as much benefit from coaching, Maynard said. Clients have to be "ready, willing, and able to be coached." In fact, she usually doesn't work with clients who've had substance abuse issues unless they've been recovered for a year. It's vital for clients to participate in psychotherapy and resolve these kinds of issues.

Tips for Finding an ADHD Coach

Search on Reputable Sites

To start researching ADHD coaches, consider checking out these sites:

- Addresources.org lets you search their national directory for providers, including coaches.

- Children and Adults with Attention-Deficit/Hyperactivity Disorder (CHADD) support groups usually have a local list of resources they give out.

- The Institute for the Advancement of AD/HD Coaching (IAAC) has a list of accredited coaches in each state.

Check Out Their Background

When selecting a coach, Maynard suggested paying attention to the number of years they've been coaching, their educational background, and their training.

Having a psychological background, she said, is helpful for picking up red flags when clients aren't ready for coaching or need help from a therapist. If you're looking for a coach for your child, a special education degree can go a long way. In other words, you want to match the qualifications of a potential coach to what you're looking for, Maynard said.

Also, certification is essential. For instance, the IAAC, where Maynard is a founding member, certifies coaches specifically in ADHD.

Go Beyond Testimonials

Don't rely on glowing testimonials that a prospective coach directly provides. "A better benchmark," according to Maynard, is "to get a referral or testimonial from another professional," such as a psychiatrist or therapist who has referred clients to that coach. You're more likely to get accurate information this way.

Interview the Coach

As part of your research, ask each coach specific questions about their background, such as: "What professional organizations do you belong to? What conferences have you attended?" These questions can help you delve deeper into their experience.

You also want to know if they specialize in what you need. Ask, "What kinds of clients have you worked with?" If you're an entrepreneur who needs help structuring your schedule and getting organized, ask if the coach has worked with other entrepreneurs. If you're looking for a coach to help your teen succeed in his last two years of high school and get college applications out on time, make sure that coach specializes in working with adolescents.

It's also a good idea to ask for a testimonial from a similar client, Maynard said (e.g., if the coach has worked with attorneys, ask to speak to one of her lawyer clients).

Understand What You Need Help With—and How the Coach Will Help

"Knowing what your needs are before you shop is important," Maynard said. Before her first appointment with clients, Maynard asks them to answer two questions: (1) "What do I need to know about you to help you?" (this gets at what your strengths and weaknesses are) and (2) "What do you hope to accomplish using my services?" (i.e., "what are your long-term and short-term goals?")

As Maynard said, some clients will be very clear on what they need, such as help with time management and organization. Others will have a general statement, such as "I'm not sure I'm using my full potential at my job." Maynard helps these clients get more specific to figure out "what's getting in the way" and how to overcome these obstacles.

Create "a brief description of what . . . you want out of coaching" and then ask the prospective coach the following: "How do you think you'll be able to help me? Have you helped someone else with this before?" This gives a better idea if that coach is best for you.

Don't Feel Pressured to Make a Rushed Decision

After your initial session, "Don't feel pressured to book the next appointment," Maynard said. Be honest and let the coach know that you have appointments with other coaches to see who's the best fit for you.

Have Reasonable Expectations

Many people have the misconception that a coach's role is to solve all the client's problems or give them the secret to swiftly change their life.

One of Maynard's clients put it perfectly in a magazine article when he said: "I am my own magic bullet." In other words, remember that an ADHD coach is there to facilitate change, Maynard said. Maynard, a former chemist, chose the word "catalytic" for her coaching practice to capture this very idea. A catalyst initiates a chemical change. But "I can't make it happen for you."

A coach will offer their support, but ultimately, the client must do the work. "The answer is within, and I help them find that answer within." It's the idea that "I'm what I've got to work with," and so you work from your strengths.

Also, remember that changes take time. Maynard works with new clients for about three months. This is usually when sustainable behavioral changes happen, she said. As time goes on, the length and frequency of sessions typically diminish—which Maynard uses as an indicator that the client is "learning how to self-initiate change and doesn't need my support and encouragement and help as much as in the beginning." She also suggested scheduling regular tune-ups (such as after six months or a year) to touch base and discuss progress.

Unsolicited Advice May Be a Red Flag

Another misconception is that coaches tell clients what to do. As Maynard said, "I'd be wary of unsolicited advice." Instead, coaches ask "those questions that need to be asked to help clients find the solution that's user-friendly for them."

Take the simple example of finding the best way to get organized. Unsolicited advice is: "What I want you to do is get an iPhone and then I want you to download these four Apps and I want you to start using XYZ for your calendar." What Maynard and other good coaches do instead is to ask whether a client is comfortable using technology or if they prefer paper and pencil. They discuss the pros and cons of each, along with what's going to be the most useful strategy for that client.

Trust Your Gut

"First impressions matter," Maynard said, so consider "your level of comfort the first time you meet" the coach. Remember that not every coach will be the right fit for you.

In addition to their credentials and experience, there needs to be a good rapport between the two of you. Not only do you need to trust your coach, but it helps to be able to laugh with them and even joke around about what went wrong, she said. So if the coach makes you uncomfortable or you just don't click, it's fine to move on to your next prospect.

Chapter 50

Special Needs Trusts

What is a "Special Needs" Trust?

"Special needs" is just a term to describe any trust intended to provide benefits without causing the beneficiary to lose public benefits he or she is entitled to receive.

What kinds of public benefits do special needs trust beneficiaries receive?

Each special needs trust can be intended to protect different public benefits. Most commonly, special needs trusts are intended to permit Supplemental Security Income (SSI) and Medicaid recipients to receive some additional services or goods.

Does the existence of a special needs trust qualify the beneficiary for public benefits?

No. The existence of a special needs trust does not itself make public benefits available; the beneficiary must qualify for the benefits program already, or qualify after the trust is established. If properly established, the special needs trust will not cause a loss of benefits (although in some circumstances the level of benefits may be reduced), but the trust does not make it easier to qualify.

What is a "supplemental benefits" trust?

Some lawyers prefer to use the term "supplemental benefits" rather than "special needs." Occasionally the term "supplemental needs" is used. All are interchangeable, and describe the purpose of the trust rather than being a limited legal term.

Who can establish a special needs trust?

Anyone can establish a special needs trust, but there are two general categories of such trusts: self-settled and third-party trusts.

What is a third-party special needs trust?

A third-party special needs trust can be established by one person for the benefit of another. The person establishing the trust, called the settlor (or grantor or, sometimes, trustor) chooses to make some of his or her own assets available for the benefit of the disabled beneficiary. Third-party special needs trusts are often established, for example, by parents for their developmentally disabled or mentally ill children.

What special rules govern third-party special needs trusts?

There are actually few rules governing third-party special needs trusts. Since the beneficiary was never entitled to the money in the trust, the most important rule is simple: the trust terms should not create any entitlement to either income or principal. If the trustee has complete discretion whether to make distributions for the beneficiary, the trust principal and income will usually not be counted as available.

What can a third-party special needs trust provide for the trust beneficiary?

The cardinal rule for special needs trusts is that the trust may not provide food, shelter, or any asset which could be converted into food or shelter (including cash), to the beneficiary. In other words, the trust can provide for physical therapy, medical treatment, education, entertainment, travel, companionship, clothing, furniture and furnishings (such as a television or computer), and some utilities (like cable television and a telephone, but not electricity, gas, or water). Distributions of cash to the special needs trust's beneficiary are almost never permitted (though even this central rule may have some limited exceptions).

I understood that a special needs trust could not pay for clothing. Has that rule changed?

Yes. As of March 2005, the old prohibition against providing clothing has been dropped by the federal government. Some state rules may still include "clothing" as a disallowed expenditure, but those should be subject to challenge in many, if not most, cases. A trust drafted before the elimination of the clothing restriction may, however, still have language prohibiting expenditures for clothing; the trust document itself should be reviewed before a final determination.

Can a special needs trust be used to purchase a home, or pay rent, for the beneficiary?

Yes. There are special rules affecting the use of special needs trusts (or any third-party payment) for shelter. Those rules are very difficult to navigate, and depend heavily on the beneficiary's situation; secure competent legal advice before making any decision about the provision of shelter.

Is it easy to establish a proper third-party special needs trust?

While the principles involved in third-party special needs trusts are simple, there are a myriad of choices involved in the actual drafting of a trust. In addition, the administration of a special needs trust can be extremely difficult. A seasoned lawyer, familiar with public benefits programs and special needs trust provisions, should always be involved in preparation of a third-party special needs trust. While many legal matters can be undertaken without a lawyer, or with a lawyer with general background, special needs trusts are complicated enough to require the services of a specialized practitioner.

What is a self-settled special needs trust?

Sometimes a public benefits recipient may have assets that prevent continued eligibility for benefits. In such a case, it may be possible and advisable to place assets into a special needs trust to regain or continue eligibility for government benefits.

What types of assets might an individual place in a self-settled special needs trust?

Self-settled special needs trusts are often established by individuals who have received a personal injury settlement (perhaps, but not necessarily, arising out of the incident that caused the disability) or inheritance. More rarely individuals with preexisting wealth determine that it would be advisable to create a special needs trust.

If the special needs trust is actually established by a guardian, or a court, is it still "self-settled?"

Yes. Federal law makes it clear that a trust established with assets which would have belonged to an individual, or his or her conservatorship, is self-settled regardless of who signs the trust instrument. (Note that in some states the term "guardian" is used instead of "conservator"—the difference does not change the result.)

Why would someone with assets want to place his or her money in a special needs trust just to qualify for government benefits?

Many benefits available from the public sector are extremely expensive when paid for privately. Some are practically unavailable except through the public system.

What restrictions are placed on self-settled special needs trusts?

Self-settled special needs trusts are much more complicated than their third-party equivalents. Usually (but not always), a self-settled special needs trust must comply with a federal law first enacted in 1993. That law requires that most self-settled special needs trusts actually be established by a judge, a court-appointed guardian, or the parents or grandparents of the beneficiary (Social Security regulations may limit creation of trusts to the first two categories in most circumstances). In addition most self-settled special needs trusts will have to include a provision repaying state Medicaid agencies for any benefits, payable at the death of the beneficiary. Such a provision is often called a "payback" provision.

Must both third-party and self-settled special needs trust include "payback" provisions?

No. Absent unusual circumstances, only self-settled special needs trusts require a provision repaying the state for Medicaid benefits.

Part Six

Additional Help
and Information

Chapter 51

Glossary of Terms Related to Learning Disabilities

accommodations: Techniques and materials that allow individuals with various disabilities to complete school or work tasks with greater ease and effectiveness. Examples include spellcheckers, tape recorders, and expanded time for completing assignments.

assistive technology: Equipment that enhances the ability of students and employees to be more efficient and successful. For individuals with disabilities, computer grammar checkers, an overhead projector used by a teacher, or the audio/visual information delivered through a CD-ROM (compact disk read-only memory) would be typical examples.

attention deficit disorder (ADD): A severe difficulty in focusing and maintaining attention. Often leads to learning and behavior problems at home, school, and work. Also called attention deficit hyperactivity disorder (ADHD).

brain imaging techniques: Noninvasive techniques for studying the activity of living brains. Includes brain electrical activity mapping (BEAM), computerized axial tomography (CAT), and magnetic resonance imaging (MRI).

brain injury: The physical damage to brain tissue or structure that occurs before, during, or after birth that is verified by electroencephalography (EEG), MRI, CAT, or a similar examination, rather than by observation of performance. When caused by an accident, the damage may be called traumatic brain injury (TBI).

collaboration: A program model in which the learning disabilities (LD) teacher demonstrates for or team-teaches with the general classroom teacher to help a student with LD be successful in a regular classroom.

developmental aphasia: A severe language disorder that is presumed to be due to brain injury rather than because of a developmental delay in the normal acquisition of language.

direct instruction: An instructional approach to academic subjects that emphasizes the use of carefully sequenced steps that include demonstration, modeling, guided practice, and independent application.

dyscalculia: A severe difficulty in understanding and using symbols or functions needed for success in mathematics.

dysgraphia: A severe difficulty in producing handwriting that is legible and written at an age-appropriate speed.

dyslexia: A severe difficulty in understanding or using one or more areas of language, including listening, speaking, reading, writing, and spelling.

dysnomia: A marked difficulty in remembering names or recalling words needed for oral or written language.

dyspraxia: A severe difficulty in performing drawing, writing, buttoning, and other tasks requiring fine motor skill, or in sequencing the necessary movements.

learned helplessness: A tendency to be a passive learner who depends on others for decisions and guidance. In individuals with LD, continued struggle and failure can heighten this lack of self-confidence.

learning modalities: Approaches to assessment or instruction stressing the auditory, visual, or tactile avenues for learning that are dependent upon the individual.

learning strategy approaches: Instructional approaches that focus on efficient ways to learn, rather than on curriculum. Includes specific techniques for organizing, actively interacting with material, memorizing, and monitoring any content or subject.

learning styles: Approaches to assessment or instruction emphasizing the variations in temperament, attitude, and preferred manner of tackling a task. Typically considered are styles along the active/passive, reflective/impulsive, or verbal/spatial dimensions.

locus of control: The tendency to attribute success and difficulties either to internal factors such as effort or to external factors such as chance. Individuals with learning disabilities tend to blame failure on themselves and achievement on luck, leading to frustration and passivity.

metacognitive learning: Instructional approaches emphasizing awareness of the cognitive processes that facilitate one's own learning and its application to academic and work assignments. Typical metacognitive techniques include systematic rehearsal of steps or conscious selection among strategies for completing a task.

minimal brain dysfunction (MBD): A medical and psychological term originally used to refer to the learning difficulties that seemed to result from identified or presumed damage to the brain. Reflects a medical rather than educational or vocational orientation.

multisensory learning: An instructional approach that combines auditory, visual, and tactile elements into a learning task. Tracing sandpaper numbers while saying a number fact aloud would be a multisensory learning activity.

neuropsychological examination: A series of tasks that allow observation of performance that is presumed to be related to the intactness of brain function.

perceptual handicap: Difficulty in accurately processing, organizing, and discriminating among visual, auditory, or tactile information. A person with a perceptual handicap may say that "cap/cup" sound the same or that "b" and "d" look the same. However, glasses or hearing aids do not necessarily indicate a perceptual handicap.

prereferral process: A procedure in which special and regular teachers develop trial strategies to help a student showing difficulty in learning remain in the regular classroom.

resource program: A program model in which a student with LD is in a regular classroom for most of each day, but also receives regularly scheduled individual services in a specialized LD resource classroom.

self-advocacy: The development of specific skills and understandings that enable children and adults to explain their specific learning disabilities to others and cope positively with the attitudes of peers, parents, teachers, and employers.

specific language disability (SLD): A severe difficulty in some aspect of listening, speaking, reading, writing, or spelling, while skills in the other areas are age-appropriate. Also called specific language learning disability (SLLD).

specific learning disability (SLD): The official term used in federal legislation to refer to difficulty in certain areas of learning, rather than in all areas of learning. Synonymous with learning disabilities.

subtype research: A recently developed research method that seeks to identify characteristics that are common to specific groups within the larger population of individuals identified as having learning disabilities.

transition: Commonly used to refer to the change from secondary school to postsecondary programs, work, and independent living typical of young adults. Also used to describe other periods of major change such as from early childhood to school or from more specialized to mainstreamed settings.

Chapter 52

Directory of Resources Related to Learning Disabilities

General

American Speech-Language-Hearing Association (ASHA)
2200 Research Boulevard
Rockville, MD 20850-3289
Toll-Free: 800-638-8255
Phone: 301-296-5700
TTY: 301-296-5650
Fax: 301-296-8580
Website: http://www.asha.org

Association for Childhood Education International (ACEI)
17904 Georgia Avenue, Suite 215
Olney, Maryland 20832
Toll-Free: 800-423-3563
Phone: 301-570-2111
Fax: 301-570-2212
Website: http://www.acei.org

Centers for Disease Control and Prevention (CDC)
1600 Clifton Road
Atlanta, GA 30333
Toll-Free: 800-CDC-INFO
(800-232-4636)
Website: http://www.cdc.gov
E-mail: cdcinfo@cdc.gov

Council for Exceptional Children (CEC)
2900 Crystal Drive, Suite 1000
Arlington, VA 22202-3557
Toll-Free: 888-232-7733
Toll-Free TTY: 866-915-5000
Website: http://www.cec.sped.org
E-mail: service@cec.sped.org

Resources in this chapter were compiled from several sources deemed reliable. All contact information was verified and updated in February 2012.

DO-IT (Disabilities, Opportunities, Internetworking, and Technology)
University of Washington
P.O. Box 354842
Seattle, WA 98195-4842
Toll-Free: 888-972-DOIT
(888-972-3648)
Toll-Free TTY: 888-972-3648
Phone: 206-685-DOIT
(206-685-3648)
TTY: 206-685-3648
Fax: 206-221-4171
Website: http://www.uw.edu/doit
E-mail: doit@uw.edu

GreatSchools
160 Spear Street, Suite 1020
San Francisco, CA 94105
Website:
http://www.greatschools.org

LD OnLine
WETA Public Television
2775 South Quincy Street
Arlington, VA 22206
Fax: 703-998-2060
Website: http://www.ldonline.org

Learning Disabilities Association of America (LDA)
4156 Library Road
Pittsburgh, PA 15234-1349
Phone: 412-341-1515
Fax: 412-344-0224
Website:
http://www.ldaamerica.org
E-mail: info@ldaamerica.org

Learning Disabilities Worldwide (LDW)
P.O. Box 142
Weston, MA 02493
Phone: 978-897-5399
Fax: 978-897-5355
Website:
http://www.ldworldwide.org
Email: info@ldworldwide.org

National Center for Learning Disabilities (NCLD)
381 Park Avenue South
Suite 1401
New York, NY 10016
Toll-Free: 888-575-7373
Phone: 212-545-7510
Fax: 212-545-9665
Website: http://www.ld.org
E-mail: ncld@ncld.org

National Dissemination Center for Children with Disabilities
NICHCY
1825 Connecticut Avenue NW
Suite 700
Washington, DC 20009
Toll-Free: 800-695-0285
Toll-Free TTY: 800-695-0285
Phone: 202-884-8200
TTY: 202-884-8200
Fax: 202-884-8441
Website: http://www.nichcy.org
E-mail: nichcy@fhi360.org

National Institute of Mental Health (NIMH)
National Institutes of Health
DHHS
6001 Executive Boulevard
Room 8184, MSC 9663
Bethesda, MD 20892-9663
Toll-Free: 866-615-6464
Toll-Free TTY: 866-415-8051
Phone: 301-443-4513
TTY: 301-443-8431
Fax: 301-443-4279
Website:
http://www.nimh.nih.gov
E-mail: nimhinfo@nih.gov

National Institute of Neurological Disorders and Stroke (NINDS)
NIH Neurological Institute
P.O. Box 5801
Bethesda, MD 20824
Toll-Free: 800-352-9424
Phone: 301-496-5751
TTY: 301-468-5981
Website:
http://www.ninds.nih.gov

National Institute on Alcohol Abuse and Alcoholism (NIAAA)
5635 Fishers Lane, MSC 9304
Bethesda, MD 20892-9304
Phone: 301-443-3860
Website:
http://www.niaaa.nih.gov

National Institute on Deafness and Other Communication Disorders (NIDCD)
NIDCD Information Clearing-house
1 Communication Avenue
Bethesda, MD 20892-3456
Toll-free: 800-241-1044
Toll-Free TTY: 800-241-1055
Fax: 301-770-8977
Website:
http://www.nidcd.nih.gov
E-mail: nidcdinfo@nidcd.nih.gov

NLD Ontario
Website:
http://www.nldontario.org
E-mail: info@NLDOntario.org

Orange County Learning Disabilities Association (OCLDA)
P.O. Box 25772
Santa Ana, CA 92799-5772
Phone: 714-638-1777
Website: http://www.oclda.org

PACER Center
8161 Normandale Boulevard
Bloomington, MN 55437
Toll-Free: 800-537-2237
Phone: 952-838-9000
TTY: 952-838-0190
Fax: 952-838-0199
Website: http://www.pacer.org

Smart Kids with Learning Disabilities
Phone: 203-226-6831
Fax: 203-226-6708
Website:
http://www.smartkidswithld.org
E-mail:
Info@SmartKidswithLD.org

Aphasia

Aphasia Hope Foundation
Website:
http://www.aphasiahope.org

National Aphasia Association
350 Seventh Avenue, Suite 902
New York, NY 10001
Toll-Free: 800-922-4NAA
(800-922-4622)
Phone: 212-267-2814
Fax: 212-267-2812
Website: http://www.aphasia.org
E-mail:
responsecenter@aphasia.org

Assistive Technology

Family Center on Technology and Disability (FCTD)
Academy for Educational Development (AED)
FHI 360
1825 Connecticut Avenue, NW
7th Floor
Washington, DC 20009-5721
Phone: 202-884-8068
Fax: 202-884-8441
Website: http://www.fctd.info
E-mail: fctd@aed.org

Attention Deficit Hyperactivity Disorder

Attention Deficit Disorder Association (ADDA)
P.O. Box 7557
Wilmington, DE 19083-9997
Toll-Free: 800-939-1019
Toll-Free Fax: 800-939-1019
Website: http://www.add.org
E-mail: info@add.org

Children and Adults with Attention-Deficit/ Hyperactivity Disorder (CHADD)
8181 Professional Place
Suite 150
Landover, MD 20785
Toll-Free: 800-233-4050
Phone: 301-306-7070
Fax: 301-306-7090
Website: http://www.chadd.org

Autism and Pervasive Developmental Disorders

Association for Science in Autism Treatment (ASAT)
P.O. Box 188
Crosswicks, NJ 08515-0188
Website:
http://www.asatonline.org
E-mail: info@asatonline.org

Autism National Committee (AUTCOM)
Website: http://www.autcom.org

Autism Network International (ANI)
P.O. Box 35448
Syracuse, NY 13235-5448
Website: http://www.autreat.com
E-mail: jisincla@syr.edu

Autism Research Institute (ARI)
4182 Adams Avenue
San Diego, CA 92116
Toll-Free: 866-366-3361
Phone: 619-281-7165
Fax: 619-563-6840
Website: http://www.autism
researchinstitute.com
E-mail: director@autism.com

Autism Society
4340 East-West Highway
Suite 350
Bethesda, MD 20814
Toll-Free: 800-3AUTISM
(800-328-8476)
Phone: 301-657-0881
Fax: 301-657-0869
Website: http://www.autism
-society.org

Autism Speaks, Inc.
1 East 33rd Street, 4th Floor
New York, NY 10016
Phone: 212-252-8584
(California: 323-549-0500)
Fax: 212-252-8676
(California: 323-549-0547)
Website:
http://www.autismspeaks.org
E-mail:
contactus@autismspeaks.org

MAAP Services for Autism, Asperger Syndrome, and PDD
P.O. Box 524
Crown Point, IN 46308
Phone: 219-662-1311
Fax: 219-662-1315
Website: http://www.asperger
syndrome.org
E-mail:
info@aspergersyndrome.org

Chromosomal Disorders

Genetics Home Reference
Website: http://ghr.nlm.nih.gov

National Human Genome Research Institute (NHGRI)
National Institutes of Health
Building 31, Room 4B09
31 Center Drive, MSC 2152
9000 Rockville Pike
Bethesda, MD 20892-2152
Phone: 301-402-0911
Fax: 301-402-2218
Website: http://www.genome.gov

Dyslexia

International Dyslexia Association (IDA)
40 York Road, 4th Floor
Baltimore, MD 21204
Toll-Free: 800-ABCD123
(800-222-3123)
Phone: 410-296-0232
Fax: 410-321-5069
Website: http://www.interdys.org
E-mail: info@interdys.org

Hearing Disorders

Children's Hearing Institute
380 Second Avenue, 9th Floor
New York, NY 10010
Phone: 646-438-7819
Fax: 646-438-7844
Website:
http://www.childrenshearing.org

National Institute on Deafness and Other Communication Disorders (NIDCD)
NIDCD Information
Clearinghouse
1 Communication Avenue
Bethesda, MD 20892-3456
Toll-Free: 800-241-1044
Toll-Free TTY: 800-241-1055
Fax: 301-770-8977
Website:
http://www.nidcd.nih.gov
E-mail: nidcdinfo@nidcd.nih.gov

Vision Disorders

All About Vision
Access Media Group LLC
1010 Turquoise Street, Suite 350
San Diego, CA 92109
Phone: 858-454-2145
Website:
http://www.allaboutvision.com

Children's Vision Information Network
Website:
http://www.childrensvision.com

National Eye Institute (NEI) Information Office
31 Center Drive MSC 2510
Bethesda, MD 20892-2510
Phone: 301-496-5248
Website: http://www.nei.nih.gov
E-mail: 2020@nei.nih.gov

Chapter 53

Sources of College Funding for Students with Disabilities

Attending college can be an exciting and enriching experience. It can also be a costly one. In addition to tuition, fees, books, and supplies, other expenses to think about include room and board, health insurance, transportation, and spending money. A combination of financial aid and other outside funding resources can help you meet college costs.

Common forms of financial aid include grants, loans, work-study, and scholarships. Some are available specifically to students with disabilities. Many students use a combination of these financial aid resources. It is important to remember that financial aid results in a partnership of the student, parents, postsecondary educational institutions, state and federal governments, and/or private organizations. Such a partnership requires cooperation, communication, and an understanding by each of their responsibilities within the financial aid process.

The financial aid office at the school you plan to attend is a good place to begin your search for financial aid information. An administrator there can tell you about student aid available from your state, the school itself, and other sources.

"College Funding for Students with Disabilities." Reprinted with permission from DO-IT (Disabilities, Opportunities, Internetworking, and Technology), © 2012 University of Washington. All rights reserved. DO-IT serves to increase the successful participation of individuals with disabilities in challenging academic programs and careers. Primary funding for DO-IT is provided by the National Science Foundation, the State of Washington, and the U.S. Department of Education. For additional information, visit the DO-IT Center website at http://www.uw.edu/doit.

Federal Student Aid Programs

The programs described below are administered by the U.S. Department of Education and provide billions of dollars each year to students attending postsecondary schools. Not all schools participate in all federal student aid programs. Check with your high school guidance counselor or the financial aid officer at a postsecondary institution to make sure your destination school participates in the federal program(s) you are interested in.

Federal Pell grants are available to undergraduate students only and they do not have to be repaid.

Federal Stafford loans are based on financial need, are available to both undergraduate and graduate students, vary in maximum value each year of study, and must be repaid. The interest rate is variable. If you qualify (based on need) for a subsidized Stafford loan, the government will pay the interest on your loan while you are in school, during grace periods, and during any deferment periods.

Federal PLUS loans are unsubsidized loans made to parents. If you are independent or your parents cannot get a PLUS loan, you are eligible to borrow additional Stafford Loan funds. The interest rate is variable.

Campus-based programs are administered by participating schools. Three of these programs are described below:

- Federal Supplemental Educational Opportunity Grants are grants available for undergraduates only and range in value.

- Federal work-study provides jobs to undergraduate and graduate students, allowing them to earn money to pay education expenses.

- Perkins loans are low-interest loans; the maximum annual loan amount is greater for graduate students than for undergraduate students.

For more information on federal student aid programs consult www.studentaid.ed.gov/ or call the Federal Student Aid Information Center at 800-433-3243 or 800-730-8913 (TTY). An online application can be found at www.fafsa.ed.gov.

Supplemental Security Income (SSI) and Plan for Achieving Self Support (PASS)

SSI is a program that pays monthly benefits to people with low incomes and limited assets who are sixty-five years of age or older, are blind, or have other disabilities. Children can qualify if they meet Social Security's definition of disability for SSI children and if their income and assets fall within the eligibility limits.

As its name implies, Supplemental Security Income supplements a person's income up to a certain level. The level varies from one state to another and may increase each year to reflect cost-of-living changes. Your local Social Security office can tell you about SSI benefit levels in your state.

Parent income and assets are considered when deciding if a child under eighteen qualifies for SSI. This applies to children who live at home or who are away at school but return home occasionally and are subject to parental control. When a child turns eighteen, parent income and assets are no longer considered when determining eligibility for SSI. Therefore, a child who was not eligible for SSI before his or her eighteenth birthday may become eligible at age eighteen.

The Social Security Administration may also approve a Plan for Achieving Self Support (PASS), in which a student is able to set aside income and resources that are being used toward a specific vocational goal (such as college tuition) and still receive SSI payments. However, be aware that earnings from employment may affect SSI benefits.

For more information on SSI and PASS, contact your local Social Security Administration office or consult www.ssa.gov/disability/.

State Vocational Rehabilitation Services

Your state vocational rehabilitation (VR) office helps people with disabilities prepare for, obtain, and retain employment. Vocational rehabilitation programs are custom-designed for each individual. Typically, you may be eligible for services if a VR counselor determines that you meet the following three conditions:

1. You have a physical or mental disability. The VR counselor must verify the disability by getting copies of medical records or by having you complete tests, examinations, or evaluations to verify the disability.

2. Your disability prevents you from getting or keeping a job.

3. You require vocational rehabilitation services to get or keep a job that matches your strengths, resources, priorities, concerns, abilities, capabilities, interests, and choices.

A state VR agency provides a wide range of services for helping clients get or keep jobs. VR services include assessment services, counseling and guidance, training (school), job-related services, rehabilitation technology (assistive technology), independent living, and a variety of support services.

To locate a state vocational rehabilitation office near you, consult the state government listings in your phone book under "Vocational Rehabilitation" or consult wdcrobcolp01.ed.gov/Programs/EROD/org_list.cfm?category_ID=SVR.

Other State Programs

Nearly all states offer financial assistance in the form of state grants and loans. Details and information can be obtained from a college financial aid office or a high school guidance counselor. To find out which agency in your state may offer financial assistance for higher education, consult wdcrobcolp01.ed.gov/Programs/EROD/org_list.cfm?category_ID=SHE.

General Scholarships and Awards

Scholarships and awards provide monetary gifts based on a student's achievements, interests, background, or other criteria. A good first step in your scholarship search is to check with your parents' employers, local organizations, your high school guidance counselor, your college or university's financial aid office, the department chairman at your chosen school, and your college or the local library. Below you'll find other resources and tips that may help you locate financial aid.

Employers: Parents can check with personnel administrators to see if their employers offer financial aid, tuition reimbursement, or scholarships for employees' children. If you are employed or volunteering, ask your company if they offer scholarships.

Organizations: Many professional or social organizations offer scholarships. The Elks Club, for example, offers millions of dollars each year in scholarships for graduating high school students. Some labor unions (American Federation of Labor and Congress of Industrial Organizations [AFL-CIO], Teamsters, etc.) offer scholarships for members and their dependent children. If you are not a member of an organization, check with organizations that are related to your chosen field of study. For example, if you plan to study aeronautical engineering, check with the American Institute of Aeronautics and Astronautics regarding college scholarships they offer.

Religious Groups: Your church or synagogue may have scholarships available. Also check with the headquarters of your religious affiliation.

Chamber of commerce: Your local chamber of commerce may offer small grants or scholarships to local students, often to those pursuing a career in business.

Take the PSAT: The Preliminary Scholastic Aptitude Test/National Merit Scholarship Qualifying Test is co-sponsored by the College Board and National Merit Scholarship Corporation (NMSC). The PSAT/NMSQT gives you practice for the SAT, as well as a chance to qualify for scholarship and recognition programs.

AmeriCorps: AmeriCorps is a network of national service programs that engage more than fifty thousand Americans each year in intensive service to meet critical needs in education, public safety, health, and the environment. AmeriCorps jobs are open to U.S. citizens, nationals, or lawful permanent residents aged seventeen or older. Members serve full- or part-time over a ten- to twelve-month period. Participants receive an education award to pay for college or graduate school, or to pay back student loans. For more information, call 800-942-2677 (TTY 800-833-3722) or consult www .americorps.org/.

Search the web: Run searches for "scholarships," "financial aid," "grants," etc.

Disability-Related Scholarships and Awards

The following opportunities are specifically available to students with disabilities.

General

Disaboom Scholarship Network
Disaboom
www.disaboom.com/scholarships

Foundation for Science and Disability Science
Student Grant Fund
Disability.gov
www.stemd.org

Incight Scholarship
Incight
971-244-0305
www.incighteducation.org/scholarship

Lime Scholarship
Google & Lime
www.limeconnect.com/opportunities/page/google-lime-scholarship
-program

Paul G. Hearne Leadership Award
800-840-8844
www.aapd.com/what-powers-us/leadership-awards

Proyecto Vision
www.proyectovision.net/english/opportunities/scholarships.html

Student Award Program
Foundation for Science and Disability, Inc.
www.as.wvu.edu/~scidis/organize/fsdinfo.html

Undergraduate Scholarship Program
Central Intelligence Agency
www.cia.gov/careers/student-opportunities/undergraduate
-scholarship-program.html

Hearing Loss/Deafness

AG Bell Financial Aid and Scholarship Program
Alexander Graham Bell Association for the Deaf
and Hard of Hearing
202-337-5220
202-337-5221 (TTY)
nc.agbell.org/document.doc?id=888

Disaboom Scholarship Network
Disaboom
www.disaboom.com/scholarships

Graduate Fellowship Fund
Gallaudet University Alumni Association
202-651-5060 (Voice/TTY)

www.gallaudet.edu/Development_and_Alumni_Relations/Alumni_
Relations/Alumni_Association_(GUAA)/The_Centennial_Fund/
GF_Fund.html

Hard of Hearing and Deaf Scholarship
Sertoma International
816-333-8300
www.sertoma.org/NETCOMMUNITY/Page.aspx?pid=344&srcid=190

Minnie Pearl Scholarship Program
The EAR Foundation
800-545-7373 (HEAR)
615-627-2724 (voice/TDD)
hearingbridges.org/images/uploads/Minnie%20Pearl%20Application
%202012.pdf

William C. Stokoe Scholarship
National Association of the Deaf: Stokoe
(301) 587-1789 (TTY)
www.nad.org

Visual Impairments

ACB Scholarship
American Council of the Blind
202-467-5081
www.acb.org

AFB Scholarships
American Foundation for the Blind
800-232-5463
www.afb.org/scholarships.asp

CCLVI Scholarships
Council of Citizens with Low Vision International
800-733-2258
www.cclvi.org

CRS Scholarship
Christian Record Services for the Blind
402-488-0981
services.christianrecord.org/scholarships/index.php

Disaboom Scholarship Network
Disaboom
www.disaboom.com/scholarships

Ferrell Scholarship
Association for Education and Rehabilitation of
the Blind and Visually Impaired
877-492-2708
www.aerbvi.org/modules.php?name=Content&pa=showpage&pid=77

Guild Scholar Award
Jewish Guild for the Blind
212-769-7801
www.jgb.org/guildscholar.asp

Lighthouse Scholarships
Lighthouse International
212-821-9428
www.lighthouse.org/aboutus/lighthouse-events/scholarships
-and-career-awards

Mary P. Oenslager Scholastic Achievement Award
Recording for the Blind and Dyslexic
609-452-0606
www.learningally.org/About-Us/National-and-Local-Award
-Opportunities/53rd-Annual-National-Achievement-Awards-Mary
-P-Oenslager-Scholastic-Achievement-Awards-SAA/914

NFB Scholarships
National Federation of the Blind
404-371-1000
www.nfb.org/nfb/scholarship_program.asp

Physical/Mobility Impairments

1800Wheelchair.com
800-320-7140
www.1800wheelchair.com/Scholarship

AmeriGlide Achiever Scholarship
AmeriGlide
800-790-1635
www.ameriglide.com/scholarship

Disaboom Scholarship Network (wheelchair user)
Disaboom
www.disaboom.com/scholarships

National Chair Scholars Scholarship
ChairScholars Foundation
813-920-1981
www.chairscholars.org/nationalprogram.htm

National MS Society Scholarship Program
National Multiple Sclerosis Society
800-344-4867
www.nationalmssociety.org/living-with-multiple-sclerosis/society
-programs-and-services/scholarship/index.aspx

SBA Scholarship Program
Spina Bifida Association of America
202-944-3285 ext. 23
www.spinabifidaassociation.org

Health Impairments

Disaboom Scholarship Network (cystic fibrosis, immunodeficiency, lupus)
Disaboom
www.disaboom.com/scholarships

HFA Educational Scholarship
Hemophilia Federation of America
800-230-9797
www.hemophiliafed.org/programs-and-services/educational-scholarships

IDF Scholarship Program
Immune Deficiency Foundation
800-296-4433
primaryimmune.org/patients-and-families/idf-scholarship-programs

Kevin Child Scholarship
National Hemophilia Foundation
800-424-2634 ext. 3700
www.hemophilia.org/NHFWeb/MainPgs/MainNHF.aspx?menuid=53
&contentid=35

Pfizer Epilepsy Scholarship Award
Intra Med Educational Group
800-292-7373
www.epilepsy-scholarship.com

Scholarships for Survivors Program
Patient Advocate Foundation
800-532-5274
www.patientadvocate.org/events.php?p=69

Solvay Cares Scholarship
Solvay Pharmaceuticals
770-578-5836
www.solvaycaresscholarship.com

Ulman Cancer Fund for Young Adults
888-393-3863 (FUND)
www.ulmanfund.org/Services/Scholarship/20092010Scholarship
Program/tabid/565/Default.aspx

Learning Disabilities

Anne Ford and Allegra Ford Scholarship
National Center for Learning Disabilities
888-575-7373
www.ncld.org/about-us/scholarships-aamp-awards/the-anne
-ford-and-allegra-ford-scholarship-award

Anne & Matt Harbison Scholarship
P. Buckley Moss Society
540-943-5678
www.mosssociety.org/page.php?id=30

Disaboom Scholarship Network
Disaboom
www.disaboom.com/scholarships

Learning Through Listening Award
Recording for the Blind and Dyslexic
609-452-0606
www.learningally.org/SiteData/docs/DC%20Scholar/0363ffc45dbf49
de/DC%20Scholarship%20Application%202011.pdf

Hydrocephalus Association
415-732-7040
www.hydroassoc.org/education_support/scholarships

Mental Health

Lilly Reintegration Scholarship
800-809-8202
www.reintegration.com

Disabled Veterans and Military Families

Disaboom Scholarship Network
Disaboom
www.disaboom.com/scholarships

Resources

The resources listed provide current information about financial aid opportunities.

Financial Aid Information

- www.collegeanswer.com
- www.collegeboard.com
- www.ed.gov
- www.fafsa.ed.gov
- www.finaid.org

Scholarship Lists

- www.collegeboard.com/student/pay/scholarshipsand-aid/index.html
- www.collegenet.com/mach25
- www.disability.gov/education/financial_aid
- www.disaboom.com/scholarships
- www.fastaid.com
- www.fastweb.com
- www.freschinfo.com

- www.internationalscholarships.com
- scholarshipexperts.com
- www.scholarship-page.com

Index

Index

Page numbers followed by 'n' indicate a footnote. Page numbers in *italics* indicate a table or illustration.

593